A Framework for Assessing Effects of the Food System

Committee on a Framework for Assessing the Health,
Environmental, and Social Effects of the Food System

Food and Nutrition Board

Board on Agriculture and Natural Resources

Malden C. Nesheim, Maria Oria, and Peggy Tsai Yih, *Editors*

INSTITUTE OF MEDICINE *AND*
NATIONAL RESEARCH COUNCIL

THE NATIONAL ACADEMIES PRESS
Washington, D.C.
www.nap.edu

THE NATIONAL ACADEMIES PRESS 500 Fifth Street, NW Washington, DC 20001

NOTICE: The project that is the subject of this report was approved by the Governing Board of the National Research Council, whose members are drawn from the councils of the National Academy of Sciences, the National Academy of Engineering, and the Institute of Medicine. The members of the committee responsible for the report were chosen for their special competences and with regard for appropriate balance.

This study was supported by a grant between the National Academy of Sciences and the JPB Foundation. Any opinions, findings, conclusions, or recommendations expressed in this publication are those of the author(s) and do not necessarily reflect the views of the organizations or agencies that provided support for the project.

International Standard Book Number-13: 978-0-309-30780-2
International Standard Book Number-10: 978-0-309-30780-5
Library of Congress Control Number: 2015903230

Additional copies of this report are available for sale from the National Academies Press, 500 Fifth Street, NW, Keck 360, Washington, DC 20001; (800) 624-6242 or (202) 334-3313; http://www.nap.edu.

For more information about the Institute of Medicine, visit the IOM home page at: **www.iom.edu.**

Printed in the United States of America

The serpent has been a symbol of long life, healing, and knowledge among almost all cultures and religions since the beginning of recorded history. The serpent adopted as a logotype by the Institute of Medicine is a relief carving from ancient Greece, now held by the Staatliche Museen in Berlin.

Suggested citation: IOM (Institute of Medicine) and NRC (National Research Council). 2015. *A framework for assessing effects of the food system.* Washington, DC: The National Academies Press.

THE NATIONAL ACADEMIES

Advisers to the Nation on Science, Engineering, and Medicine

The **National Academy of Sciences** is a private, nonprofit, self-perpetuating society of distinguished scholars engaged in scientific and engineering research, dedicated to the furtherance of science and technology and to their use for the general welfare. Upon the authority of the charter granted to it by the Congress in 1863, the Academy has a mandate that requires it to advise the federal government on scientific and technical matters. Dr. Ralph J. Cicerone is president of the National Academy of Sciences.

The **National Academy of Engineering** was established in 1964, under the charter of the National Academy of Sciences, as a parallel organization of outstanding engineers. It is autonomous in its administration and in the selection of its members, sharing with the National Academy of Sciences the responsibility for advising the federal government. The National Academy of Engineering also sponsors engineering programs aimed at meeting national needs, encourages education and research, and recognizes the superior achievements of engineers. Dr. C. D. Mote, Jr., is president of the National Academy of Engineering.

The **Institute of Medicine** was established in 1970 by the National Academy of Sciences to secure the services of eminent members of appropriate professions in the examination of policy matters pertaining to the health of the public. The Institute acts under the responsibility given to the National Academy of Sciences by its congressional charter to be an adviser to the federal government and, upon its own initiative, to identify issues of medical care, research, and education. Dr. Victor J. Dzau is president of the Institute of Medicine.

The **National Research Council** was organized by the National Academy of Sciences in 1916 to associate the broad community of science and technology with the Academy's purposes of furthering knowledge and advising the federal government. Functioning in accordance with general policies determined by the Academy, the Council has become the principal operating agency of both the National Academy of Sciences and the National Academy of Engineering in providing services to the government, the public, and the scientific and engineering communities. The Council is administered jointly by both Academies and the Institute of Medicine. Dr. Ralph J. Cicerone and Dr. C. D. Mote, Jr., are chair and vice chair, respectively, of the National Research Council.

www.national-academies.org

COMMITTEE ON A FRAMEWORK FOR ASSESSING THE HEALTH, ENVIRONMENTAL, AND SOCIAL EFFECTS OF THE FOOD SYSTEM

MALDEN C. NESHEIM (*Chair*), Provost Emeritus, Professor of Nutrition Emeritus, Cornell University, Ithaca, NY
KATHERINE (KATE) CLANCY, Food Systems Consultant, Visiting Scholar, Center for a Livable Future, Johns Hopkins Bloomberg School of Public Health, Baltimore, MD
JAMES K. HAMMITT, Professor of Economics and Decision Sciences, Harvard University School of Public Health, Boston, MA
ROSS A. HAMMOND, Director, Center on Social Dynamics and Policy, Senior Fellow, Economic Studies, Brookings Institution, Washington, DC
DARREN L. HAVER, Director and Advisor, Division of Agriculture and Natural Resources, University of California Cooperative Extension, Orange County
DOUGLAS JACKSON-SMITH, Professor, Department of Sociology, Social Work, and Anthropology, Utah State University, Logan
ROBBIN S. JOHNSON, Senior Advisor, Global Policy Studies, Humphrey School of Public Affairs, University of Minnesota, Minneapolis
JEAN D. KINSEY, Professor Emeritus, Department of Applied Economics, Director Emeritus, The Food Industry Center, University of Minnesota, St. Paul
SUSAN M. KREBS-SMITH, Chief, Risk Factor Monitoring and Methods Branch, National Cancer Institute, Bethesda, MD
MATTHEW LIEBMAN, Professor of Agronomy, Henry A. Wallace Chair for Sustainable Agriculture, Iowa State University, Ames
FRANK MITLOEHNER, Professor, Department of Animal Science, University of California, Davis
KESHIA M. POLLACK, Associate Professor, Johns Hopkins Bloomberg School of Public Health, Baltimore, MD
PATRICK J. STOVER, Professor and Director, Division of Nutritional Sciences, Cornell University, Ithaca, NY
KATHERINE M. J. SWANSON, President, KMJ Swanson Food Safety, Inc., Mendota Heights, MN
SCOTT M. SWINTON, Professor, Department of Agricultural, Food, and Resource Economics, Michigan State University, East Lansing

IOM and NRC Study Staff

MARIA ORIA, Study Director
PEGGY TSAI YIH, Senior Program Officer
ALLISON BERGER, Senior Program Assistant
ALICE VOROSMARTI, Research Associate
FAYE HILLMAN, Financial Associate
GERALDINE KENNEDO, Administrative Assistant
ANA VELASQUEZ, Intern (until August 2013)
WILLIAM HALL, Mirzayan Science & Technology Policy Fellow (until April 2014)
ANN L. YAKTINE, Director, Food and Nutrition Board
ROBIN SCHOEN, Director, Board on Agriculture and Natural Resources

Reviewers

This report has been reviewed in draft form by individuals chosen for their diverse perspectives and technical expertise, in accordance with procedures approved by the National Research Council's Report Review Committee. The purpose of this independent review is to provide candid and critical comments that will assist the institution in making its published report as sound as possible and to ensure that the report meets institutional standards for objectivity, evidence, and responsiveness to the study charge. The review comments and draft manuscript remain confidential to protect the integrity of the deliberative process. We wish to thank the following individuals for their review of this report:

William H. Dietz, The George Washington University
George M. Gray, The George Washington University
Michael W. Hamm, Michigan State University
Shiriki K. Kumanyika, University of Pennsylvania Perelman School of Medicine
Paul J. Lioy, UMDNJ–Robert Wood Johnson Medical School Piscataway
Stephen Polasky, University of Minnesota, Minneapolis
Mark A. Rasmussen, Iowa State University, Leopold Center for Sustainable Agriculture
Angela Tagtow, U.S. Department of Agriculture, Center for Nutrition Policy and Promotion
Lori Ann Thrupp, University of California, Berkeley

Wallace E. Tyner, Purdue University
Laurian J. Unnevehr, University of Illinois at Urbana-Champaign
John H. Vandermeer, University of Michigan
Patricia Verduin, Colgate-Palmolive Company
Rick Welsh, Syracuse University
Parke E. Wilde, Tufts University

Although the reviewers listed above have provided many constructive comments and suggestions, they were not asked to endorse the conclusions or recommendations nor did they see the final draft of the report before its release. The review of this report was overseen by **Diane Birt,** Iowa State University, and **Mark R. Cullen,** Stanford University. Appointed by the National Research Council and the Institute of Medicine, they were responsible for making certain that an independent examination of this report was carried out in accordance with institutional procedures and that all review comments were carefully considered. Responsibility for the final content of this report rests entirely with the authoring committee and the institution.

Preface

Food is a topic that has become central to practically all aspects of modern life. Its centrality raises questions as to what constitutes a healthy diet, how is food produced, and what kind of food production is best for the environment. Will there be sufficient food in response to rising world population? Are there segments of the U.S. population that are food insecure? Are food animals raised humanely? Who is involved in food production? Are workers treated fairly and do they earn a decent living? Today, chefs are celebrities and our society increasingly outsources food preparation and service. Food studies has become a part of diverse academic curricula from the sciences to the humanities and has produced an expanding literature about the food system and its relationship to modern life. Health professionals and the public have come to realize that food is not merely a source of nourishment, it also reflects individual values and culture.

This increased interest in food follows a time of intense change in how food is produced, who produces it, and where it is produced. Over the past century, the United States has gone from being an overwhelmingly agrarian nation to a highly industrialized, urban nation where only a small portion of the population is involved in the actual production of food. The U.S. food system provides a remarkably varied food supply to the U.S. consumer at lower cost than nearly anywhere else in the world. Many are concerned, however, that the cost of food in the marketplace may not reflect its true cost. Some of the costs of food production and distribution are not reflected in the marketplace price of food but are "externalized," borne by other aspects of the health, environmental, and social domains of our society.

Agriculture now represents a bioeconomy that produces not only food but also raw material for a variety of nonfood industrial purposes, including biofuels that power our vehicles. Food production, a core of this bio-economy, competes with other societal demands for raw materials. Food components enter a supply chain that transports, manufactures, distributes, and markets food to consumers through a wide a variety of outlets. The interconnectivity of the components of the bioeconomy means that policies meant to affect one aspect of the system may affect other components in a manner often not anticipated. A committee was appointed by the Food and Nutrition Board of the Institute of Medicine (IOM) in collaboration with the Board on Agriculture and Natural Resources of the National Research Council (NRC) to develop an analytical framework to assess the health, environmental, social, and economic aspects of the U.S. food system to take into account the complexity of the system. The committee recognizes that the U.S. food system is embedded in a global system that is broadly interconnected but the report concentrates on the U.S. component.

In carrying out this task the committee needed to define and characterize the current U.S. food system and to consider its evolution over time. The committee drew on the potential effects of the current system on health, the environment, and the social and economic domain that are described and documented in current published literature. The chapters that describe the effects provide insights into how aspects of the food system influence modern life in ways not always appreciated or accounted for. In producing this report, the committee has considered both positive and negative effects of the food system, without making overall value judgments about any particular aspect. The report is not intended as a critique of the U.S. food system but instead recognizes the numerous trade-offs embedded in current agricultural and food system practices. This report considers these trade-offs in examples that illustrate the interconnections between the food system, health, environment, and quality of life and demonstrate the analytical challenges of assessing new policies or practices.

During the committee's deliberations, it became apparent that the food system is highly complex, with many drivers and actors. This realization led the committee to determine that analytical methods aimed at understanding complex systems are most appropriate for understanding configurations of the food system and the policies that affect it. The committee views the analytical framework as generic, one that can be used to investigate many different questions about the food system using a wide variety of methodologies, but requires that any analysis consider the implications of the health, environmental, social, and economic aspects of the question. The report identifies situations in the food system where such analyses are essential, as their effects go beyond a particular policy or recommendation aimed at improving one area.

The committee hopes that the analytical framework outlined in this report will be broadly used by researchers and policy makers considering or evaluating alternative policies or potential configurations that project changes in the U.S. food system. The full use of the framework across all domains may require development of new methodologies or models that can deal with the full scope of the system. In the committee's view, such analyses can help assure that the U.S. food system supports the health and the quality of life of our citizens and the sustainability of the environment.

The committee responsible for the report is unusually varied in expertise, with members chosen for their experience in agriculture, public health, nutrition, food safety, sociology, economics, complex systems, and the food industry. The chapters are authored jointly by committee members who contributed their expertise to appropriate areas, subject to review and comment from the entire committee. Committee members volunteered countless hours to the research, deliberations, and preparation of the report. Many other individuals contributed significant time and effort to address the subject matter of the report during an open committee session and through presentations at a workshop. We are grateful for their efforts.

The committee is especially thankful to the IOM and the NRC staff team for their continued support, particularly to the Study Director, Maria Oria, and Senior Program Officer, Peggy Tsai Yih, who ably shepherded the preparation of this very complex report; Alice Vorosmarti, who was invaluable for her information-gathering and drawing skills; and Allison Berger for her administrative support. The committee also benefited from the overall guidance of Robin Schoen, Director of the Board on Agriculture and Natural Resources, and from Ann Yaktine, Director of the Food and Nutrition Board.

I am personally impressed by and grateful for the dedication and hard work of the committee members and staff in support of this project.

Malden C. Nesheim, *Chair*
Committee on a Framework for Assessing the Health, Environmental, and Social Effects of the Food System

Contents

Summary

The nation's food system historically has seen remarkable success in providing the U.S. population with a varied, relatively inexpensive, and widely available supply of food. It has done so through a supply chain of producers, processors, and distributors that provides food to consumers (see Figure S-1). The food system also represents one of the most significant components of the U.S. economy.

The U.S. food system has extensive connections to the global food system and exercises important influences in the global community. It is also embedded within a diverse, ever-changing, and broader economic, biophysical, and sociopolitical context (see Figure S-2).

A myriad of actors with diverse goals that are interested in specific aspects of improving health, protecting the environment, or increasing productivity make decisions that shape the food system every day. Those decisions, however, may have unexpected consequences beyond their original intent both in the United States and abroad. The results of those decisions may impact the environment (e.g., effects on biodiversity, water, soil, air, and climate), human health (e.g., direct effects on diet-related chronic disease risk, and indirect effects associated with soil, air, and water pollution), and society (e.g., effects on food accessibility and affordability, land use, employment, labor conditions, and local economies).

To date, most studies that address changes within the food system have taken a relatively narrow approach with limited consideration of the system's complexity. However, such approaches can often miss important interconnections and may not capture the full set of impacts flowing from any particular change in the food system.

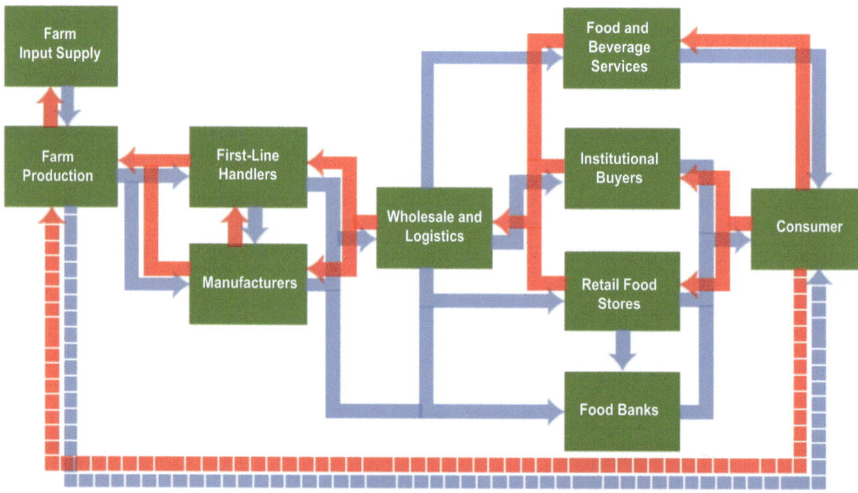

FIGURE S-1 Conceptual model of a food supply chain. Elements or actors in this supply chain in one area (e.g., region or country) also have interactions (e.g., international trade) with actors in other areas.

In considering any changes, decision makers need the right tools for analyzing intended and unintended effects, understanding how to weigh those potential effects, and being able to recognize the need for trade-offs.[1] For example, recommendations to increase the consumption of fruits and vegetables to promote healthier diets raise questions about the potential consequences of expanding their supply, such as increased irrigation water or farm labor. Deciding among various options can be challenging because there could be a large number of trade-offs that are difficult to compare. However, any solutions will need to integrate a multifaceted approach for measuring and weighing various consequences.

The committee proposes an analytical framework as a tool for decision makers, researchers, and other stakeholders to examine the possible impacts of interventions and evaluate the collective health, environmental, social, and economic outcomes of specific changes in the food system. The framework provides a conceptual and an empirical structure consisting of four

[1] A trade-off is a situation that involves losing one quality or aspect of something in return for gaining another quality or aspect.

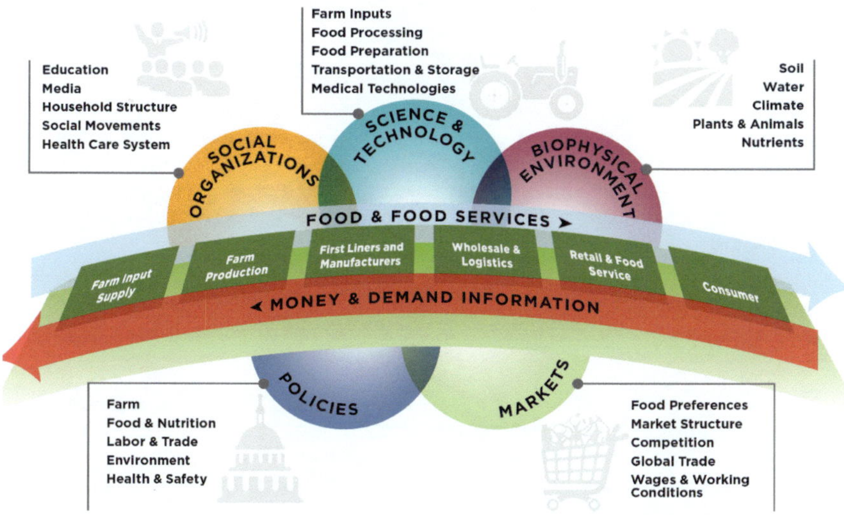

FIGURE S-2 Links between the food supply chain and the larger biophysical and social/institutional context.

principles and six steps, as described later. This framework will be useful for (1) identifying and potentially preventing unintended effects of an intervention; (2) promoting transparency among stakeholders about decisions; (3) improving communication and providing a better understanding of values and perspectives among scientists, policy makers, and other stakeholders; and (4) decreasing the likelihood of misinterpretation of results from any particular analysis.

The intent of the framework is to provide guidance when conducting evaluations within food and agriculture. The committee recognizes that, as with any tool, analysis using the framework would simply be one input into any decision-making processes. Many other factors come into consideration (e.g., judgments) that are beyond the scope of this report.

THE TASK

The Institute of Medicine and the National Research Council convened an expert committee to develop an analytical framework relevant for the food system (see the Statement of Task in Box S-1). The ultimate aim of the study is to (1) facilitate an understanding of the environmental, health, social, and economic effects associated with all components of the food system and how these effects are linked; (2) encourage the development of

BOX S-1
Statement of Task

The expert committee will develop a framework for assessing the health, environmental, and social effects (positive and negative) associated with the ways in which food is grown, processed, distributed, marketed, retailed, and consumed within the U.S. food system. In developing the framework, the committee will undertake the following activities:

1. Examine available methods, methodologies, and data that are needed to undertake comparisons and measure effects. Examples of such needs that the committee will examine are:

    - Defining comparable characteristics of different configurations of elements within the food system.
    - Mapping the pathways through which different configurations of elements of the food system create or contribute to health, environmental, and social effects.
    - Determining the contribution of those configurations to effects relative to those from other influences.
    - Characterizing the scale of effects (e.g., individual, national).
    - Quantifying the magnitude and direction of effects.
    - Monetizing effects, when appropriate.
    - Addressing uncertainty, complexity, and variability in conducting comparisons and measuring effects.

improved data collection systems and methodologies to identify and measure these effects; and (3) inform decision making in food and agricultural practices and policies in ways that minimize unintended health, environmental, social, and economic consequences.

Approach of the Committee

In order to provide some context, this report describes the U.S. food system and gives a brief history of how the current system evolved and how the system can be viewed as a complex adaptive system. The report describes the most salient effects of the food system in the health, environmental, and social and economic domains. Understanding the relationships among components of the food system and their effects on health, the environment, and society are essential prerequisites for attempting any evaluation of costs and benefits of the health, environmental, social, and economic effects of the food system.

2. Describe several examples of different configurations of elements within the food system and describe how the framework will be applied, step by step, to compare them. Examples should be drawn from different parts of the food system (production, harvest, processing, distribution, marketing, retailing, and consumption). The emphasis will be on those effects that are generally not recognized (i.e., they may not be fully incorporated into the price of food). Different configurations for the committee to consider might include regionally based food systems and a global food system; free-range production of poultry and caged housing practices; and reduced retail presence of processed food and current availability of processed food.
3. In constructing examples, describe the strengths and weaknesses of the framework in different contextual situations and suggest how and when adjustments to the framework may lead to more accurate comparisons. The goal of the examples is to illustrate the potential use of the framework to analyze a variety of questions and compare, measure, and, in some cases, monetize the effects of different scenarios on public health, the environment, and society. The focus of these exercises should be in explaining the elements of the framework, not in attempting the analyses.
4. The committee will also identify information needs and gaps in methods and methodologies that, if filled, could provide greater certainty in the attribution and quantification of effects related to food system configurations and improve the predictive value of the framework for evaluating how changes in and across the food system might affect health, the environment, and society.

The committee has written its report from a U.S. perspective while recognizing the global nature of the food system and its effects. The committee focused primarily on the domestic effects due to time, expertise, and page limit constraints. Consequently, discussions in this report preclude U.S. food-related interactions and consequences with the rest of the world, yet the committee's proposed framework is still valid for examining those global interactions and effects.

Six examples were selected to illustrate how the framework might be used when comparing current versus alternative configurations within the food system. By applying the framework to these six examples, it revealed how features of the food system are intricately tied to one another. The committee did not take it one step further with these examples in conducting assessments which would be outside the scope of the Statement of Task.

BOX S-2
Characteristics of the Food System as a Complex Adaptive System

The following are characteristics of the food system that makes it a complex adaptive system:

Individual adaptive actors. The food system is composed of a variety of actors, including human actors (e.g., farmers, workers, researchers, consumers), institutions (e.g., governments, corporations, universities, organizations), and organisms (e.g., microorganisms or insects). The decentralized behavior and interaction of these actors shapes and modifies the food system; at the same time, actors respond and adapt to changes in the system around them. For example, consumer behavior shapes market demand, but may change in response to new products, information, or social forces. Consideration of adaptive responses (by multiple types of actors) can be important in a sufficient understanding of likely effects over time that result from any change to the food system.

Feedback and interdependence. Many mechanisms at work within the food system cross multiple levels (e.g., the biological level, physical food environment, and social or market context are all involved in food preferences and eating behavior). Multiple interacting mechanisms across levels of scale can lead to interdependence among actors, sectors, or factors. Feedback loops can also arise, through which initial changes to one component of the food system that affect a second component may "feed back" to further alter the first component after a time lag. For example, limited pesticide introduction may initially control pests, but over time resistance may arise, leading to increasing pesticide usage to maintain control.

THE FOOD SYSTEM: A COMPLEX ADAPTIVE SYSTEM

The food system is woven together as a supply chain that operates within broader economic, biophysical, and sociopolitical contexts. Health, environmental, social, and economic effects are associated with the U.S. food system, often with both beneficial and detrimental aspects. For instance, in the area of health, the U.S. food system supplies a wide variety of foods in sufficient quantity and at low cost for most, but not all, of the population. However, unhealthy dietary patterns are identified as a risk factor in the etiology of several leading causes of mortality and morbidity. Other effects of the food system involve climate, land, and water resources. Depletion of resources (e.g., water) and flow of outputs (e.g., nitrogen from fertilization, pesticides, and greenhouse gases) to the environment as a result of food system activities can be significant and disturb the ecosystem dynamic. The U.S. food system also carries social and economic effects that are mediated

Heterogeneity. Actors and processes in the food system differ from each other in important ways that can shape local dynamics and lead to divergent adaptive responses to changes in the system. For example, corporations will likely have constraints, goals, and information that differ from those of individual consumers. An intervention designed to increase intake of fruits and vegetables will affect farmers, workers, manufacturers, consumers, and retailers in different ways, and each type of actor may respond differently to any change.

Spatial complexity. Spatial organization shapes many dynamics within the food system, both directly affecting the local context experienced by actors and governing impacts across time and space. In agriculture production, a key factor determining the impacts of agricultural production systems on water, wildlife, and other natural resources is the spatial organization of the components. For example, the concentration of agricultural production can magnify environmental effects in a particular location if not managed appropriately.

Dynamic complexity. The presence of feedback, interdependence, and adaptation can produce dynamics in the food system with characteristics such as nonlinearity (a small change yielding a large effect), path dependence (dynamics strongly shaped by early events), and resilience (the ability to bounce back after a shock to the system). The reduction of soil sediment redistribution as a result of prairie reconstruction is an example of nonlinearity. A clear case of path dependence is the strong association between early life nutrition and diseases later in life. Resilience can be the result of farmers' behaviors to minimize their risks, such as providing irrigation systems to prepare for precipitation deficits.

by policy contexts and responses. Notable effects are described and categorized in the report under levels of income, wealth, and distributional equity; quality of life; and worker health and well-being.

The committee identified both direct and indirect consequences, and it found interactions across the various health, environmental, social, and economic domains (e.g., health effects that are due to environmental exposures; interdependency between socioeconomic status and health outcomes). The committee also found heterogeneity in the distribution of effects (e.g., obesity rates and food security that differ based on population characteristics). As a result of its structure (see Figures S-1 and S-2) and characteristics (see Box S-2), the committee concluded that the food system can be conceptualized as a complex adaptive system.[2] As a result,

[2] A complex adaptive system is a system composed of many heterogeneous pieces, whose interactions drive system behavior in ways that cannot easily be understood from considering the components separately.

study of the food system requires an analytical framework and appropriate methodologies that can capture key interactions and features.

THE FRAMEWORK

The committee developed an analytical framework that could be used to assess a vast array of possible configurations conceived for the food system. One single analytical tool to answer questions about the food system does not exist; however, the use of several validated tools can be helpful in addressing questions. The framework consists of a series of steps that are common in any assessment. Within that process, the core of the committee's framework consists of a set of principles to be considered throughout all of the steps.

Steps of the Framework

The six steps of the framework are (1) identify the problem; (2) define the scope of the problem; (3) identify the scenarios; (4) conduct the analysis; (5) synthesize the results; and (6) report the findings. The steps are meant to be followed in an iterative, not linear, manner. Figure S-3 shows the six steps as circles to the left of the figure.

Step 1: Identify the Problem

This step identifies the problem and goal(s) of the assessment. Assessments are generally motivated by broad problems and are often based on interactions with stakeholders and reviews of relevant literature. The problem statement should guide the direction of the assessment, including its goals, objectives, and research questions and all future assessment decisions.

Step 2: Define the Scope of the Problem

This step defines the boundaries and level of detail of the assessment. To analyze all effects on the entire food system across all possible dimensions may be intractable. Defining the relevant scope for analysis entails using the framework to identify meaningful changes along the food supply chain—in various effect domains and dimensions, in the time horizon, in interacting processes, and in system feedbacks. The scope defines the elements of the food system to be analyzed. The boundaries may enclose a subset of the larger food system (e.g., a particular food commodity, time, or geographic area). Boundaries for the system under analysis can be shaped by the nature of the problem and often depend on input from stakeholders

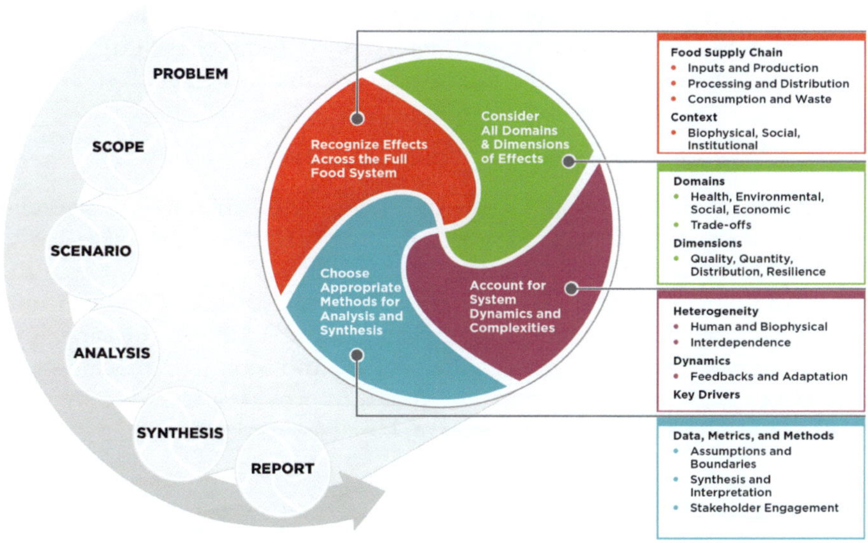

FIGURE S-3 Conceptual illustration of the analytical framework. The four principles of the framework are represented in the larger circle, the core of the framework. These principles need to be considered throughout the assessment steps, represented in the figure as six small circles.

and on budget limitations. Outside the boundaries, the assessment may assume constant conditions, even though potential far-reaching effects are possible beyond the boundaries. Within the defined boundaries, the assessment seeks to describe interactions and relationships among key actors along the relevant parts of the food supply chain; the impact of changes on a range of health, environment, social, and economic effects; and the processes and pathways that produce the outcomes of interest.

Step 3: Identify the Scenarios

This step identifies the food system scenarios (or configuration[s][3]) being analyzed. Most assessments compare system performance to one or more baseline scenarios. Alternative scenarios typically specify potential

[3] Configurations are elements within the food system, such as policy interventions, technologies, market conditions, or organizational structure of different segments of the food system, that can be modified to achieve a particular goal or to explore how potential drivers (e.g., growth in demand for foods with particular traits) might impact the distribution of health, environmental, social, and economic effects.

changes or interventions, such as a new policy or a new technology. Assessments should be explicit about each intervention being considered, including when, where, and how the intervention occurs.

Step 4: Conduct the Analysis

In this step, appropriate data and methods of analysis are selected. Multiple datasets, metrics, or analytical tools, including qualitative analysis, may be used to assess the range of scenarios and questions. Given the intended scope of a particular assessment, an analysis should draw on suitable methodologies to interpret measurements and build relevant models to assess the likely health, environmental, social, and economic effects associated with food system scenarios. The goal is to provide a scientifically valid basis for public and private decision making (see Appendix B).

Step 5: Synthesize the Results

In this step, synthesis and interpretation of findings and evidence is undertaken. Analyses of the complex food system are unlikely to offer simple answers, but rather may aim to provide insight into the range of outcomes resulting from any action, both beneficial and harmful, and their potential magnitude. Ultimately, value judgments of stakeholders and decision makers are often required to determine how to weight the various outcomes.

Step 6: Report the Findings

The goal of this step is to communicate findings to key stakeholders. Reporting involves sharing the assessment and recommendations with key stakeholders, broadly defined as the end-user of the assessment, members of affected communities, and the general public. The reporting step typically involves creating a report that clearly documents how the assessment was conducted; data sources and analytical tools, including the assumptions; interaction with stakeholders; findings; and recommendations.

Principles of the Framework

The framework consists of the following principles that would guide a team of assessors throughout an analysis (see Figure S-3): Consider effects across the full food system; address all domains and dimensions of effects; account for system dynamics and complexities; and choose appropriate methods.

Principle 1: Recognize Effects Across the Full Food System

Positive and negative health, environmental, social, and economic effects occur all along the food supply chain illustrated in Figure S-1 and also within the economic, biophysical, and social/political context. Both the food supply chain and its surrounding biophysical and institutional context should be recognized in any assessment.

Principle 2: Consider All Domains and Dimensions of Effects

Any single assessment should consider all four important domains of food system effects (health, environmental, social, and economic) and recognize that trade-offs among the different effects both within each domain and across them will often be necessary. Within each domain, four dimensions of effects[4]—quantity, quality, distribution, and resilience—measure how much of what the food system provides, where and to whom it goes, and how sustainably it can do so. Judgments about the relative importance of these dimensions for any particular assessment may be normative as well as empirical, and different assessors of the food system may disagree about their relative importance.

Principle 3: Account for System Dynamics and Complexities

An assessment should account for the characteristics of the food system as a complex adaptive system, as explained in Box S-2. For example, the food system is heterogeneous in terms of the variety of the actors and processes at each step of the food chain. Heterogeneity applies to the range of actors involved; to difference within a type of actors in resources, relationships, and knowledge; and to biophysical settings, including terrain, climate, and other natural resources. These heterogeneous actors interact within the system, and may adapt their behavior as system changes take place. Given the tendency of complex interactions to trigger dynamic repercussions, assessments should, to the extent feasible, account for effects across time, space, and heterogeneous populations. They should also acknowledge the potential role of underlying drivers and interacting

[4] Quantity, quality, distribution, and resilience measure how much the food system provides, where and to whom the production goes, and how sustainably it can produce. *Quantity* in the food system often matters relative to a benchmark because too little or too much can be problematic. *Quality* characterizes an outcome, such as the nutrition, taste, or safety of a food. *Distribution* measures where an outcome goes, such as the incidence of obesity across different consumer populations. *Resilience* measures the food system's ability to bounce back from sudden shocks and long-term pressures. For example, in response to honeybees dying of disease, resilience measures the food system's ability to continue to supply crops that rely on bee pollination.

pathways. The committee recognizes that any research or assessment team may be limited in terms of human and economic resources. Therefore, many assessments will be simplified (e.g., will only explore a specific question or effect). While scope limitations may preclude a specific study from careful consideration of *all* effects and drivers, it is important for *any* study to define the boundaries (i.e., what is the scope of the study) and assumptions (i.e., the potential role of relevant aspects not included). Also important is that the team of assessors has expertise in various disciplines related to the questions to be answered and that they have a plan for consulting with relevant stakeholders.

Principle 4: Choose Appropriate Methods for Analysis and Synthesis

Careful choice of metrics and methods is fundamental to conducting a meaningful assessment. Prevailing standards of evidence govern the choice of metrics and methods. They vary across health, environmental, social, and economic effects because of measurement challenges specific to each domain. The assumptions, limitations, accuracy, sensitivity, and other relevant factors for methods used should be clearly stated in the assessment. The committee has identified selected metrics, data sources, analytical techniques, and simulation models that might be used in an assessment of a policy or action affecting the food system (see Appendix B). As mentioned above, regardless of the method used, clearly framing the scope of the assessment and assumptions are important steps, given the complexity of the food system. In such cases, the committee recommends that any assessment at least acknowledge the existence of some potentially important effects or drivers that are outside the scope of the specific assessment.

LESSONS LEARNED

The committee was charged with providing examples from various parts of the food system to demonstrate how the framework could be applied for evaluating the effects of an alternative configuration (see Box S-3). The committee followed the first three steps as prescribed by the framework to illustrate how it could identify and define the problems in these examples. The last three steps (analysis, synthesis, and reporting) were excluded from those examples because conducting the assessment would have been beyond the committee's task. Therefore, readers should not take any of the specific analysis or configurations as recommendations, but rather as examples for future consideration.

Within these examples, there were several instances in which a proposed

BOX S-3
Examples of Food System Configurations Selected to Illustrate the Application of the Framework

The use of antibiotics in agriculture. The wide use of antibiotics in agriculture may contribute to the development of antibiotic-resistant organisms with implications for human and animal health. Analysis of historical and/or current configurations of the system may yield insights about the relative contributions of the food system and of human medicine to current growth in antibiotic resistance.

Recommendations for fish consumption and health. Consumption guidelines for fish have not considered the availability of sufficient fish to meet them and the potential environmental impacts. Several alternative scenarios could entail a change in dietary recommendations or the application of new technologies (e.g., sustainable farming production methods).

Policies mandating biofuel blending in gasoline supplies. Biofuel policies intended to increase the country's energy independence and decrease greenhouse gas emissions compared to fossil fuel were implemented without consideration of wider environmental effects and effects on domestic and global food prices.

Recommendations to increase fruit and vegetable consumption. The purpose of this assessment could be to understand the barriers and inducements to fruit and vegetable consumption so that better interventions to increase consumption can be implemented.

Nitrogen dynamics and management in agroecosystems. The use of high levels of nitrogen fertilizer to increase crop yields has environmental, health, and economic consequences that go beyond immediate concerns with crop yields. A baseline scenario could be one that is mostly reliant on mineral fertilizers without the use of methods to increase nitrogen uptake and retention. For comparison, an alternative cropping system could be less reliant on mineral nitrogen fertilizer and emphasize biological nitrogen fixation, manure and organic matter, amendments, cover crops, and perennial crops.

Policies on hen housing practices. This case study presents an assessment that is currently being conducted to analyze the implications for productivity, food safety, and workers' health of changing egg production practices. Data for the assessment are currently being collected on three types of hen management systems.

change (in recommended policy or practice to achieve a specific objective) within the food system could lead to unintended and unexpected consequences in multiple domains. These examples demonstrate the complexity of issues and confirm the need for the committee's analytical framework, which considers health, environmental, social, and economic domains.

CONCLUSIONS

Although no assessment was conducted, the examples and a literature review on effects of the food system did provide the committee with some insights. The committee provides the following conclusions:

1. *Comprehensive studies of food systems that use all principles of the committee's framework are rare in published literature. For example, the committee could not find a single example where all four domains (health, environment, social, and economic effects) and the four key dimensions (quantity, quality, distribution, and resilience) were considered. More importantly, most studies lack clear statements of boundaries and assumptions about the affected domains, their interactions, or dynamic feedbacks.*
2. *Studies that consider the entire food supply chain and address multiple domains (and dimensions) of effects of an intervention and its drivers can identify outcomes and trade-offs that are not visible in more narrowly focused assessments.*
3. *Policies or actions that aim for an outcome in one domain of the food system (e.g., health) can have consequences not only in the same domain but also in other ones (e.g., environmental, social, and economic domains). These consequences may be positive or negative, intended or unintended. They can be substantial and are often not proportional to the change incurred. That is, what might appear as a small intervention may have disproportionately large consequences in various domains across time and space.*
4. *The data and methodologies used to study the food system have been collected and developed both by public and by private initiatives, depending on the questions they help to address (e.g., public health or climate change questions versus questions related to the environmental effects of a specific company). Methodologies include not only those to describe and assess the effects of the system but also those that serve to synthesize and interpret the results. Publicly collected data and publicly supported models have been and continue to be critically important in assessing and comparing the effects of the food system in various domains and dimensions. The lack of access to data collected by industry can be a major challenge for public research aimed at understanding the drivers and effects of the food system.*
5. *Stakeholders are important audiences of any assessment exercise, but they also can play an important role throughout the process by contributing to, identifying, or scoping the problem or potential effects that may not have been apparent to the researchers. They*

also can be important sources of data when public sources are not readily available. Effectively engaging stakeholders has challenges, such as avoiding conflicts of interest, ensuring equitable engagement, and addressing potential lack of trust by the public. Therefore, this type of participatory process requires careful planning about whom to involve, when to involve them, and how much involvement is appropriate.

6. *Even though major improvements in the U.S. food system have resulted in the past from the introduction of new technologies, needed future improvements in the system may not be achievable solely through technological innovation. Achieving them may require more comprehensive approaches that incorporate non-technological factors to reach long-term solutions. Systemic approaches that take full account of social, economic, ecological, and evolutionary factors and processes will be required to meet challenges to the U.S. food system in the 21st century. Such challenges include antibiotic and pesticide resistance; chemical contamination of air and water; soil erosion and degradation; water deficits; diet-related chronic disease, obesity, domestic and global hunger, and malnutrition; and food safety.*
7. *To discover the best solutions to these problems, it is important not only to identify the effects of the current system but also to understand the drivers (e.g., human behavior, markets, policy) and how they interact with each other and with the observable system effects. Such understanding can help decision makers to identify the best opportunities to intervene and to anticipate the potential consequences of any intervention.*

A CALL TO ACTION

Use of the Framework

The committee provides an analytical framework that should be used to examine policies or proposed changes in the food system that may have wide implications. The committee intends for the report to stimulate broad thinking among policy makers, researchers, and other stakeholders about the consequences of food system policies and actions beyond a single dimension. The proposed framework is relevant for researchers who are interested in examining the health, environmental, social, and economic effects of aspects of food production, processing, distribution, and marketing. Applying the framework also will help to identify uncertainties and identify and prioritize research needs. Other stakeholders can use the framework to develop evidence that will be helpful in understanding the costs and benefits of alternative configurations within a food system. Moreover, the framework provides a tool for all interested stakeholders to deliberate about challenging issues in a transparent manner by considering multiple sources of data and information. Given that other factors, such as value judgments, underlie many choices for interventions, the committee strongly urges decision makers to use this framework to analyze the best available information about system-wide effects, trade-offs, and dynamics and to guide their selection of interventions.

This framework is sufficiently general and flexible for analyzing various configurations of the current and future food system. The committee recognizes that in some cases limited resources might preclude a comprehensive analysis of the food system. Also, discrete questions may not require a full systemic analysis. In such instances, not all steps of the framework or methods will apply equally, depending on the scope and topic chosen by a researcher. Regardless of the scope of the analysis, assessors still need to recognize boundaries and implications and to take into account the various interrelationships of the food system.

The description of the food system and its effects has intentionally been presented from a U.S. perspective, and it omits important interactions and effects for the rest of the world. However, its application is aimed not only at those attempting to understand the U.S. food system and its consequences but also at others outside the United States who are conducting similar research and making similar decisions about their food systems.

Critical Needs for Using the Framework

The committee identified two general areas that need urgent attention to make the best use of the framework: the need for data collection (as well as development of validated metrics and methodologies), and the need for increased human capacity. The committee did not specify areas of research that should be prioritized, as one expected outcome of applying the framework would be identification of the most important research needs for a particular area.

Organized and systematic collection of data on local, state, regional, national, and international bases is vital to improving the ability to answer critical questions on U.S. food system impacts. The U.S. government maintains major datasets that are useful for assessing the health, environmental, social, and economic effects of the food system. These include the U.S. Department of Agriculture's (USDA's) Food Availability Data System and Loss-Adjusted Food Availability; the Centers for Disease Control and Prevention's National Health and Nutrition Examination Survey; the National Agricultural Statistics Service's Agricultural Chemical Use Program; the U.S.

Department of Labor's National Agricultural Worker Survey; and USDA's National Agriculture Statistics Service data series (e.g., the Farm Labor Survey; the Census of Agriculture; and the Agricultural Resource Management Survey). Many other databases are also crucial for conducting assessments (see Appendix B).

The design, collection, and analysis of data should be reviewed periodically so that it matches the needs of researchers and decision makers as new questions arise. Specific needs for data collection could be identified in all domains, but some general areas of concern are the overall lack of segregated datasets (e.g., data by sociodemographic factors at regional or local levels) and, for some variables, the lack of validated metrics, such as the well-being of individuals or groups.

The committee recommends that Congress and federal agencies continue funding and supporting the collection (and improvement) of datasets that can be used for food system assessment studies along with giving consideration to creating new data collection programs as priorities arise. Likewise, continued support to develop and advance validated methods and models is necessary for a comprehensive understanding of the U.S. food system effects across all domains.

Government, academic, and private sectors have recognized the need to share data. The committee supports federal government efforts to share data and recommends further development of improved methods for more efficiently sharing data and models across disciplines and agencies and with the private sector. The committee recommends that government–industry collaboration mechanisms be developed to make industry-collected information more readily available for use in research and policy analysis.

Efforts to build human capacity are needed for the recommended framework to be used appropriately. As this report has pointed out, a fuller understanding of the implications of changes to the food system could be gained by integrated analyses, yet much research in these domains remains narrowly focused and linear in its design. Scientists in academia, the private sector, and government agencies need to be trained in all aspects of complex systems approaches—including systems research design, data collection, and analytical methodologies—and the use of models would remove some barriers impeding progress. Continued support for research on and demonstration of systems analysis methodologies will be important to ensure that innovation in this field continues. It is particularly important that federal agencies such as USDA, the Food and Drug Administration, the Environmental Protection Agency, and the U.S. Department of Labor—as well as other relevant federal agencies— have the human and analytical capacity to undertake assessments using the principles of the framework as they consider policies with domestic and global consequences.

PART I

The U.S. Food System

1

Introduction

From the earliest developments of agriculture, a major goal has been to attain sufficient foods to provide the energy and nutrients needed for a healthy, active life. Food production has adapted to changing demographics; consumer preferences; ideas about health, social, and economic conditions; environmental concerns; and advances in science and technology. As a result, the U.S. food system today has many actors and processes, affecting numerous areas of our lives that go beyond providing nutritious foods. Over time, food production has evolved and become highly complex. This complexity takes many forms, such as (1) interconnected markets that function at global, regional, national, and local levels; (2) the diversity of public interventions in those markets, from information and research through subsidies, regulations, and standards to taxes, mandates, quotas, and requirements; and (3) the varying needs, perceptions, and values among all actors. The result is a multilayered, dynamic, multipurposed food system. The behavior of actors can lead to unforeseen, unintended, or unwanted results, even with the best analytical techniques. Other characteristics of the system—its permeable borders that connect it both to a global food system and to a diverse, changing broader economy and society and the different tolerances for risk and values as well as changing individual and societal priorities—add further dynamism to the food system and uncertainty to its analysis.

Due to limited time and resources, the committee made the following simplifying decisions that should be borne in mind by those using the framework:

- The extensive connections of the U.S. food system to the global food system, and the effects of changes in the U.S. system on other countries, are not included in the committee's review of effects of the food system; and
- The extensive connections to labor markets and social structures that have significant behavioral (e.g., habits and lifestyle choices) and socioeconomic (e.g., working conditions) effects and are important to consider in assessing causality between the food system and its effects are not explored in detail.

Policy or business interventions involving a segment of the food system often have consequences beyond the original issue the intervention was meant to address. Because of these consequences, when considering actions affecting a segment of the food system, decision makers must think broadly about potential intervention options and effects. They will also need to make trade-offs, that is, situations that involve losing one quality or aspect of something in return for gaining another quality or aspect.

Making decisions is typically challenging as the number of trade-offs among potential options is large, comparisons among trade-offs are not always clear, and measuring the effects resulting from decisions is complicated. To add to the challenge, individuals differ in their values and in how they weigh trade-offs. This study examined the U.S. food system from the perspective of its domestic health, environmental, social, and economic effects. Its aim is to develop an analytical framework that will enable decision makers, researchers, and others to examine the possible effects of alternative policies on agricultural or food practices.

This introductory chapter discusses the origins and justification of the study, describes the charge and formation of the committee, and outlines the general approach to accomplishing the task. The chapter also describes the organization of the report.

ORIGINS AND NEED FOR THE STUDY

The U.S. food system is a dynamic, fast-changing, multidimensional enterprise. Through many technological advances, policies, market forces, and other drivers, it has managed to provide abundant food at relatively low cost in the midst of a growing world population. Yet, it also affects the environment (e.g., biodiversity, water, soil, air, and climate, both domestically and globally), human health (e.g., direct health effects, such as nutrition and hunger, foodborne illnesses or diet-related chronic disease risk, and indirect health effects, such as those associated with hunger and stunted development or soil, air, and water pollution), and society (e.g., effects on food accessibility and affordability, land use, labor, and local economies). Some of these consequences are not captured in the price of food, but rather, are incurred by society at large in the form of health care costs, environmental remediation, and other "hidden" costs. Other consequences are intensified by changes in food price levels or price volatility. If ignored, these costs will continue to compromise health and food security, the environment, and the resilience of the food system. Finding the best solutions that minimize costs to society can only be achieved when the options are well considered and their differing effects are measured and weighed. In addressing these issues, questions arise as to how to measure the effects and consider trade-offs resulting from agricultural and food system practices, what current methodologies can be used to analyze and compare the trade-offs, and what data gaps and uncertainties exist to hamper decision making.

As the population continues to grow, important questions about the future of the food system have been raised (see Box 1-1). In many different ways and from many different perspectives, various groups (e.g., U.S. Department of Agriculture, U.S. Agency for International Development, Food and Agriculture Organization, UN Environment Programme, World Food Program) have expressed concerns and made serious calls and efforts

BOX 1-1
Selected Concerns About the Food System

- Availability, accessibility, affordability, and quality of the food supply.
- Effects of global climate change on agricultural productivity.
- Emissions of greenhouse gases that result from the activities in the food system.
- The prevalence of antibiotic-resistant bacteria in food or the environment, with serious consequences in human health.
- Levels and quality of water and other natural resources that are important for sustaining life.
- The prevalence of obesity and diet-associated chronic diseases.
- Global and U.S. food security and malnutrition, particularly when the global population is predicted to increase to 9 billion by 2050.
- Exposure to chemical contaminants occurring in the environment and to chemical residues as a result of agriculture and food-producing activities.
- The social and economic viability of livelihoods of rural or fishing communities.
- The balance of natural ecosystems and biodiversity.
- Workers' quality of life characteristics, including access to health, safety concerns, and adequate wages.

to address a range of world food problems. The report elaborates on many of them.

The idea for this study originated at a 2012 Institute of Medicine (IOM)/National Research Council (NRC) workshop, *Exploring the True Costs of Food*. The workshop was designed to spur interdisciplinary discussion about the domestic environmental and health effects of the food system. It brought together expert stakeholders who rarely explore these questions together, and individual speakers who stressed the need for an evidence-based, integrated framework that could systemically examine the complex relationships among domestic environmental and health effects of the U.S. food system. At a meeting immediately after the workshop, attendees generated key questions about emerging challenges in food and agriculture. Those ideas led to many conversations that resulted in the current study.

To inform business and management decisions, a first task when addressing these challenges is to understand and measure the various costs and benefits of the food system. At the 2012 IOM/NRC workshop, the speakers shared tools and methodologies, and these presentations highlighted two important problems that limit a comprehensive approach to addressing the complex relationships that exist within the U.S. food system. The first is that current methods designed to examine impacts, such as life cycle assessment (LCA) and health impact assessment (HIA), are limited in a variety of ways. LCA—the evaluation of the environmental costs and benefits across a product's life span—has been used to compare the effects of alternative practices and for business/management decision-making processes. However, an LCA rarely includes health or socioeconomic effects and often only accounts for a limited number of environmental effect categories (e.g., greenhouse gas emissions). HIA is a systematic process to assess the potential health effects of proposed policies and programs that have historically not been recognized as related to health; however, HIA has not been broadly used in the context of agriculture and food. Other analytical tools, such as risk assessments, continue to be improved, but they are generally used only to assist in making decisions about chemical and microbiological safety. These methodologies work well in some situations but may have critical limitations when measuring the complex relationships within the food system. Their limitations have led to disagreements about their proper use, which hinders potential improvements in decision-making processes.

A second problem that was highlighted at the workshop is that although a siloed approach (taking one effect at a time) to making decisions might be clearer at communicating with others, it may also lead to potential unintended and undesirable effects. For example, evaluations about the merits of various farm animal housing designs can lead to unintended consequences if important dimensions (health, environmental, social, or economic effects) are absent from the decision-making process. Several reports also have recommended improved consistency and alignment between agriculture and health and nutrition policies, which highlight the need for improved approaches (Hawkes, 2007; IOM, 2012). Such challenges become even greater when the effects of U.S. actions on the global food system are added to the equation.

Understanding the relationships among components of the food system and their effects on health, the environment, and society are essential prerequisites for attempting any quantitative evaluation of costs and benefits of the food system. Building on the methods mentioned above, a common analytical framework for decision makers, researchers, and practitioners is needed to systemically consider and evaluate contentious topics.

STATEMENT OF TASK AND APPROACH OF THE COMMITTEE

The Task

The IOM and the NRC convened an expert committee to develop an analytical framework for assessing the health, environmental, social, and economic effects (whether positive or negative, intentional or unintentional) associated with the ways in which food is grown, processed, distributed, and marketed in the United States. It was desired that the framework would provide a systemic approach that would examine the effects of activities, practices, or policies within the U.S. food system and across its broader global and societal settings. This framework would use a variety of methods that could enable decision makers, researchers, and others to understand the potential impact of a proposed change. To assist readers in understanding the framework, the committee was also charged with selecting examples to illustrate the potential utility of the framework, and to identify gaps in areas where further information is needed for more accurate assessments (see the Statement of Task in Box 1-2).

Because of the tight timeline, early on the committee decided to focus primarily on the domestic effects of the U.S. food system. Consequently, the discussions about the effects of the food system do not include discussion of important consequences of U.S. food-related actions for the rest of the world, or feedbacks from global responses to changes in the U.S. food system. Those discussions need to be understood with that limitation in mind.

This study has three major aims: (1) facilitating understanding of the environmental, health, social, and economic effects associated with the food system and how these effects are interlinked; (2) encouraging the development of improved metrics to identify and measure these effects; and (3) enhancing decision making about agricultural and food policies and practices

BOX 1-2
Statement of Task

The expert committee will develop a framework for assessing the health, environmental, and social effects (positive and negative) associated with the ways in which food is grown, processed, distributed, marketed, retailed, and consumed within the U.S. food system. In developing the framework, the committee will undertake the following activities:

1. Examine available methods, methodologies, and data that are needed to undertake comparisons and measure effects. Examples of such needs that the committee will examine are:

    - Defining comparable characteristics of different configurations of elements within the food system.
    - Mapping the pathways through which different configurations of elements of the food system create or contribute to health, environmental, and social effects.
    - Determining the contribution of those configurations to effects relative to those from other influences.
    - Characterizing the scale of effects (e.g., individual, national).
    - Quantifying the magnitude and direction of effects.
    - Monetizing effects, when appropriate.
    - Addressing uncertainty, complexity, and variability in conducting comparisons and measuring effects.

so as to minimize unintended consequences across the health, environmental, social, and economic dimensions.

The committee envisions the framework to be useful in many ways and to be used by different audiences (e.g., policy makers, researchers, practitioners, other stakeholders). For example, policy makers could use the framework to compare the effects and trade-offs of alternative food system policies or practices. The proposed framework is also relevant for researchers who are interested in examining the health, environmental, social, and economic effects of food production, processing, distribution, and marketing. Practitioners and other stakeholders working in agriculture, health, and the environment can use the framework to develop evidence that would be helpful in understanding the costs and benefits of alternative configurations[1] (e.g., activities, practices, or policies) within a food system.

[1] Configurations are elements within the food system, such as policy interventions, technologies, market conditions, or organizational structure of different segments of the food system,

2. Describe several examples of different configurations of elements within the food system and describe how the framework will be applied, step by step, to compare them. Examples should be drawn from different parts of the food system (production, harvest, processing, distribution, marketing, retailing, and consumption). The emphasis will be on those effects that are generally not recognized (i.e., they may not be fully incorporated into the price of food). Different configurations for the committee to consider might include regionally based food systems and a global food system; free-range production of poultry and caged housing practices; and reduced retail presence of processed food and current availability of processed food.
3. In constructing examples, describe the strengths and weaknesses of the framework in different contextual situations and suggest how and when adjustments to the framework may lead to more accurate comparisons. The goal of the examples is to illustrate the potential use of the framework to analyze a variety of questions and compare, measure, and, in some cases, monetize the effects of different scenarios on public health, the environment, and society. The focus of these exercises should be in explaining the elements of the framework, not in attempting the analyses.
4. The committee will also identify information needs and gaps in methods and methodologies that, if filled, could provide greater certainty in the attribution and quantification of effects related to food system configurations and improve the predictive value of the framework for evaluating how changes in and across the food system might affect health, the environment, and society.

General Approach

An ad hoc, expert committee of 15 experts was convened to conduct the study and develop a consensus report. The committee members have expertise in agricultural production systems; food system analysis; food and nutritional sciences; environmental effects of food and agriculture; HIA; LCA; health, agriculture, and food economics; and complex systems modeling. The composition of the committee reflects the fact that the main goal of the Statement of Task is to develop an analytical framework to assess the food system (which requires highly technical skills and knowledge of methodologies) and not to evaluate food system configurations.

The committee met five times in closed session to gather information,

that can be modified to achieve a particular goal or to explore how potential drivers (e.g., growth in demand for foods with particular traits) might impact the distribution of health, environmental, social, and economic effects.

assess literature and other evidence sources, and deliberate, and they had numerous other interactions by telephone and e-mail. In addition, the committee conducted two public sessions and one 1.5-day workshop. The public sessions and workshop provided an opportunity for the committee to obtain information helpful to accomplishing its tasks (see Appendix A for public sessions and workshop agendas).

Before developing its framework, the committee believed it was necessary to define critical terms to provide context for its task. In that vein, the committee first undertook an exercise to describe the U.S. food system and to examine how the current system has evolved. In examining the domestic food system, the intricacies and nuances of the system were revealed, along with its numerous interactions across multiple dimensions, confirming the need for a comprehensive assessment that would consider these complexities.

Boundaries and Clarifications About the Task

Although the task of the committee is clear in delineating the scope of the committee's work, a few aspects of the task deserve further explanation so that the reader has the appropriate expectations about the report.

The committee carried out its task from the U.S. perspective, which was used in the description of the U.S. food system and a brief historical overview of how it evolved. Similarly, the descriptions of the effects and its complexities have focused on the U.S. population and environment. Given the level of international trade, investment, and institutional relationships of the U.S. food system and the global nature of the food and agriculture industry as a whole, the committee recognizes that any actions in the United States will have effects not just at the domestic level, but globally as well. Given widely different levels of economic and food system development worldwide, effects of similar policies or practices elsewhere could be both important and very different. Such variations and trade-offs are important considerations when crafting effective interventions.

In addition to developing a framework, the committee was asked to provide different examples within the food system on how proposed changes in one area could affect others. These examples would demonstrate how the framework could be applied to assess different configurations within the food system. Although it was outside the committee's task to conduct any actual assessments, the examples reiterate how decisions may have unanticipated consequences across the food system. The six examples chosen by the committee are relevant for the current U.S. food system because they raise important and complex questions. The issues touch on healthy and safe diets, food security, animal welfare, environmental health, and natural resource use. In presenting the examples, the committee strove to provide contextual information and evidence relative to the potential effects. The examples have global effects that in some cases were not assessed; still, the intention of the committee was that any user of the framework would also consider effects at the global level. The committee did not conduct any analysis or make recommendations on how to improve any aspect of the food system by new processes or policy interventions. In addition, the committee did not make recommendations on how the framework could be used in the policy-making process. Because the committee did not conduct actual assessments, it did not attempt to gather all of the necessary data or review the evidence in a systematic manner. Therefore, these applications of the framework are conducted in relatively brief and theoretical terms.

The framework is intended to be an analytical tool to evaluate discrete components of the food system and their interplay with the broader food system. When analyzing specific areas of the food system, users of this framework will need to be aware of as many effects as possible, even when they cannot all be included in an analysis. The committee recognizes that for many of the effects mentioned, the data are scarce and assessments are difficult to conduct. In such circumstances, decisions still need to be made about agriculture and food and data or analytical deficiencies should be noted. However, with enough interest and urgency from stakeholders, data can be collected and analyzed and scientific assessments can be conducted to strengthen analyses and decisions.

As noted earlier, the U.S. food system is embedded in a broader social, biophysical, and economic context within American society. Within that context, many factors play a role in shaping the health, environmental, social, and economic effects of the food system. The committee recognizes that neither all of the factors nor all of the effects and complexities of the food system were identified in the report. For example, significant factors that need to be considered, such as the anthropological and cultural aspects of populations, were omitted. Important effects such as genetic biodiversity, food waste, and others are also not mentioned. Furthermore, the committee made no attempt to assess levels of causation to attribute to these factors or to provide guidance for what will constitute various levels of evidence, but it does refer to other authoritative reports and papers that have addressed this difficult question.

In addition, there are many other important scenarios (or configurations) of the food system that could have been used as examples to show the application of the framework. For example, the framework could be used by private companies or public institutions to help guide decisions about management of food waste or of food defense concerns, but none of these aspects (or many others) are elaborated in the report.

ORGANIZATION OF THE REPORT

This introductory chapter has described the origins of the study, the Statement of Task, and the approach taken by the committee to address its charge. Chapter 2 describes the U.S. food system and highlights the evolutionary process that has led to its current configuration. The next series of chapters discuss important effects in four dimensions of interest, namely, health (Chapter 3), environmental (Chapter 4), and social and economic (Chapter 5) dimensions. Chapter 6 discusses the food system as a "complex adaptive system"[2] and Chapter 7 describes the committee's analytic framework. In describing the utility of the framework, Chapter 7 takes the issue of antibiotics to illustrate steps for applying the framework. Chapter 7 also illustrates the use of the framework with five additional examples (Annexes 1 through 5): (1) recommendations for fish consumption; (2) biofuels; (3) recommendations for fruit and vegetable consumption; (4) nitrogen use in agriculture; and (5) hen housing practices. The committee notes that some readers might want to go directly to Chapter 6 ("The U.S. Food and Agriculture System as a Complex Adaptive System") and Chapter 7 ("A Framework for Assessing the Food System and Its Effects"), but other readers might find the effects of the food system (Chapters 3, 4, and 5) useful as they provide valuable details demonstrating the complexities. The report ends with concluding comments in Chapter 8. Finally, the appendixes present the open sessions' agendas (Appendix A); tables of selected metrics, methodologies, data, and models (Appendix B); a list of acronyms (Appendix C); and short biographies of the committee members (Appendix D).

REFERENCES

Hawkes, C. 2007. Promoting healthy diets and tackling obesity and diet-related chronic diseases: What are the agricultural policy levers? *Food and Nutrition Bulletin* 28(2 Suppl):S312-S322.

IOM (Institute of Medicine). 2012. *Accelerating progress in obesity prevention: Solving the weight of the nation.* Washington, DC: The National Academies Press.

---

[2] A complex adaptive system is a system composed of many heterogeneous pieces, whose interactions drive system behavior in ways that cannot easily be understood from considering the components separately.

2

Overview of the U.S. Food System

To develop a framework for assessing the effects of a food system, it is essential to define the internal components and boundaries of the system, as well as its linkages to an "external" world. Previous scholars have operationalized a definition of the U.S. food system in many ways (Kinsey, 2001, 2013; Oskam et al., 2010; Senauer and Venturini, 2005). Nearly all contain some notion of a "food supply chain" through which raw materials and inputs are turned into edible food products that are consumed by end-users. Other definitions include significant attention to the biophysical and social/institutional environments within which the supply chain operates. The committee has used this more comprehensive approach in developing its framework. But today's food system has been shaped historically by different internal and external drivers (e.g., policy, markets, environmental change) that have evolved with time as well. To view the food system in this historical context, the chapter describes the current system followed by a brief history of its evolution as it has been shaped by those drivers. Because the focus of this report is to develop a framework and not to represent a historical account of events, the committee treats the history and evolution of the food system succinctly, avoiding extensive descriptions of events or identification of all of the drivers and their interactions. Furthermore, to assess the effects of the food system, it is necessary to have a good understanding of its drivers (see Chapter 7). Because the food system is dynamic and the drivers will likely be different in the future, the intent of this chapter is simply to expose the readers (and future assessors of the food system) to ideas for potential drivers. Some of the drivers, however, are elaborated further in other chapters to exemplify the complexities of the food system.

DEFINING AND MAPPING THE CURRENT U.S. FOOD SYSTEM

Food Supply Chain

In a simple subsistence agricultural society, the number of actors, inputs, flows, processes, and outputs in a food supply chain might be relatively few because most producers and consumers of food are the same. In the modern U.S. food system, however, the food supply chain is extremely complex, and the delivery of a single type of food to a consumer involves many actors. Here, we describe a system that has experienced significant changes over the past 50 years, with multiple positive and negative effects on health, the environment, society, and the economy.

Food Supply Chain Components

Figure 2-1 illustrates the core components of the modern U.S. food supply chain.[1] Primary production of food commodities usually originates in the farm production sector, in which farmers, fishers, and ranchers combine their land, water, and labor resources with capital, machinery, and manufactured inputs from an input supply sector to produce raw agricultural commodities (crops and livestock).

Although food sold directly from farmers to consumers is a small but growing segment of the market, the overwhelming bulk of food is handled by several other sectors before being consumed. Initially, many commodities are sold by farmers to first line handlers or primary processors who aggregate, store, and provide initial processing of commodities before shipping them to wholesalers or the processing and manufacturing sectors. First line handlers include both for-profit commodity trading companies and farmer cooperatives that aggregate the output of individual farms to gain economies of scale and market access to the rest of the food supply chain. First line handlers also include companies that wash, wax, wrap, and pack fruits and vegetables, as well as flour millers, oilseed processors, and other firms that prepare raw materials for use in the processing and manufacturing of finished food products. By-products from this sector often are fed to livestock or used in industrial processes. The food processing and manufacturing sector includes meat packers, bakeries, and consumer product

[1] A more detailed description of the key actors within each subsector is provided in Chapter 5.

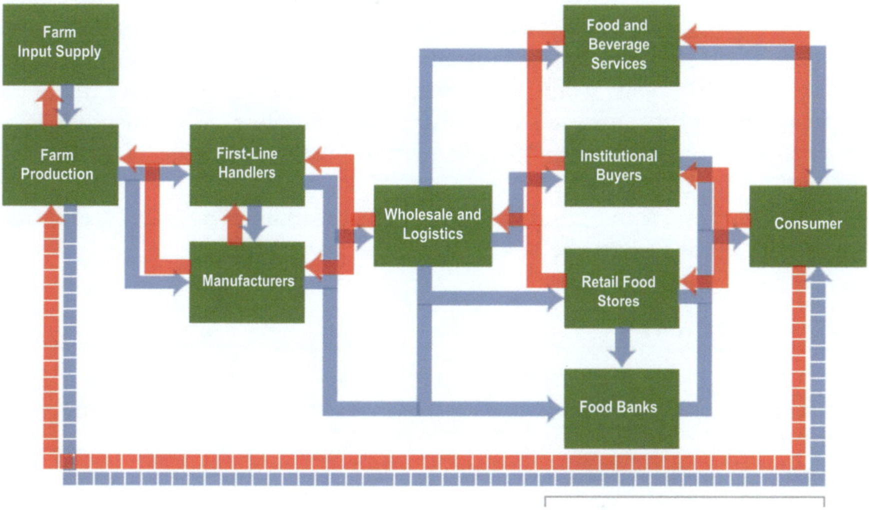

FIGURE 2-1 Conceptual model of a food supply chain. Elements or actors in this supply chain in one area (e.g., region or country) also have interactions (e.g., international trade) with actors in other areas.

goods companies that turn raw materials into higher-value packaged and processed food products.

The food products provided by first line handlers and the processing and manufacturing sector are often passed along to a wholesale and logistics sector. The wholesale food industry consists of companies that purchase and store food products in a network of warehouse facilities and then sell and distribute these products to retail outlets using an extensive transportation infrastructure. A logistics firm refers to a company that does not actually assume ownership of the food products but is paid to provide the service of logistical distribution and inventory coordination.

Ultimately, most food products are passed along to the retail food and food service sectors, where most consumers in the United States purchase their food. The retail food sector includes grocery stores, convenience stores, vending machines, and other retail outlets where individual consumers buy food products for home preparation and consumption. The food service sector includes restaurants, fast-food outlets, eating and drinking establishments, and institutional cafeterias where individuals purchase both food and the service of having that food prepared and served. This sector represents a growing percentage of the retail food supply.

In most graphic depictions of the food supply chain, consumers represent the final actors. Consumers are individuals who purchase (and store) food to be prepared or eaten at home or elsewhere, or who eat in a food service establishment. Some consumers receive food assistance through governmental programs such as the Supplemental Nutrition Assistance Program (SNAP) and the Special Supplemental Nutrition Program for Women, Infants, and Children (WIC).

Others may receive food through school feeding programs or through private food banks and shelves.

Supply Chain Material Flows

Figure 2-1 also highlights the flows of food, services, and information about food (orange arrows), which begin at the input and farm production sector and extend along the food supply chain until they reach the consumer. This information includes grades, brands, nutritional labels, and advertising. At the same time, the figure illustrates the flows of information about consumer preferences (blue arrows) expressed in terms of market demand (purchases) or pressure on policy makers that move back up the chain and influence the types of foods that are grown, processed, distributed, and sold.

To put the material flows in perspective, the approximate volumes of different types of food that flow through the U.S. food system are highlighted in Figure 2-2. All quantities are converted to billions of pounds and are based on 2009 numbers from the U.S. Department of Agriculture (USDA). The first observation is that about one-third of the 1,260 billion pounds (b. lbs) of all field crop production in the United States is used directly for animal feed. Livestock are also fed a considerable amount of forages (from harvested hay, pastures, and rangelands) that is not included in the figure. As a rough approximation, U.S. producers harvested 130-155 million tons of hay and forage for livestock feed in 2007 and 2012 (USDA, 2009, 2014). Statistics about the total volume of forages consumed by livestock grazing on pasture and rangeland are not systematically gathered by USDA, but estimates of average intake for grazing livestock suggest an equal or larger share of total beef, dairy, and sheep livestock forage intake (USDA, 2003). Another 18 percent of field crops (230 b. lbs) are exported as bulk commodities. This export market has been a source of economic growth and stability for producers. Because the United States imports only 67 b. lbs of food products (both crops and livestock), the U.S. food system has contributed to moving the overall U.S. balance of trade toward the positive side.

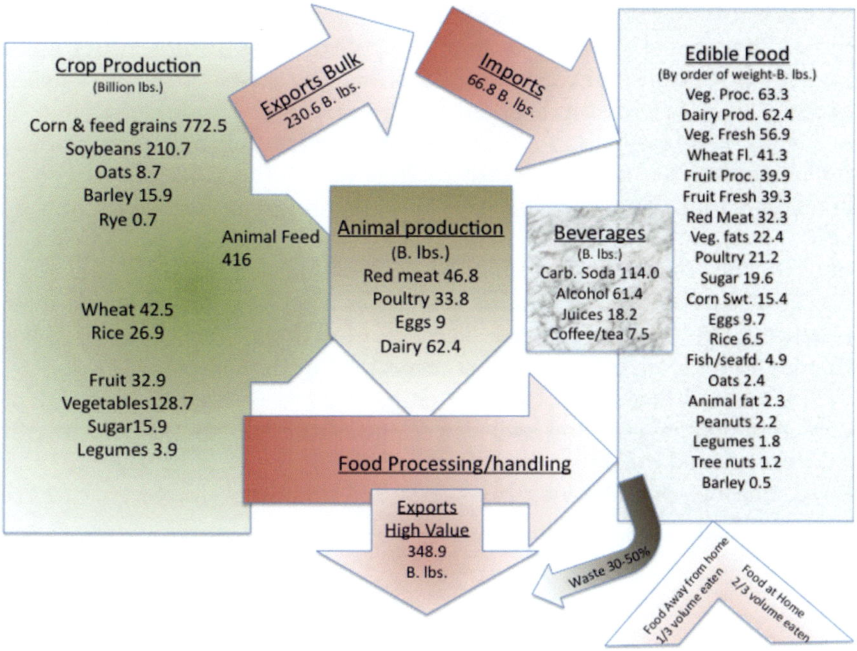

FIGURE 2-2 Flow of food in the U.S. food system.
NOTE: Approximations based on 2009 data from http://www.ers.usda.gov/data-products.aspx (accessed April 2, 2015).
SOURCE: Adapted from Kinsey, 2013, p. 22. Reprinted with permission from Springer.

Most of the field crop production in the United States that is not exported or fed to livestock (roughly half the total) goes through some type of food processing and manufacturing before being consumed by people. Although many fruits and vegetables are consumed in raw form, most are still subjected to washing, sorting, waxing, storing, and transportation through the commercial supply chain.

Some representations of the food supply chain that are based on "full life cycle accounting" approaches also include the actors and subsectors that deal with food loss, waste, and recovery. Food loss and waste occur all along the food supply chain, from farm to fork. Examples of loss[2] include farmers finding it economically unfeasible to send all of their product to market; food producers deciding not to use products that fail to meet qual-

[2] Loss is the edible, post-harvest food available for human consumption but not consumed for any reason.

ity standards; quality of product not meeting standards at retail; households discarding food that is out of date or spoiled; and consumers not always saving leftover food for future consumption. The waste stream also includes products that result from food consumption.

The roughly 1 trillion lbs of crop products (1,260 b. lbs minus 230 b. lbs of exports) are converted into roughly 664 billion pounds of beverages and edible food. This implies a one-third loss in weight between production and retail. Some of this weight loss is due to field trimming and storing, but much of the volume is recycled as by-products used in animal husbandry or industrial applications. Other weight losses come in processing and manufacturing, as raw products are trimmed of fat and bone, peeled, cooked, dried, and stored. Spoilage occurs, especially in fresh product.

Retail and household losses of edible food are estimated to be 31 percent of the pounds of food available for consumption and 33 percent of the calories in food available for consumption (Buzby et al., 2013, 2014). In 2010, this aggregate loss/waste equaled $161.6 billion (Buzby et al., 2014),

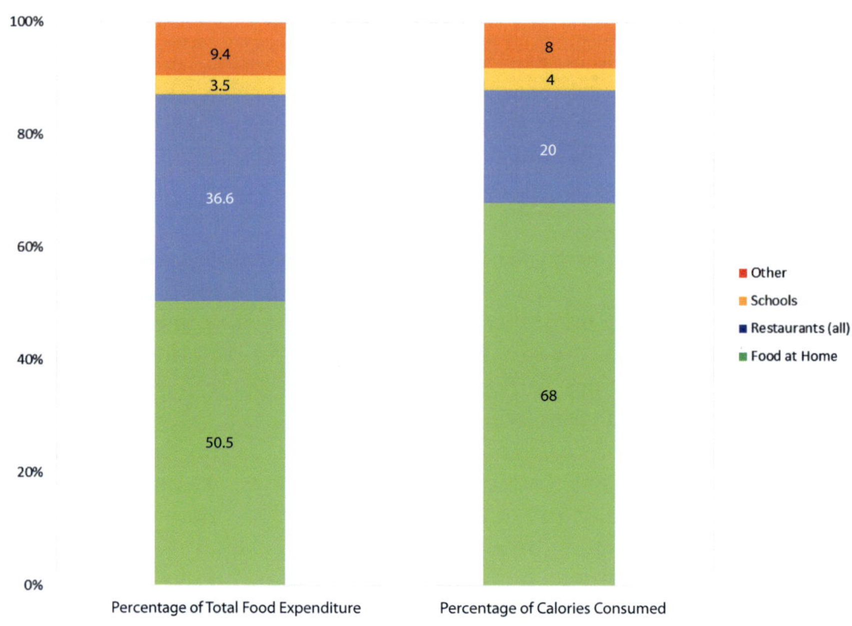

FIGURE 2-3 Percentage of calories and food expenditures for food consumed at home and away from home.
SOURCES: ERS, 2013a; Lin and Guthrie, 2012.

which is about 11 percent of the total value of food and beverage sales in 2013 dollars ($1,624 billion) (Food Institute, 2014).

The 664 billion pounds of beverages and edible food available to consumers can be further subdivided to illustrate the relative importance of different retail outlets. Figure 2-3 uses data from the 2005-2008 National Health and Nutrition Examination Survey (NHANES) and 2012 data from the USDA Economic Research Service (ERS) to show that about two-thirds of the volume of the available edible foods and beverages and about half of the dollars spent on food were consumed at home, with the remainder consumed away from home (Lin and Guthrie, 2012).

Economic Importance of U.S. Food Chain Components

The percentage of income spent on food is approximately 10 percent (ERS, 2013a), although it varies somewhat depending on household income (see Chapter 5). Overall, however, the food system represents one of the most significant components of the U.S. economy. It affects the social and economic well-being of nearly all Americans and plays a significant role in the well-being of the global community. The USDA/ERS estimates that agriculture and food contributed nearly $776 billion to the U.S. gross domestic product (GDP) in 2012 (nearly 5 percent of the total) (ERS, 2014a).

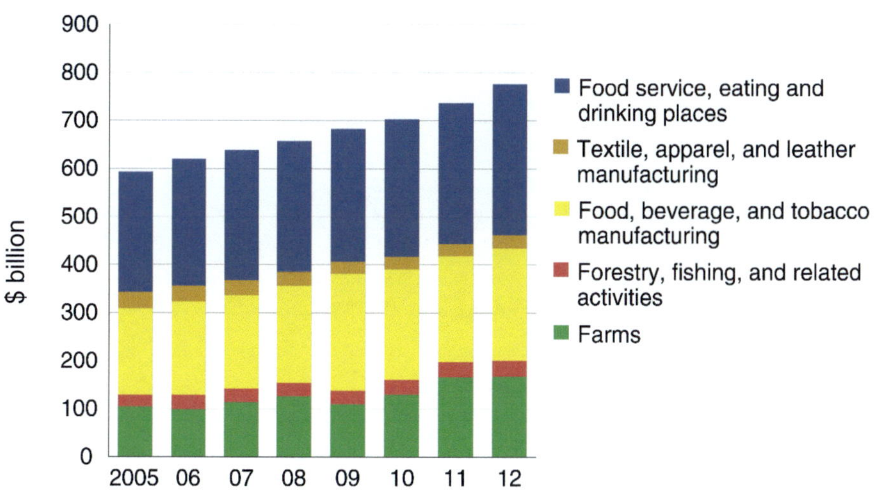

FIGURE 2-4 Estimated value added to GDP by sectors of U.S. food supply chain, 2005-2012.
NOTE: GDP = gross domestic product.
SOURCE: ERS, 2014a.

Although production agriculture generates slightly less than 1 percent of GDP, the food processing and manufacturing as well as the food service industries (including retail stores) each account for an additional 2 percent of U.S. economic output (see Figure 2-4). The U.S. food and fiber system accounted for 18 percent of employment (King et al., 2012), 4 percent of imported goods, and 11 percent of exports in 2011 (ERS, 2014c).

The relative economic contribution of each various step of the U.S. food supply chain has changed significantly over the past 100 years. Generally speaking, the economic importance of the farm production subsector has steadily diminished relative to the shares of the other components of the food supply chain. This reflects the increasing role of processing, distribution, and marketing activities in transforming raw agricultural commodities into food products and services and transferring them to consumers in an increasingly national and global marketplace. USDA regularly estimates what the typical consumer's food dollar is used to pay for, according to three perspectives (Canning, 2011). Figure 2-5 shows how the consumer dollar was divided between the farm and marketing sectors between 1993 and 2012. The marketing share in 2012 illustrates the fact that more than

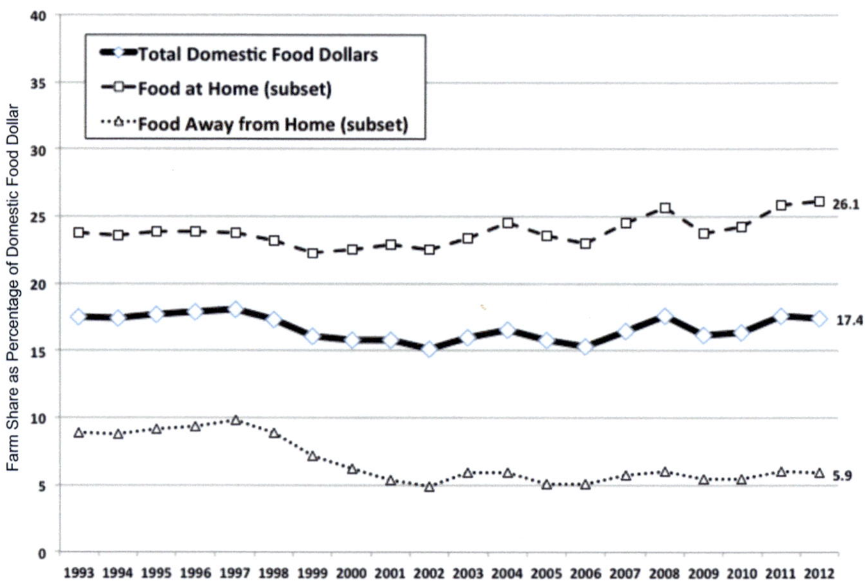

FIGURE 2-5 Farm share of consumer food expenditures, 1993-2012.
SOURCE: ERS, 2014b.

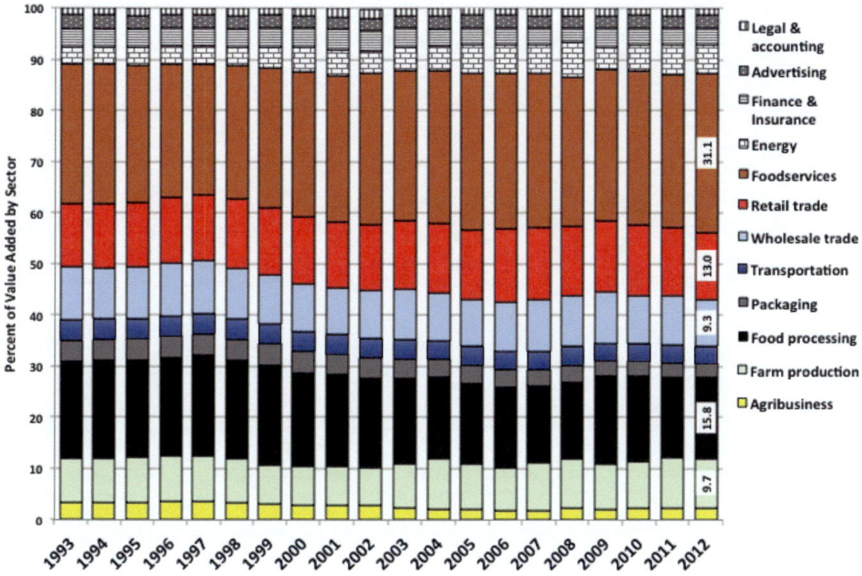

FIGURE 2-6 Distribution of value added across subsectors of food supply chain, 1993-2012.
SOURCE: ERS, 2014b.

80 percent of consumer food dollars pay for services throughout all of the post-harvest segments of the food supply chain; the remaining 17 percent is returned as gross receipts to farm producers. As a point of historic comparison, in 1950 more than 40 percent of consumer food expenditures went to farm producers (Schnepf, 2013). Much of the change in the farm share of food expenditures over time also reflects the growing consumption of food away from home (where, by definition, food service industries capture a larger share of dollars). Still, in recent years, the farm share of home-consumed food expenditures has actually increased to more than 26 percent.

Figure 2-6 looks at the consumer food dollar from a second aspect, namely, the distribution of consumer food dollars based on the value added (or marginal economic contribution) made by each successive step in the food production and distribution process. "Value added" is defined as proceeds from the sale of outputs minus the outlays for goods and services purchased from other establishments. Using value added measures for 2012, farming and agribusiness input firms are responsible for just 12 percent of total economic value created in the food system (9.7 percent and 2.4 percent, respectively). Food processing and packaging together represent roughly 19 percent of value, while the food retail and food services sectors

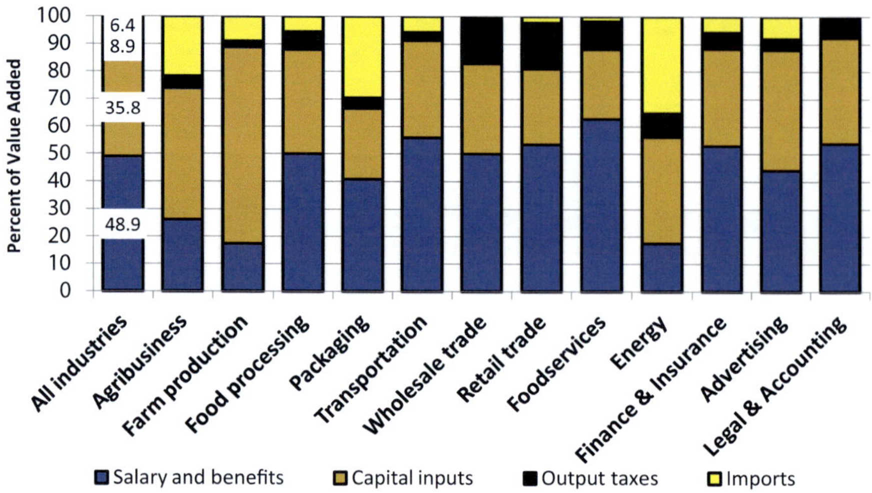

FIGURE 2-7 Distribution of value added by factor of production across subsectors of the U.S. food supply chain, 2012.
SOURCE: ERS, 2014b.

contribute the greatest economic value added, with more than 44 percent of the total (ERS, 2014b).

A third approach to understanding the distribution of the consumer food dollar among different sectors captures this distribution based on an allocation of economic value to the primary factors of production: domestic labor, capital, output taxes, and imports (see Figure 2-7). Approximately one-third of all spending on food covers the capital costs associated with ownership or rental of property (land, machinery, buildings, and other capital inputs) required for food production. Half of all spending goes to compensate workers and managers (through net returns to labor and management, wages, salaries, and benefits). This reflects the fact that transforming raw commodities into safe and edible food products requires a variety of tasks and that consumers now depend on various food industry sectors for much of this labor. Figure 2-7 also shows the distribution of value added to various factors of production for each subsector in the food supply chain. The farm production sector is notable for allocating most of its economic returns to capital inputs, while the food service sector is most focused on labor expenses.

Biophysical and Social/Institutional Contexts

Up to this point, the report has focused on the food supply chain as the core of the U.S. food system. Yet this economic system of producing, processing, distributing, marketing, and consuming food developed and operates within a broader biophysical and social/institutional context. Figure 2-8 provides a visual illustration of the connections among the various components of the U.S. food system and this broader context.

Biophysical Environment

Initially, it should be obvious that the natural resource base (e.g., land, water, nutrients, sunlight, energy, biodiversity, and genetic diversity) provide critical inputs to the farming sector that make possible the productivity and output that enter the rest of the food supply chain. In terms of the sheer size and quality of our farmland, water resources, and the variety of favorable climatic growing zones, the United States is one of the two most fertile areas in the world, according to a 2006 study by the Potsdam Institute for Climate Impact Research (Dutia, 2014). These natural endowments have been augmented by public and private investments in productivity-enhancing research and development: fertilizers and agricultural chemicals,

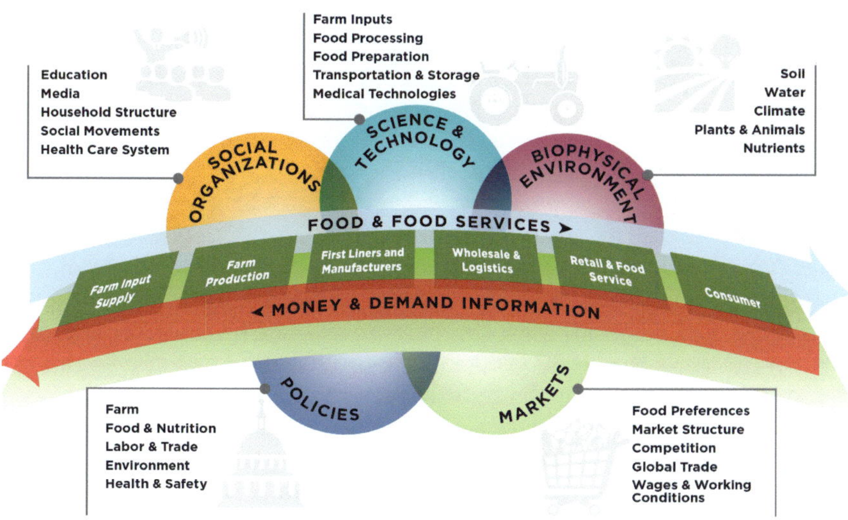

FIGURE 2-8 Links between the food supply chain and the larger biophysical and social/institutional context.

mechanization, efficient plant and animal breeding, information management systems, and constantly evolving handling and processing systems. As a result, the United States has a global comparative advantage in producing many types of agricultural products for both domestic use and export.

Despite these advantages, the development and performance of the food supply chain also can diminish the natural resource base by consuming scarce resources (like energy or nutrients), contaminating resources, or generating outputs (often waste products) that diminish the quality of the biophysical environment. These negative effects can be reduced through public and private investments to mitigate or ameliorate harms, and such investments have taken an increasing share of research and development (R&D) funding in recent decades. Today, soil degradation in North America affects only 25 percent of cropland, compared to roughly two-thirds in Africa and more than 50 percent in Latin America (Wiebe, 2003). Consequently, the United States also has an environmental comparative advantage in producing land-intensive crops and livestock products.

As both a source of critical inputs and a recipient of the waste stream and by-products of farm and food production, the biophysical environment is an integral component of the U.S. food system, and its quality and condition is critical to the long-term sustainability of the food system. Key biophysical elements of the food system are illustrated in Figure 2-8.

Social/Institutional Context

A wide range of social and institutional factors also shapes the ways in which the U.S. food system evolves and operates. These factors can be grouped into four categories: (1) markets, (2) policies, (3) science and technology, and (4) social organizations. Examples of the kinds of forces at work in each category are illustrated in Figure 2-8.

Markets The food system is clearly driven by the structure of markets, changes in supply and demand, and shifts in the economic status of U.S. consumers through time. Shifts in the size, number, and organization of farm and food businesses over the past 50 years also have dramatically reshaped the ways that food products are produced and economic returns are distributed throughout the food supply chain. These changes are tied to shifts in consumer preferences and food consumption patterns. The food system also interacts with other sectors of the U.S. economy through exchanges of inputs or outputs and competition for raw materials and consumer dollars. For example, land as a resource is critically important for producing food, but it also grows fiber, energy crops, and trees, and it serves as a carbon sink. Land also is a critical resource for residences, businesses, roads, recreation, and amenities. At the consumption link, nutritional patterns interact with lifestyles to shape health outcomes. So, while the food system has boundaries, those boundaries are permeable and often overlap with other important human systems. As a result, to understand any food system, it is important to include a careful analysis of how markets shape and are shaped by the behaviors of farmers, processors, handlers, manufacturers, marketers, and consumers.

Policies Many local, state, and federal policies directly affect U.S. farming activities, food processing and marketing practices, nutrition guidance, and food consumption behaviors. These include farm commodity and risk management policies, nutrition programs, food safety regulations, labor regulations, environmental laws, and programs to promote or shape patterns of international trade in farm commodities and food products. The trajectory of change and performance of any food system requires an understanding of the configuration of public and private policies and the politics and resources behind them, and new laws, regulations, and changes in public spending can be major levers used by societal actors to alter food system behaviors.

Science and technology Research and innovations shape the trajectory of technological change in the farm and food industry sectors. In the United States, drivers of technological innovation in food and agriculture include the extensive network of public agricultural research institutions (e.g., land-grant universities, the Agricultural Research Service) as well as the significant R&D programs implemented by private-sector agribusiness and food industry firms. With their mission to integrate research, education, and extension, land-grant universities have been especially critical for agricultural R&D by creating an effective avenue of communicating the most pressing concerns from farmers to researchers, and communicating solutions from researchers to farmers through the extension network. Together, the public- and private-sector institutions determine the information that key food system actors have about the performance of alternative approaches to farming and food provision and affect the relative economic viability of different farm production and food processing systems. At this time, budgets for public research in agriculture and food are declining, in many instances replaced by R&D funding from the private sector for the development of commercial products (Buttel, 2003b; Pardey et al., 2013).

Social organizations Many actors, organizations, and stakeholder groups actively seek to change consumer and producer behaviors and to shape "the structure and behavior of public and private institutions" (NRC, 2010, p. 272). Private firms, government agencies, and nonprofit organizations regularly disseminate information to consumers in the hope of influencing their food consumption behaviors. Other actors are only indirectly engaged in the food system, but their interests and preferences directly influence food-system dynamics. These include farm and food interest groups, government agencies, community civic organizations, media commentators, and academics. The activities of these groups shape (and respond to) the behaviors of individual actors and firms in the farm's production and food system, altering markets and, often, public policies.

Boundaries of the U.S. Food System

As described above, the committee's working definition of the U.S. food system includes both the core components of the food supply chain as well as key features of the broader biophysical and social/institutional context within which food production, processing, distribution, marketing, and consumption activities take place. Any assessment of the effects of alternative configurations of the U.S. food system will require specification of the boundaries of the system of interest (see Chapter 7). Depending on the questions of greatest interest, this approach may require a local, sectoral, national, or global approach.

At one level, it is possible to conceive of the entire U.S. food system as a single national system. This would include all of the segments of the food supply chain that exist within U.S. borders as well as the biophysical resources on which farm and food production depend and the social and institutional components that most directly shape the dynamics of farm and food system activity.

Many analyses will choose to focus on a smaller scale, perhaps by examining the dynamics of the food system in particular regions of the United States, or by focusing on the production of a particular commodity or class of commodities (say the poultry production system, or the fruit and vegetable system). In these cases, the general conceptual model that includes both the supply chain and the biophysical and social/institutional components is still helpful in pointing to the key components that an assessment would need to include. In these cases, the physical and economic boundaries of the components that are considered to be "inside" or "outside" the system may differ, depending on the focus of the study.

Although drawing a bright line at the U.S. border when defining the food system can be analytically helpful, it is impossible to ignore the fact that the U.S. food system is increasingly integrated within a much larger global food system. The boundaries of the U.S. food system are highly permeable to the rest of the world's food system (see Figure 2-9). People migrate, agricultural inputs and food products are traded, and policies and markets create price and behavioral repercussions elsewhere. Changes in global environmental conditions also affect food system dynamics across

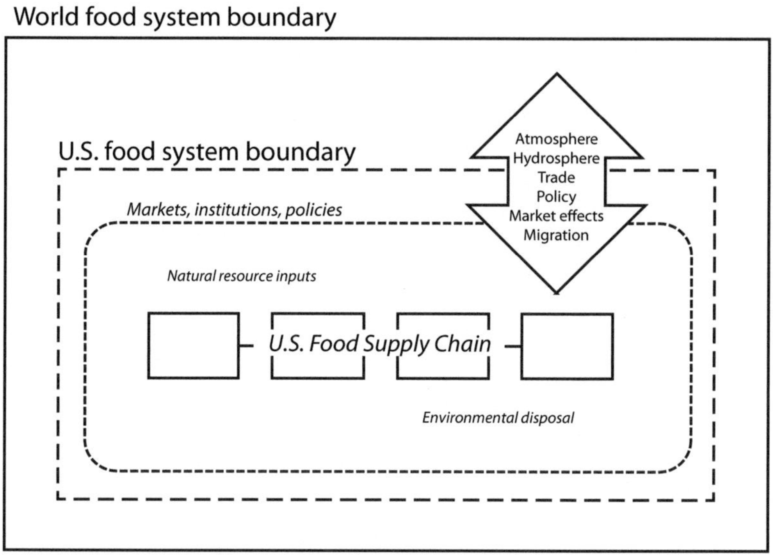

FIGURE 2-9 Conceptual model of connections between the U.S. food system and the global food system.

national boundaries. Some of these interactions are episodic, but many have become deeply embedded interdependencies. As a result, any analysis of the effects of changes in the U.S. food system would be incomplete without accounting for responses and feedbacks related to global markets, policies, technology, and influencers.

EVOLUTION OF THE U.S. FOOD SYSTEM

This section provides a brief history of food and agriculture in the United States by highlighting events that shaped the development of the current food system. It points to the core drivers and major trends that will continue to shape this constantly changing and evolving system in the future. As the committee discusses in more depth in Chapter 6, the food system is a good example of a complex adaptive system where changes in one part (or outside the system) often generate unexpected outcomes in other parts of the food system. Assessing the effects of different configurations of the food system needs to integrate considerations of how key drivers and feedbacks will affect outcomes.

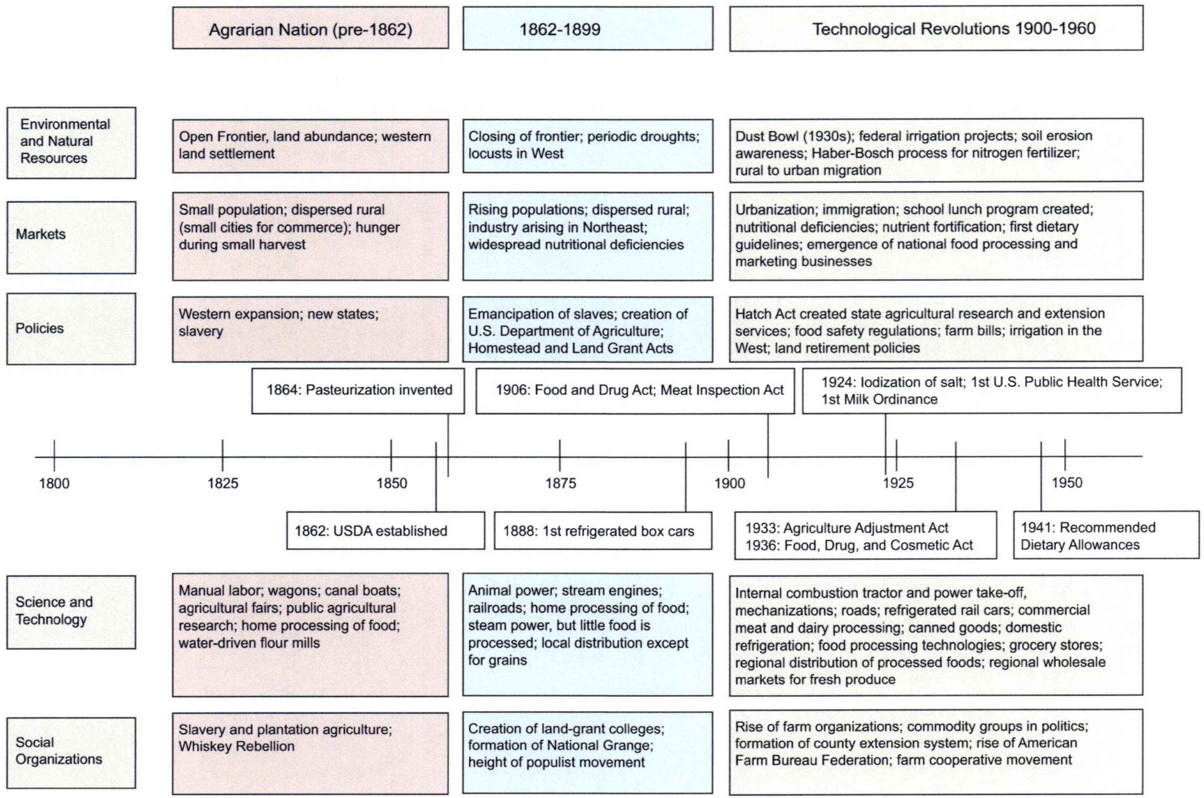

FIGURE 2-10 Major drivers and changes in food and agriculture in the United States from 1800s to 1960.
SOURCES: ARS, 2014; Backstrand, 2002.

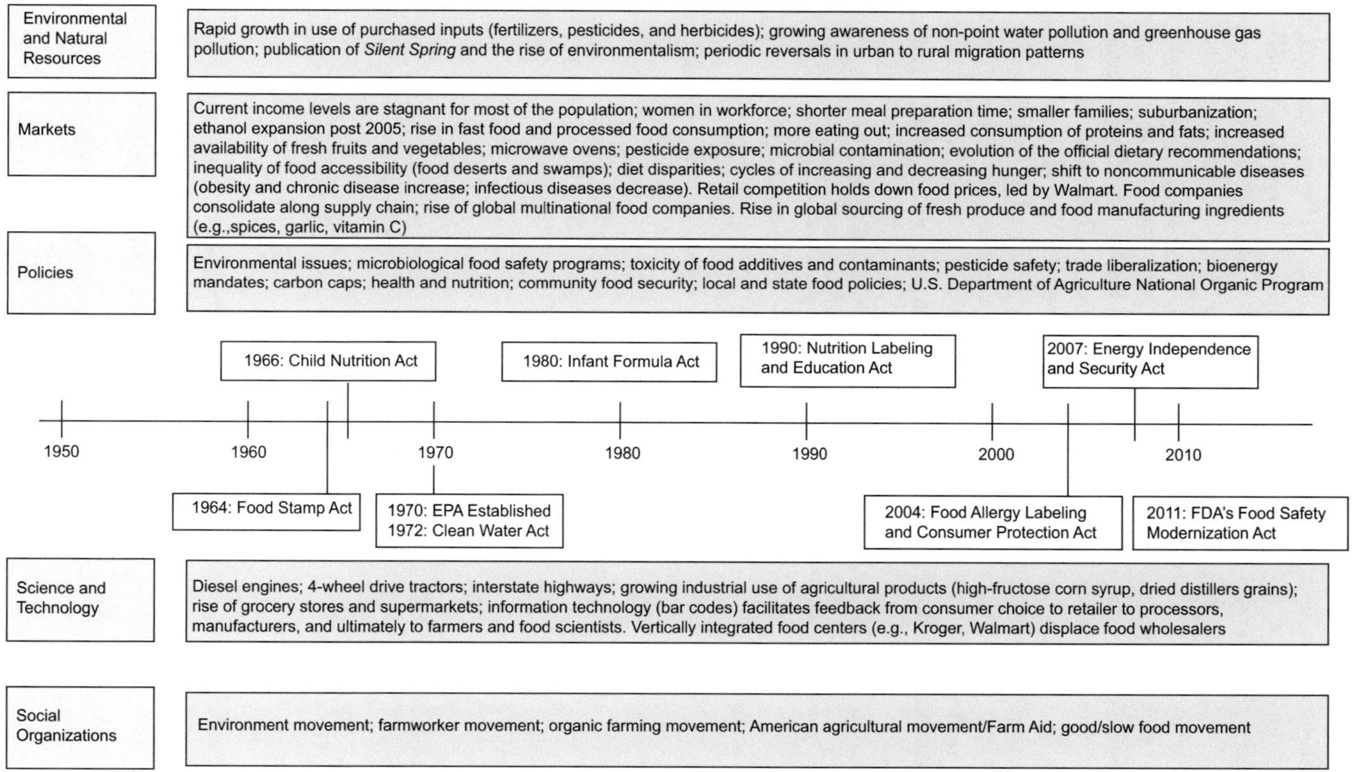

FIGURE 2-11 Major drivers and changes in food and agriculture in the United States from 1960 to present.
SOURCE: Gardner, 2002.

The timeline shown in Figures 2-10 and 2-11 provides a very general chronological guide to some of the key events or changes in natural resources, markets, policies, science, and technology, as well as the social organizations that shaped the evolution of the U.S. farm and food system from 1800 to 2014. Taking a long view, the current U.S. food system clearly bears little resemblance to the food system that sustained the nation's population throughout the 19th century. Figure 2-12 shows how the farm sector witnessed dramatic growth (in both farm numbers and farm acreage) throughout the 19th century, as high rates of immigration and the rapid expansion of frontier land settlement contributed to the growth of the nation. During the 20th century, output continued to rise, but technological change and growth in farm size was associated with a steady drop in farm numbers and the size of the hired farm labor force. Meanwhile, total acres used in farming remained relatively stable, though the total available prime farmland has declined slowly as urban and suburban areas have expanded onto former farm fields at the outskirts of cities and small towns.

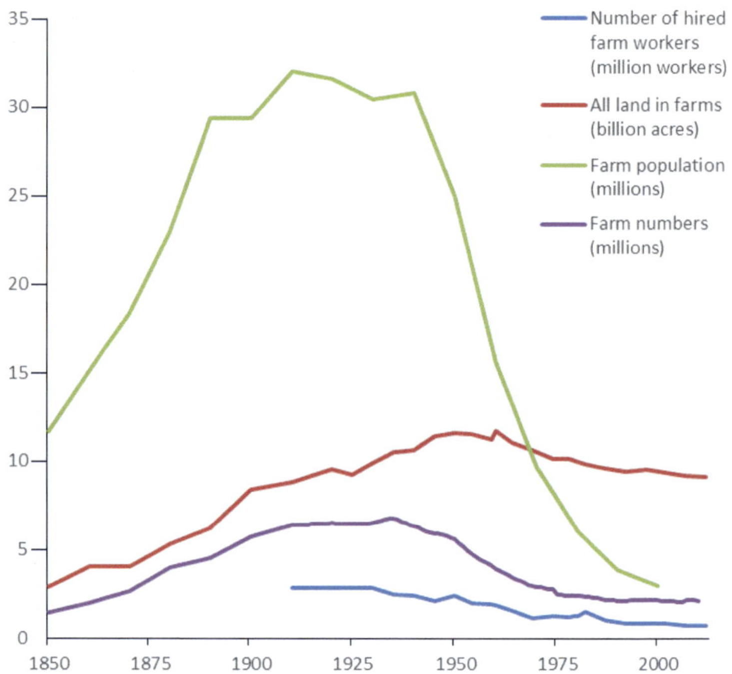

FIGURE 2-12 Number of acres of farmland, farm numbers, farm population, and number of hired farm workers in the United States from 1850 to 2012.
SOURCES: Agriculture in the Classroom, 2014; BLS, 2014; NASS, 2014a,b; U.S. Census Bureau, 2014a,b; USDA, 2012.

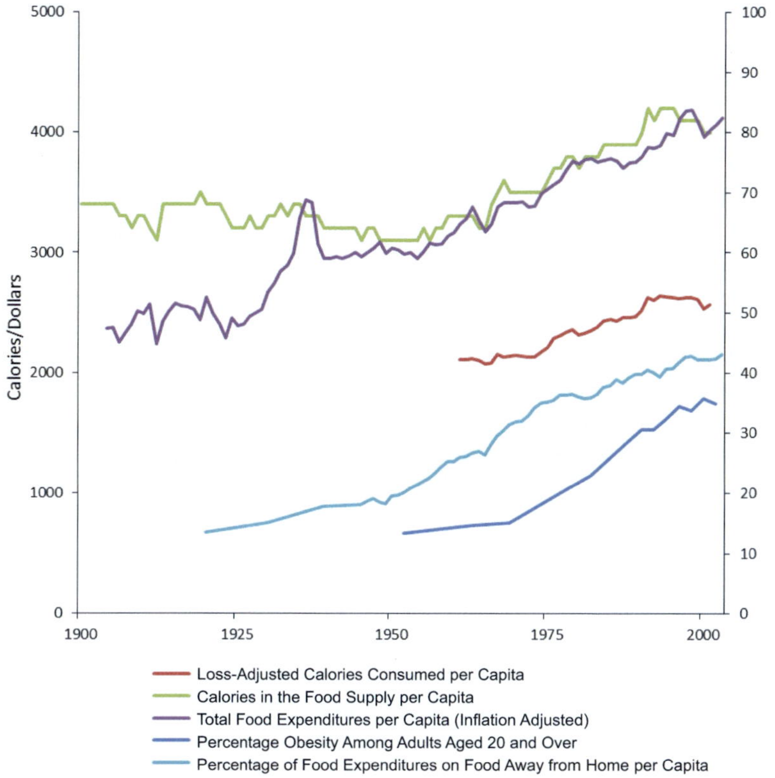

FIGURE 2-13 Trends in major indicators of food supply, expenditures, and nutrition in the United States, 1900-present.
SOURCES: CDC/NCHS, 2014; CNPP, 2014; ERS, 2013a.

Similar dramatic changes have occurred throughout the food supply chain, with dramatic impacts on the nutrition and health status of the population. Figure 2-13 illustrates a steady growth in the availability of calories (on a per-capita basis) since the middle of the 20th century. The graph also shows a steady rise in the inflation-adjusted volume of food expenditures in the United States, possibly due in part to improvements in diets, increased consumption of livestock products, and a shift toward consumption of food away from home. On the down side, an increase in obesity and in the loss-adjusted calories consumed per capita also has occurred since the middle of the 20th century.

Although these figures provide some highlights of overall trends, they do not fully explain the environmental, farm, off-farm, and societal developments that both resulted from and shaped this agricultural transformation. In the next few sections, we explore the importance of these developments in more detail. This discussion is organized around the five major drivers of change introduced above: (1) environmental change; (2) markets; (3) policies; (4) technology; and (5) social organizations. Each of these forces represents dynamic processes that will continue to shape the health, environmental, social, and economic effects of the U.S. food system.

Environmental Change

The quality and spatial distribution of our natural resources—soils, water, and climate—have contributed to the overall development and regional character of farm production across the United States. Over the past 100 years, changes in resource conditions (e.g., soil quality and water availability) and growing awareness of the environmental effects of agricultural activities (and associated policy responses) have been important drivers of change within the U.S. farm sector.

Frederick Jackson Turner, an eminent American historian, argued that the early 20th century represented an important turning point in American society and culture (Cronon, 1987). Before that time, the growth and development of the nation was based on the availability of relatively large quantities of untapped land and natural resources on the nation's frontier. Early settlers discovered a relatively rich agricultural land with good soils and a favorable climate. A series of migrations westward ensued as farmland in the original 13 colonies began to be depleted because of intensive cultivation there as well as competition from farmers who had moved into newly opened lands (e.g., the Ohio River Valley and Corn Belt states) with climates and soils more suited to crop production.

Regional differences in climate, land quality, and the availability of labor led to the development of distinctive farming systems (Pfeffer, 1983). Patterns of settlement in the Midwest during the mid-1800s also were shaped by large numbers of northern European immigrants, who had extensive experience with mixed crop–livestock systems. The southeastern United States was dominated by a slave-supported plantation agriculture that produced export crops (cotton, tobacco) and led to little investment in social infrastructure. California after Spanish settlement had a hacienda system in place where large landowners established elaborate irrigation systems and farming operations that spread over extensive land. Differences in the original natural resource base and changes in resource conditions associated with different farming systems shaped patterns of land management and population movement. One major factor in this evolution was that the availability of land in most areas of the United States was much greater than the availability of labor, except where slaves were used. In Iowa and much of the Midwest, the U.S. government gave away quarter sections (160 acres)[3] to those who could show they used it effectively.

The closing of the American frontier occurred simultaneously with the rise of industrialization and concentration of economic activity in the urban centers of the growing nation. A process of outmigration from agriculture was associated with a time when the amount of land available for farming was at its peak (see Figure 2-11), leading to growth in farm size and rapid technical changes that allowed greater productivity and production by a smaller number of people.

The availability and quality of natural resources continues to be a primary driver behind management decisions within the U.S. food system, particularly at the farm level. Farmers make crop decisions based on the availability of water, climate appropriateness, and soil quality. As a result, prime farmland tends to be located where natural resources are plentiful (i.e., rich, deep soils; available surface and groundwater sources; and favorable climates). During the early decades of the 20th century, in many parts of the United States, prime farmland was replaced by urban centers reliant on natural resources, especially water, and favorable climatic conditions. This forced food production to lands characterized by fewer natural resources and less satisfactory growing conditions. The agriculture sector overcame this obstacle by substantially increasing yields on both prime and marginal farmland through the development and implementation of technological advances in the 1930s and 1940s, such as new genetics (e.g., hybrid corn), the use of synthetic fertilizers, investment in large water projects to irrigate the West, greater use of pesticides to combat pest outbreaks, and a widespread shift to mechanical traction and tillage.

These technologies led to the successful production of food for a growing population, but not without significant environmental consequences. In the 1930s, U.S. agriculture in the Great Plains and the West faced severe drought and widespread soil erosion (known as the "Dust Bowl"), leading to a focus on soil conservation policies and practices. Growing concerns over the impacts of pesticide and synthetic fertilizer use on soil quality, species biodiversity, and water and air quality in the latter half of the 20th century, as well as overpumping of groundwater in several parts of the country, sparked the development of additional conservation policies, environmental protection regulations, and a renewed interest in the production of food, fiber, and fuels that used management strategies having minimal impact on the environment. Conservation policies and environmental regulations enacted at the federal, state, and local levels—mainly since the 1970s, in response to the degradation of air and water quality—sought to protect

[3] Homestead Act of 1862, Public Law 37-64, 37th Cong., 2nd sess. (December 2, 1861).

natural resources while at the same time meeting the growing demands for a safe, affordable, and plentiful food supply.

The 1960s brought further concerns over the impact of pesticides on the environment. The publication of *Silent Spring* by Rachel Carson in 1962 is credited with initiating the development of such landmark policies as the formation of the Environmental Protection Agency (EPA) in 1970, the 1972 Federal Insecticide, Fungicide, and Rodenticide Act,[4] and the 1972 Federal Water Pollution Control Act[5] (commonly known as the Clean Water Act). In more recent years, the development and adoption of integrated pest management strategies continues to increase in an effort to address pest problems while reducing pest resistance, protecting water quality, and reducing human and wildlife exposure to potentially toxic chemicals. Additionally, widespread eutrophication of freshwater systems and hypoxia zones in the Gulf of Mexico over the past 30 years, attributed to nutrient loading mainly from agriculture, has heightened the call for increased regulations on non-point source pollution in several U.S. states.

Recently, consumer demands for environmentally friendly products are shaping agricultural management decisions. For example, the increase in the demand for organic foods and humanely raised animals is a result of consumer choice and attendant changes in corporate buyer standards (a phenomenon known as "market pull"). Additionally, climate change will most likely become a significant driver of U.S. farming practices, as changes in temperature and rainfall patterns may limit the types and quantity of crops grown in what is now the most productive agricultural land in the United States.

Markets

A major driver of the U.S. food system's evolution—one that continues today—is market forces, especially the competitive pressure to produce more, ever more efficiently. Market forces reflect decisions by economic actors seeking to maximize their well-being, and always take place within broader institutional, political, and technological contexts (discussed in more detail in the next sections), which in turn shape the distribution of economic costs and benefits. Over the past century, intense market competition, globalization, and changes in consumer preferences have contributed to a dramatic restructuring of the organization of both farm and food production, and to the development of new and rapidly evolving food markets and technologies. Some of these interdependent changes are described briefly below.

---

[4] Federal Insecticide, Fungicide, and Rodenticide Act, 7 U.S.C. § 136 et seq. (1996).

[5] Federal Water Pollution Control Act, Public Law 92-500, 92nd Cong., 2nd sess. (October 18, 1972).

Restructuring of Farm and Food Production

Competition to be productive and profitable and the development of new technologies and management practices have contributed to significant farm consolidation in the United States. In 1850, roughly half of the U.S. population lived on farms; today, less than 1 percent of Americans earn their livelihoods from farming (BLS, 2014; U.S. Census Bureau, 2014a). This has been termed the "great agricultural transition" of the 20th century; farming was abandoned as a household livelihood strategy (Lobao and Meyer, 2001). The mass decline of the farm population resulted in fewer and larger farms. The concentration of farm sales and assets, the specialization of farm enterprises and regions, and agribusiness concentration increased greatly over the last half of the 20th century (Buttel, 2003a) and continue to this day.

Roughly 80 to 90 percent of U.S. food production is now provided by the 10 to 20 percent of farmers who farm full-time (Hoppe and Banker, 2010). They are typically well educated and run commercial businesses with sales often well above USDA's $350,000 threshold for "large commercial farms" (Hoppe and MacDonald, 2013). Parallel to this, the number of farming-dependent counties has fallen to fewer than 500 today, with such off-farm activities as manufacturing, services, and amenities becoming more important sources of local well-being in rural counties (ERS, 2006, 2012). Where rural communities have lost off-farm activities, many services, such as hospitals and schools, have closed.

Concentration also has occurred in the hog and beef industries, where production has shifted to large specialized farms (MacDonald and McBride, 2009). For example, in 2004, 80 percent of the hog farms had more than 2,000 animals, up from 30 percent in 1992 (Key and McBride, 2007). Vertical integration of production, processing, and marketing has remade many animal protein supply chains. An example is the poultry industry, where integrators (companies that resulted from the integration of feeding, hatching, and processing poultry) and growers have altered their reciprocal business relationships. The integrators now own the birds and feed and control the production process. This structure, combined with the fact that a few integrators control an increasing market share, has resulted in a greater power over poultry growers, with important social consequences. (For research data on concentration of meat markets, see Ward and Schroeder, 1994.)

The seed industry provides a good illustration of the broader pattern of agribusiness firm consolidation in the latter 20th century. The small circles in Figure 2-14 were each independent seed companies that sold inputs to farmers well into the 1970s and 1980s. However, a series of mergers and acquisitions in the 1990s (prompted mainly by the entry of pharmaceutical

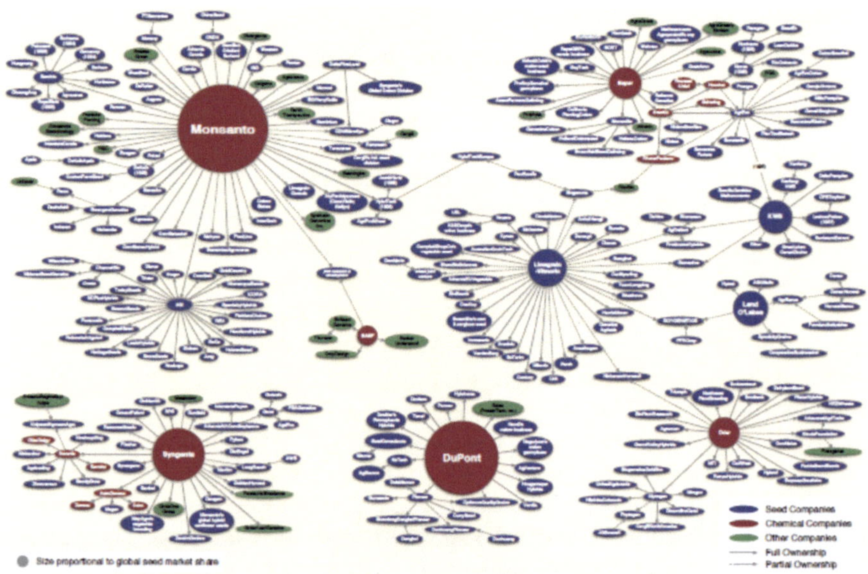

FIGURE 2-14 Seed industry structure, 1996-2013.
SOURCE: Howard, 2014. Reprinted with permission. https://www.msu.edu/~howardp/seedindustry.html (accessed January 8, 2015).

and chemical companies into the sector and with the rise of biotechnology methods to genetically engineer seeds) led to rapid consolidation in the seed industry. In 2013, this sector was under the control of eight major firms (Howard, 2009, 2014).

As a result of these mergers, the crop seed/biotechnology input sector now has what is termed a "four-firm concentration ratio" of 53.9, meaning that the four largest firms have nearly 54 percent of the global market sales for these types of products. The four largest firms in each of the other input industries (agricultural chemicals, farm machinery, animal health, and animal genetics) also have more than 50 percent of the global market sales (Fuglie et al., 2012). In 2012, the U.S. Department of Justice organized a series of workshops that allowed farmers and others to voice their concerns about competing in a highly consolidated market (USDOJ, 2012). (For a selection of potential effects due to industry restructuring, see Chapter 5.)

Similar changes—consolidation, use of new technology, vertical integration, market expansion, and market differentiation—have occurred in the organizational structure of many other parts of the food supply chain. Although some vibrant alternative food systems are emerging, most of the food produced today relies on the logistical coordination of elaborated supply chains. The competitive pressure to reduce prices has been a key goal stimulating greater efficiencies and organizational changes in the supply chain, from the retailer back to the farmer.

The food processing sector provides a good illustration of the concentration of the material flows within the food supply chain in the United States. The 12 percent of plants with more than 100 employees ship 77 percent of all of the value of food, and mergers and acquisitions continue to occur often (ERS, 2014d). Concentration is not limited to food manufacturing. The top four beef processing companies increased their share of the slaughter market from 36 to 79 percent between 1980 and 2005, while the four firm concentration ratio in hog and poultry reached 64 and 53 percent by 2005 (Macdonald and McBride, 2009). The most concentrated food processing sectors continue to be beef packing and soybean crushing (see Figure 2-15). By 2007, the concentration ratio in poultry reached 58 percent (see Figure 2-15). The most dramatic increase in the concentration of food processing sectors since 1990 may be in pork packing, where the four-firm concentration ratio increased from 40 to 66 percent in 2007 (Hendrickson and Heffernan, 2007; Sexton, 2013).

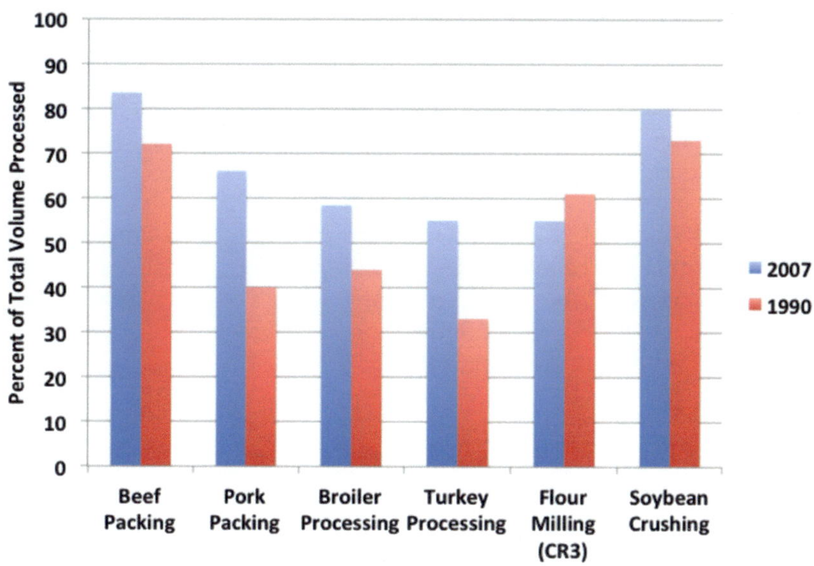

FIGURE 2-15 Four-Firm Concentration Index (CR4): Percentage of total processed volume controlled by top four firms, 1990 and 2007.
SOURCE: Data from Hendrickson and Heffernan, 2007.

Farm and Food System Labor

The evolution of the U.S. farm and food sector also is shaped by the skills and availability of the labor force. Farm production suffers from the particular challenge of requiring large amounts of labor at critical times (e.g., during crop harvest), followed by extended periods of low labor demand. Regional differences in the structure of U.S. farming have been linked to the relative abundance or scarcity of labor (Pfeffer, 1983). Family-run farms have survived in part because unpaid family members were able to provide flexible labor to the operation without the fixed costs of a hired workforce (Reinhardt and Barlett, 1989). In recent years, U.S. farmers and the food manufacturing and food service industries have come to rely more heavily on hired workers, many of whom are believed not to be authorized to work in the United States (Martin, 2013; Martin and Jackson-Smith, 2013). Immigration policies, access to land for independent operators, efforts to organize or unionize hired workers, and competition from non-farm sectors offering better income or benefits have all contributed to the degree to which farm and food production has been able to rely on unpaid family labor and inexpensive hired workers (Findeis et al., 2002; Martin, 2009).

The availability of a flexible labor force willing to work for relatively low wages and minimal benefits has been an important factor in the evolution of farming and food system industries (FCWA, 2012). On the other hand, the farm and food sectors have seen dramatic increases in labor productivity related to mechanization and other technological changes. For much of the 20th century, mechanization has facilitated the growth in scale and productivity on most U.S. farms, and it has freed labor to flow to non-farm industries in urban areas (Gardner, 2002; Lobao and Meyer, 2001). The pace and direction of mechanization in farm production and food processing have been linked to situations where global competition is intense and domestic labor costs are relatively high due to scarcity, changes in labor law, or efforts to unionize workers (Calvin and Martin, 2010; Fidelibus, 2014; Friedland et al., 1981).

Restructuring of Food Sales Sector

The retail–wholesale sector also has evolved dramatically since the 1980s with the advent of self-distribution centers by large retail food companies (those with more than 100 stores). Traditionally, wholesalers have bought foodstuffs (and other consumer product goods) from processors and manufacturers, held the inventory in their warehouses, and resold and delivered them to retail stores or other buyers. In recent years, many of these wholesalers have gone out of business, shrunk to providing these services to smaller stores, or become logistics companies. This evolution came about as part of retail business strategies designed to hold as little inventory as possible, which in turn induced wholesale warehouses to shrink their inventory and switch to a faster turnover model. The ideal, though not attainable, goal is to have a just-in-time delivery model.

The 1990s saw the creation of retail "supercenters" and big box stores that also offer nonfood products. Key operational changes that made these stores possible were (1) the increased collaboration between retailers and suppliers with the development of retailer-owned distribution centers; (2) the acquisition and analysis of consumer purchasing data at each store;[6] (3) lower food prices (and less profitability in the food segment) that could be sustained by retailers with more profitable sales in general merchandise; and (4) restructuring of operations, closing older stores and focusing on core areas to further cut costs. Other strategies to stay competitive have been (1) globalization, which lowers the costs of marketing and provides year-round availability of fresh produce; (2) product differentiation, such as organics or private labels; (3) perks for consumers (nonfood products, e.g., gas, electronics, car washes); and (4) new technologies, such as self-checkout lines.

Smaller retailers and midsize consumer package goods firms have not been able to compete with the supercenters' ability to negotiate low prices. Because of the economies of scale, the costs of technology, and the speed of the changes, the big retailers and suppliers have been able to buy or merge with other companies while smaller firms have been bought or simply disappeared.

Structural changes in this sector have led to a situation in which the largest 20 retail food companies have 64 percent of all of the sales. The top four have nearly 40 percent of retail food sales, and the top one has almost 20 percent of retail food sales. Ninety-one percent of retail food sales are in some type of supermarket (ERS, 2014f). Figure 2-16 illustrates the growing share of sales captured by the top 4, 8, and 20 retail food companies between 1992 and 2013. The 2007-2009 recession, however, slowed the rise in the share of sales.

Evolution of Other Food System Sectors

In contrast to the sales sector, consolidation has not happened as quickly in the food service sector. In fact, the number of companies in this

[6] This practice of sharing information about sales was started by large food retailers in the early 1990s and it resulted in inventory efficiencies for processors/manufacturers, wholesalers, and retailers. It was later adopted by other retailers domestically, then internationally.

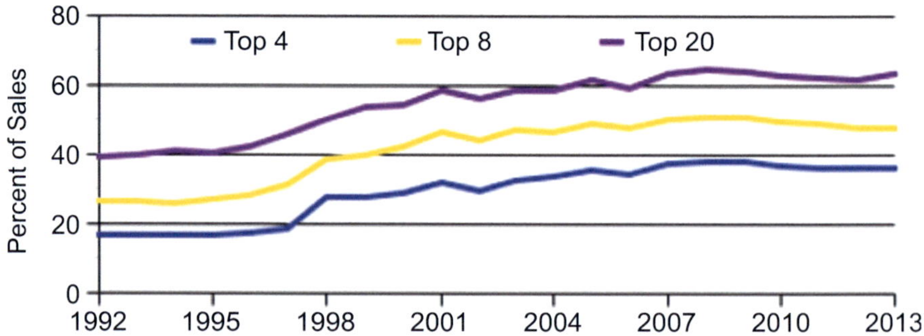

FIGURE 2-16 Top 4, 8, and 20 firms' share of U.S. grocery store sales, 1992-2013.
SOURCE: ERS, 2014f.

sector has increased. Small venues can perform well when they can differentiate themselves based on products and services offered.

The development of a national infrastructure also has affected the evolution of the food supply chain. Improved cold chain and transportation economics have opened the potential for national markets for fresh meats, seafood, and fruits and vegetables, which can sometimes supplement and sometimes displace local, seasonal production. Freeze-drying and ultra-high temperature techniques have had similar effects for coffee and dairy products. Completion of the interstate highway system has made truck delivery of both fresh and packaged goods possible to virtually every city and town. This has facilitated development of national brands and consolidation among food processors and manufacturers, and it has had a similar effect on retail, with the growth and then consolidation of supermarket chains. Infrastructure developments also have underpinned the uniform product offerings and quality controls that have facilitated the growth of fast-food chains.

Falling costs also have resulted in offsetting developments. For example, private labels seek to offer a comparable product to national brands at a lower price point. Their market share now approaches 25 percent (IRI, 2013). Lower costs also make premium brands and offerings available to larger markets, giving rise to supermarkets and restaurants that are priced between discount houses/fast-food chains and deluxe establishments. With food costs overall declining toward 10 percent of the average American's disposable income, more meals eaten away from home also have become accessible to more people (ERS, 2013a).

One of the most important market developments has been the emergence of futures markets[7] traded on centralized exchanges. This has made price discovery more transparent, brought national and international supply/demand factors to bear on local markets, facilitated forward sales and contracting, and given farmers, handlers, processors, distributors, and users new tools for managing price risks in future time periods. Moreover, clearinghouses at these centralized exchanges have eliminated the risk of default, making futures markets an attractive way to hedge or unload unwanted price risks.

Changes in Food Prices

Food prices are a function of the interaction of supply and demand, which are, in turn, functions of major drivers involving bioavailability (land and climate), income of both producers and consumers, the productivity (efficiency) of crop and livestock production, and the growth in population. On the supply side, crop production and productivity respond to technology (e.g., seed, fertilizer, and capital equipment) as well as the availability of land. The more efficient the production is (more output per acre of land), the lower the price of the commodity. The caveat on this price is that the productive units (e.g., farmers, processors, and distribution companies) must cover at least their average variable costs and provide a margin for profit. If the prices that these suppliers can receive in the market are less than their costs, they will go out of business. Public policy that encourages more crop production can act to decrease the costs and therefore the price (corn and soybeans) or decrease competition and increase the price (sugar). Increased demand for the crops and livestock will increase the price when demand exceeds the supply.

On the demand side, consumer income, population growth, and changing tastes and preferences influence food demand. The willingness to pay for more or better quality food rises as income rises. The feedback loop from consumer markets is critical to informing food producers all along the supply chain about the quantity and quality of food that will sell on the market. Heterogeneous consumer tastes and lifestyles heavily influence the types of food that are demanded in the market. As incomes rise in low- to middle-income populations globally, consumers demand more animal protein and the raising of more livestock demands greater crop production and generally higher prices. The demand for animal feed is a driver for increased crop production, yet as crop production becomes more efficient, the price per bushel can actually drop. In addition, the demand for crops used to

---

[7] A futures market is a central financial exchange where people can trade standardized *futures contracts*, that is, a contract to buy specific quantities of a *commodity* at a specified price with *delivery* set at a specified time in the future.

produce fuel or other nonfood products incents greater supply at higher prices, which also increases the price of the commodity used for food.

An important point to understand is that the consumer of raw agricultural commodities is generally not the final consumer, but the supply chain customer (e.g., processor/manufacturer, wholesaler, or retailer). These agents provide the feedback from final consumers about final demand and willingness-to-pay at the retail point of sale. Retail competition plays an important role in holding down final prices to consumers, reducing profit margins all along the supply chain.

As clearly demonstrated in Figure 2-6, the price of food is shaped by many economic sectors beyond agricultural production. Changes in food processing, marketing, transportation, packaging, and retail sectors now have more impact on consumer food prices than do changes in production practices or variation in farm yields and output. As the complexity of the food supply chain increases, the price of food consumed by the public will reflect the gains from greater production efficiencies and the costs associated with increased processing and handling. When food choices are abundant, consumers are likely to substitute among alternatives as the relative prices change. This price and cross-price elasticity of demand[8] influences the intersection of supply and demand and the final food price. In addition, a cycle of over- and undersupply of basic crops and livestock occurs as farmers respond to higher and lower prices in the market. Typically, they overshoot their estimates of next year's prices, creating an oversupply in the years after prices have been high, which suppresses prices in the current year. This continual adjustment occurs and responds to both global and domestic demands.

Price competition among food retailers is one reason why short-term price fluctuations in commodity prices are not fully reflected in the retail store, although over the long run, inflationary pressures will affect consumer food prices. Food price inflation has traditionally been followed with overall inflation. Figure 2-17 illustrates the relative stability of food price increases since 1975.

Changes in Consumer Preferences

Changes in U.S. consumer behaviors also are reshaping markets and the food system (see "Factors Influencing Food Purchase Decisions" in Chapter 5). During the 1960s, with many women entering the workforce for the first time, the food industry used this opportunity to market to

[8] Elasticity of demand is a measure used in economics to show the responsiveness of the quantity demanded of a good or service to a change in its price. It gives the percentage change in quantity demanded in response to a 1 percent change in price.

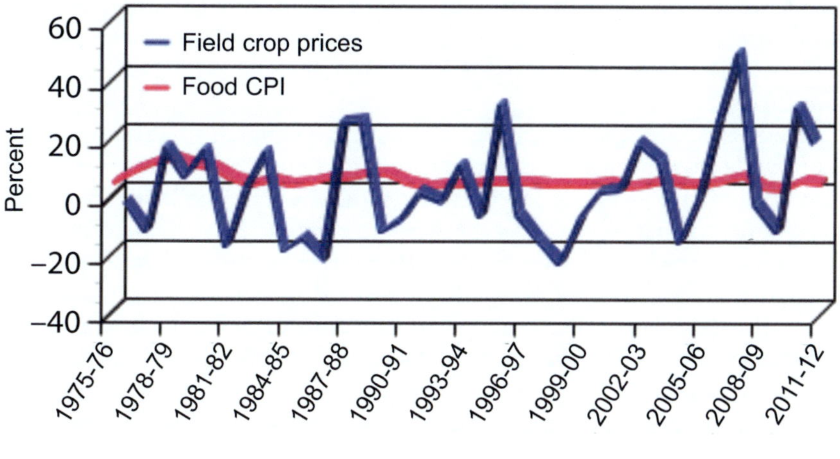

FIGURE 2-17 Percentage change in the annual CPI for food and prices for field crops, 1976-2012. CPI is a measure of the average change over time in the prices paid by consumers for a market basket of consumer goods and services. Field crop prices are represented by the production-weighted average farm price of corn, wheat, and soybeans in the United States.
NOTES: Calculated by the Economic Research Service, based on Bureau of Labor Statistics and National Agricultural Statistics Service data. CPI = Consumer Price Index.
SOURCE: http://www.ers.usda.gov/data-products/food-price-outlook/charts.aspx#fieldcrop (accessed January 8, 2015).

women who had less time to cook for their families. Advances in domestic technologies (e.g., refrigerators and microwaves) and in packaging increased shelf life and made preparation more convenient (Bell and Valentine, 1997; Mintz and Du Bois, 2002). As a result of this and other social trends and changes in consumer attitudes and behavior, over the past 60 years a growing percentage of food in the United States is consumed away from home (ERS, 2013a). Altogether, these changes have likely led to increasingly individualized consumption patterns and larger amounts of added sugars, sodium, and fats in diets.

Many changes in food distribution and consumption have been due to the automobile (Jakle and Sculle, 1999; Schlosser, 2001). The car quickly transformed the architecture of cities and towns across the country—and gradually located supermarkets in the suburbs and away from urban areas. Additional transformations induced by the car were quick-service restaurants and stores with drive-through windows to speed up sales. Although the restaurant industry as a whole steadily grew, fast-food businesses in particular exploded during the late 20th century (Jakle and Sculle, 1999;

Schlosser, 2001). More recently, a study found that the percentage of calories consumed from fast food in adults was lower in 2007-2010 (10 percent of calories) as compared to 2003-2006 (13 percent of calories) (Fryer and Ervin, 2013).

Although some 20th-century trends have contributed to a smaller number of foods in American diets, recent decades have seen a resurgence in diversification. The types of food products and markets available are driven by consumer demands, as they become stimulated by sellers. Alongside commodity, convenience, and staple products, conventional food companies have provided new offerings built around market segmentation and product differentiation. Perhaps the most significant change in consumption patterns in the 21st century has been remarkable growth in demand for food produced or marketed in ways that are perceived to support the health, environmental, or social equity goals of farmers and consumers, such as organic, free range, fair trade, local, and natural. Animal welfare concerns have encouraged the development of free-range, cage-free, and grass-fed products. New interests, such as gluten free, high fiber, and omega-3, have burst onto the market as a result of consumers' desires for a healthful diet. For example, demand for organic foods in the United States has grown at roughly 20 percent annually (ERS, 2014e). Despite potential benefits and safety protections, some customers—especially in Europe—have expressed preferences for food products grown without the use of genetically modified organisms (GMOs). Concurrently, new alternative food marketing and distribution systems have emerged and grown to deliver such products, including farmers' markets, community cooperatives, alternative restaurants, or specialized supermarkets.

The role of "risk" in the food system also has changed in response to increased consumer attention and sensitivity to this issue. Some consumers seem to be paying more attention to perceived risks and giving more weight in buying decisions to suspect sources, processes, or future dangers. As per-capita incomes rise, the threshold of acceptable risk has appeared to escalate, moving from risk reduction toward avoidance. At the same time, techniques for detecting chemical residues or foreign substances have become more sensitive (from parts per million to parts per billion or trillion). Although this led to the Food Quality Protection Act[9] and effectively repealed the Delaney Clause for pesticides, it also has heightened consumer awareness of and sensitivity to foodborne risks. As described below, government safety policies and risk management strategies by industry (e.g., labeling and certification systems and traceability) also have expanded substantially and become increasingly expensive.

---

[9] Food Quality Protection Act of 1996, Public Law 104-170, 104th Cong., 2nd sess. (August 3, 1996).

Globalization

As indicated earlier, the U.S. food system has strong connections to the global food system. As recently as the mid-1980s, U.S. agricultural exports and imports were valued at less than $30 billion each (ERS, 2013b). By 2012, exports were worth about $135 billion, and imports were approaching $105 billion, more than a threefold increase for each (Flake et al., 2013). At the same time, global trade of grains, rice, oilseeds, meat, and other commodities has grown dramatically, causing interregional interdependencies.

Global food trade also is beginning to reflect more specialization along lines of relative resource endowments and comparative advantage. Regions with abundant land resources (e.g., North and South America) are shipping hundreds of millions of tons of food per year to densely populated or resource-stressed regions (e.g., the Middle East, North Africa, and Asia) (Portnoy, 2013). Labor-intensive agricultural production, such as fruits, vegetables, aquaculture, and horticulture, are being produced in larger amounts for domestic use and for export to labor-scarce regions, such as the United States.

Changes in food supply and demand in other countries promise to be a major driver of commodity prices and marketing opportunities for U.S. farmers and food processing and distribution firms. For example, a serious problem in many countries is continuing food insecurity, which can take the form of chronic hunger, periodic food crises, or malnutrition among vulnerable population groups. During much of the 20th century, the drive for greater efficiency in agricultural production yielded a steady decline in inflation-adjusted food prices. These falling real food prices, in turn, were a major factor in reducing chronic global hunger. By contrast, rising real commodity prices in the first decade of the 21st century has reversed this decline, and it will add as many as 600 million people to the list of the chronically hungry by 2025 if the trend continues (Runge and Senauer, 2007). Moreover, tight supplies produced serious, temporary food crises in 2008 and 2012, which were aggravated by market-disrupting price-control and export-control policies.

The problem of food insecurity for some has been compounded by economic development and increases in per-capita incomes, which have generated an increased preference for animal protein in the diet. Although these dietary shifts reflect strong preferences as disposable income rises, they also add to the challenge of feeding 9 billion people by 2050. In addition, urbanization is proceeding at the fastest rate in human history; Africa and Asia are likely to be two-thirds urban within two decades. In addition, virtually all of the projected global population growth between now and 2050 will occur in low-income countries, many of them already crowded.

This combination of forces will reshape the food security challenge in critical ways.

Policies

The unfolding of market forces in U.S. agriculture has always been shaped by the policies and institutions that were developed to accomplish a wide range of public goals. The development of local, state, and federal policies to address farm production, food safety, and other public goals has played a pivotal role in the evolution of the current U.S. food system.

Farm Policy

Modern farm policy has its roots in the federal response to the Great Depression through the Agricultural Adjustment Act of 1933 and its successors. A collapse in both domestic food demand and exports had led to price-depressing surpluses. U.S. farm policy responded by supporting prices of designated commodities at levels thought to be fairer than market prices. The main commodities covered were grains, oilseeds, cotton, rice, and dairy, although marketing orders came to be available for some fruits and vegetables. This quickly resulted in accumulation of surpluses for those commodities.

The farm policy response involved paying farmers and warehousers to store surpluses, paying farmers to reduce their production by idling land or culling herds and paying for surplus disposal through domestic food programs (e.g., 1964 Food Stamp Act[10] and 1966 Child Nutrition Act[11]) and through exports, both as food aid (e.g., Public Law 83-480[12]) and as subsidized commercial sales. As costs of this strategy mounted, the Kennedy administration conducted a farm referendum in 1963 to see whether farmers would accept mandatory production controls (Cochrane and Runge, 1992). When that referendum failed, farm policy began a process of separating income supports from commodity prices in the marketplace. In the 1960s, political support for farm programs was sustained by broadening the scope of an omnibus legislation to include support for farmers as well as food and nutrition programs designed to address problems and priorities of urban legislators.

The ensuing decades witnessed a sequence of policy shifts that shaped

[10] The Food Stamp Act of 1964, Public Law 88-525, 88th Cong., 2nd sess. (August 31, 1964).

[11] Child Nutrition Act of 1966, Public Law 89-642, 89th Cong., 2nd sess. (October 11, 1966).

[12] Agricultural Trade Development and Assistance Act of 1954, Public Law 83-480, 83rd Cong., 2nd sess. (July 10, 1954).

the development of the nation's farm and food industries. During the 1970s, rapid growth in global market opportunities and rising commodity prices led to policy reforms to remove caps on acreage that could be planted with particular crops. When production exceeded demand, market prices for farm commodities were allowed to fall, which benefited food processors and consumers. Meanwhile, federal payments were mainly used to compensate producers for the gap between the market and a designated target price for their products. In the 1980s, efforts to renew farm programs faltered, and environmental advocates succeeded in tying support for farmers to the expansion of programs to incentivize conservation of soil and natural resources. By the early 1990s, the balance of farm output and market demand appeared to be stabilizing, and a desire to reduce government intervention in the decisions of farm producers ("freedom to farm") led to a shift toward fixed "direct payments" to farmers that were based on historic planting practices rather than annual variation in production or market prices (Gardner, 2000). This experiment was short lived, as severe market downturns led to the restoration of price supports, emergency payments, and other income protection programs for farmers (on top of the continued direct payment programs). Farm policy changed course with passage of the Agricultural Act of 2014[13] (2014 Farm Act), which was signed on February 7, 2014, and will remain the law until 2018. It makes major changes in commodity programs, adds new insurance options, consolidates conservation programs, and expands programs for specialty crops, organic farmers, bioenergy, rural development, and beginning farmers and ranchers. Price and income support for farmers is now provided primarily through an elaborate suite of subsidized insurance programs. The Act also eliminates the controversial direct payments to farmers and most countercyclical price programs. Although the law reauthorizes SNAP, it tightens the criteria for participation. The Act passed after a 2-year delay, in part as a compromise between rural and urban interests and in part because a reversion to so-called permanent farm law was feared to be highly disruptive.

Environmental Policies

Environmental policies are an increasingly important driver of the evolution of the U.S. food system, particularly with respect to the practices used in production agriculture. The two lead federal agencies responsible for writing and implementing environmental policy are USDA and EPA. Traditional farm policies have tended to subsidize farm production while reducing the risks of farming on marginal lands and drought- or flood-prone areas. These approaches have tended to aggravate the environmental

[13] Agricultural Act of 2014, Public Law 113-79, 113th Cong., 2nd sess. (February 7, 2014).

stresses that agriculture imposes on land and water resources, and the costs of these externalities are not usually captured in the price consumers pay for their food (Buttel, 2003b).

USDA's approach has focused on voluntary programs and public investments that provide technical and financial assistance to encourage farmers to adopt practices that minimize soil erosion and other environmental impacts. Since the 1980s, federal policy has tied receipt of commodity payments to the adoption of conservation plans (called "conservation compliance") and paid farmers to retire the most environmentally sensitive lands from active production (under the Conservation Reserve Program and the Wetland Reserve Program). Current programs also provide cost-share incentives for adopting or maintaining environmentally sound practices under the Environmental Quality Incentives and the Conservation Stewardship Programs. The funding of these initiatives often has lagged behind the intent of the authorizing measures (Cochrane and Runge, 1992). Still, some success can be appreciated in the expansion of land under restoration initiatives, the investments in joint ventures where USDA helps with technical assistance and capacity building in sustainable practices, and investments in research. The 2014 Farm Act reduced funding for the Conservation Reserve Program, consolidated conservation programs, and linked crop insurance premium subsidies to conservation compliance.

Debates among agricultural producers, environmental groups, and rural communities in regard to the strictness of the policies to manage animal waste by concentrated animal feeding operations (CAFOs)[14] continue. EPA started regulating CAFOs under the Clean Water Act[15] in 2003. As with other environmental policies, national guidelines are set up by EPA whereas the states are charged to address specific issues and are responsible for preventing and reducing environmental pollution. Under the National Pollutant Discharge Elimination System (EPA, 2014a), EPA grants states jurisdiction to implement programs to regulate CAFOs to protect surface water. This decentralized approach allows flexibility to respond to unique local industry and resource conditions, but also allows standards to vary from state to state. Recently, EPA has been asked by environmental groups to consider regulating CAFOs under the Clean Air Act,[16] but it is unclear whether their emissions exceed established statutory thresholds. In the absence of federal rules, some local governments (notably in California,

---

[14] CAFOs are agricultural enterprises where animals are confined on a small land area and feed is brought to the animals. The EPA has delineated three categories of CAFOs, ordered in terms of capacity: large, medium, and small. The relevant animal unit for each category varies depending on species and capacity.

[15] Federal Water Pollution Control Act, Public Law 92-500, 92nd Cong., 2nd sess. (October 18, 1972).

[16] The Clean Air Act, 42 U.S.C. § 7401 et seq. (1970).

the leading agricultural producer in the country) have adopted their own regulations to ensure that agricultural operations do not affect air quality.

Health and Safety Policies

Agriculture and food operations are subject to regulations to prevent the release of potentially hazardous chemicals into the environment. The initial Federal Insecticide, Fungicide, and Rodenticide Act[17] sought to ensure that such chemicals performed as advertised. First passed in 1947, changes in the 1970s shifted the focus to protecting humans, including farm workers, and wildlife from harm. The Food Quality Protection Act of 1996[18] heightened safety standards, especially for infants and children, and required a complete reassessment of tolerances. Initial guidance on appraising the toxicity of chemicals in food was published in 1949 and revised in 1982 with guidance on toxicological considerations for food additives (this guidance is called the "Redbook" [FDA, 2007]). The Food Allergen Labeling and Consumer Protection Act[19] (2004) was enacted to ensure accurate labeling of food products relative to allergens present, as this is the only way that consumers can avoid consuming potentially life-threatening food allergens.

Food safety policy also has focused on managing the risks from pathogen contamination. Microbial contamination can originate on farms or food handlers and can be introduced as food is stored, transported, or processed. Regulations to prevent and control pathogen contamination began with the Pure Food and Drug Act of 1906[20] and were supplemented by a number of laws dealing with milk (1924), shellfish (1925), and restaurants (1934), culminating in the 1938 Food, Drug, and Cosmetic Act.[21] Other important laws are the Federal Meat Inspection Act,[22] the Poultry Products Inspection Act,[23] and the Egg Products Inspection Act,[24] administered by USDA's Food Safety and Inspection Service. In the 1960s, the Hazard Analysis and

[17] Federal Insecticide, Fungicide, and Rodenticide Act, 7 U.S.C. § 136 et seq. (1996).

[18] Food Quality Protection Act of 1996, Public Law 104-70, 104th Cong., 2nd sess. (August 3, 1996).

[19] Food Allergen Labeling and Consumer Protection Act of 2004, Public Law 108-282, 108th Cong., 2nd sess. (August 2, 2004).

[20] Pure Food and Drug Act of 1906, Public Law 59-384, 59th Cong., 1st sess. (June 30, 1906).

[21] Federal Food, Drug, and Cosmetic Act, Public Law 75-717, 75th Cong., 3rd sess. (June 25, 1938).

[22] Federal Meat Inspection Act, 21 U.S. Code Chapter 12 § 601.

[23] Poultry Products Inspection Act, Public Law 85-172, 85th Cong., 1st sess. (August 28, 1957).

[24] Egg Products Inspection Act, Public Law 91-597, 91st Cong., 2nd sess. (December 29, 1970).

Critical Control Points (HACCP) risk-based approach to food safety was initiated, first for the U.S. space program but subsequently for the broader food supply. The HACCP's prevention-focused approach for pathogens and chemical and physical hazards has expanded voluntarily throughout many segments of the food industry. In response to significant outbreaks and concerns, HACCP-based regulations have been introduced, including the Food and Drug Administration's (FDA's) Low Acid Canned Foods regulations (1970), USDA's Pathogen Reduction/HACCP rule (1996), and FDA's HACCP regulations for seafood (1999) and juice (2001). The 2010 Food Safety Modernization Act[25] (FSMA) extended this preventive strategy for food safety to foods not covered by HACCP regulations. Other important provisions of FSMA currently under consideration by FDA are first-time mandatory preventive controls at the farm level and stricter controls of imported foods. FSMA also placed more responsibility on food companies to record and report food safety issues.

FDA and USDA food safety regulations apply only to products in interstate commerce, while food service and retail food safety considerations are managed by state and local jurisdictions. FDA's Food Code, updated every 2 years, provides a model for adoption by these jurisdictions. This consensus-based process, managed by the Conference for Food Protection, involves government, academic, industry, and consumer delegates and leads to science-based requirements to minimize biological, chemical, and physical hazards in foods.

In addition to health and safety policies, two types of nutrition policies have been key drivers of the food system. The first is the Recommended Dietary Allowances (RDAs) for key nutrients, which were established in 1941 because of concerns about nutrition deficiencies among many recruits during World War II. In 1989, the National Research Council published the 10th (and last) edition of the RDAs. The Dietary Reference Intakes (DRIs), first published in 1997, represented a new methodological approach to the development of nutrient reference standards. The most recent edition of the DRIs was released in 2010. Developed by expert committees, they are used to plan and assess diets for healthy people, including the standards for government nutrition assistance programs (e.g., WIC and SNAP), and to estimate the percent of recommended nutrients on the Nutrition Facts panel of packaged foods.

A second nutrition policy is the *Dietary Guidelines for Americans* (DGA), which has been published jointly by the U.S. Department of Health and Human Services and USDA every 5 years since 1980. The Guidelines are based on the recommendations of a panel of experts (USDA and HHS,

---

[25] FDA Food Safety Modernization Act, Public Law 111-353, 111th Cong., 2nd sess. (January 4, 2011).

2010). The DGA provides guidance about reducing consumption of foods that are believed to increase the risk of chronic disease and increase consumption of foods that promote health. In addition to advice for the general population, the DGA represents a statement of federal nutrition policy and forms the basis of all federal nutrition programs.

The importance of nutrition assistance programs in relieving food insecurity cannot be overemphasized. For example, in 2013 SNAP helped more than 47 million participants with their food purchases each month. In 2010, it reached approximately 75 percent of eligible individuals in a month (Rosenbaum, 2013). Other programs, such as WIC and the School Breakfast and Lunch programs, have a similarly large impact on the ability of individuals and families to access a nutritious diet. Fifty-one percent of infants born in the United States participate in WIC during the first year of life (Betson et al., 2011). The National School Lunch Program serves more than 30 million children per day. The School Breakfast Program has 13.5 million participants (FNS, 2014). Many private feeding initiatives, including Feeding America and its local food banks, local food shelves, and institutional feeding programs for the homeless, play a critical role in reducing food insecurity.

Energy Policies

Early in the 21st century, major changes to energy policy began to affect the food system. Prompted by concerns about dependence on oil imports and risks from climate change, the Energy Policy Act of 2005[26] and the subsequent Energy Independence and Security Act of 2007[27] mandated the blending of renewable fuels (especially ethanol) into the national automobile fuel supply. Associated farm policy added subsidies and tariffs to favor domestic U.S. ethanol production. As a result, grain ethanol production quickly came to consume 40 percent of the U.S. corn crop, though some of the by-products returned to the food system as livestock feed (see Chapter 7, Annex 2).

Other Policies

Two final broader policy arenas that continue to shape the evolution of the modern U.S. food system have been trade and climate policies. Agricultural protection has persisted through a number of trade-negotiating rounds, both in the United States and in key customer countries. This is

[26] Energy Policy Act of 2005, Public Law 109-58, 109th Cong., 1st sess. (August 8, 2005).
[27] Energy Independence and Security Act of 2007, Public Law 110-140, 110th Cong., 1st sess. (December 19, 2007).

because much governmental support for agriculture is through high and protected domestic prices rather than through direct subsidies, and it has resulted in lower exports of commodities in which the United States has a comparative advantage (especially grains, oilseeds, and livestock products) and lower imports of commodities in which other countries—particularly developing countries—have a comparative advantage (e.g., sugar, seafood, and fruits and vegetables) (Josling et al., 1996).

Climate change concerns have ushered in more attention to farming practices, as agriculture is estimated to contribute to greenhouse gas (GHG) emissions (EPA, 2014b; IPCC, 2014; Vermeulen et al., 2012). On the other hand, agriculture also is a potentially important carbon sink, so its overall carbon footprint has become more important in policy debates and production and marketing practices (Clay, 2004). Still, comprehensive national legislation to curtail GHG emissions is just starting to be developed. Progress has been made on adaptation, however, where the federal government has made some efforts to support local communities. For example, as part of President Obama's initiative to reduce methane emissions, USDA has created seven new "climate hubs" to help farmers adapt their operations to a changing climate. In addition, in September 2014 Obama announced the launch of the Global Alliance for Climate Smart Agriculture to promote solutions in agriculture that can help decrease the impact of climate change. Future climate policy initiatives will undoubtedly be a driver of how the food system will develop.

Technology

Technology has exerted an enormous influence on the food system, both in lifting resource constraints and in ushering in new issues and concerns. At the production end, hybrid seeds, synthetic fertilizers, chemical pesticides, mechanical innovations, information technologies, genetics, bioengineering, and precision agriculture have transformed the face of conventional farming. Together, they have continued to lift the productivity of land and labor; reduced losses to pests, diseases, and waste; increased resilience of plants and animals to weather variations; and produced an abundant quantity and variety of food choices. At the same time, they have given rise to new concerns about chemical residues in foods; pollution of air, land, and, especially, water; and worker exposure to new hazards.

Some of the most significant technological changes that have transformed production agriculture over the past 100 years include

- Mechanization, which freed up land from producing feed for draught animals for use to produce food while enabling individuals to farm more land;

- Synthetic fertilizers and pesticides, which increased yields per acre and reduced losses to pests and diseases;
- Plant and animal breeding, which increased land, feed, animal, and human productivity and shortened time to market; and
- Information and management practices, which made agronomics and animal husbandry increasingly science based and data driven.

At the processing and distribution levels, technology has enabled better control of pathogens and spoilage organisms, a larger range of product offerings, the substitution of capital and machinery for labor (especially in repetitive tasks), and the minimization of loss or waste. Because new technologies can convey a competitive advantage to early developers or adopters, however, they also have further facilitated industry consolidation and growth in market reach of firms to national and international levels while resulting in dislocations of workers and communities (see Chapter 5).

Consumption of food also has been reshaped by technologies. Packaging improvements have prolonged the useful life of many foods. Appliances—especially the microwave—have changed food preparation and use. Our mobile society has created huge markets for ready-to-eat and handheld items. Declining real food costs, demands for fresh (not frozen or canned) foods, and ease of disposal have increased waste at points of consumption. Bar codes have facilitated inventory management as well as an awareness of consumer behavior, giving added impetus to some market segmentation and product differentiation. Concentration, vertical integration,[28] and inventory management have not only lowered food costs and expanded choices but also contributed to an environment in which obesity and other unhealthy behaviors have increased.

Modern genetic engineering techniques also have been a powerful force for change. Genetically engineered corn and soybeans have led to the most rapid transformation of global cropping patterns in history. In the United States, 90 percent of all cotton, corn, and soybean acres have genetically engineered traits (Fernandez-Cornejo et al., 2014), and globally they are planted in 28 countries (James, 2012). From a global perspective, the Food and Agriculture Organization acknowledges that biotechnology can be a useful tool to address the issue of food security when applied appropriately (FAO, 2014). Potential benefits of GMO food applications include improved nutritional value (e.g., the incorporation of the vitamin A precursor, β-carotene, to rice), increased fish yield (e.g., aquaculture tilapia), and tolerance of poor environmental conditions (e.g., drought-resistant

---

[28] Vertical integration is a form of business organization in which all stages of production of a good, from the acquisition of raw materials to the retailing of the final product, are controlled by one company.

and salt-tolerant crops). Although 60 percent of the area planted to bioengineered seeds is in the United States and Canada, adoption in developing countries is expanding rapidly, and 90 percent of the 14 million farmers planting transgenic crops live in developing countries (James, 2012). This rapid adoption is driven by higher yields and lower pesticide costs that more than offset higher seed costs, with these benefits captured by small and large farmers alike (Raney and Pingali, 2007).

Since their first commercial introduction in 1996, the costs and benefits of genetically engineered plants and animals have generated controversy among consumers, farmers, advocates, and scientists. Potential risks that need to be managed include inadequate control (e.g., GMO genes transferring to non-GMO crops), transfer of allergens, displacement of native species, and other unpredicted issues. Some stakeholders are concerned about the emergence of super-weeds, reliance of farmers on agrichemical inputs, reduced biodiversity, or other environmental and trade issues (Benbrook, 2012; Garcia and Altieri, 2005; Gurian-Sherman, 2009; Liberty Beacon Staff, 2013). As a result, the technology has been taken up very unevenly. For example, in the United States, no wheat or rice is genetically modified. Globally, Western Europe has imposed strict labeling and tracking requirements that have essentially banned products of the technology there, while Canada, China, Brazil, and Argentina grow genetically modified crops, especially for animal feed. Differing standards and timing of approvals for genetically engineered products has disrupted trade patterns and led to disputes. Overall, genetic engineering continues to struggle for acceptance among some consumers and for additional applications, such as in animal and aquaculture production. Past National Academy of Sciences (NAS) reports have examined these questions, but with the limited data available at that time, the reports were only able to provide informed advice about the potential unintended consequences on health and environment (NRC, 2000, 2002; NRC and IOM, 2004). Currently, another NAS study is being conducted to examine the data and critically evaluate the issues.

Social Organizations

The demand for food products is driven by consumer preferences as they are shaped by marketing and advertising, but important social organizations also contribute to product demand (and changes in policies). These include public and private educational institutions where many U.S. children are first exposed to information about diet, nutrition, and health (Golden and Earp, 2012; St. Leger, 2001), as well as the extensive food advertising and marketing efforts by the food industry (Brownell and Horgen, 2003). Changes in the structure of the family and related shifts in the role of women in the workforce also have been important drivers of food system changes. Social movements—historically built around issues of food safety, but more recently related to how food is produced in the United States—have always been important drivers of change in policy and dietary practices. Finally, changes over time in the structure and organization of the U.S. health care industry can have significant effects on the incentives and disincentives to consume food in particular ways.

Whether food marketing is based on the way foods are presented at a grocery store, labeling on the food itself, or various forms of advertising, the food industry (like other industries) is aggressive in its marketing strategies. Some of these practices have been sharply criticized. For example, a 2006 Institute of Medicine report concluded that "food and beverage marketing practices geared to children and youth are out of balance with healthful diets, and contribute to an environment that puts their health at risk" (IOM, 2006, p. 10). Chandon and Wansink (2012) also proposed that food marketing has contributed to obesity by increasing the accessibility to large portions of inexpensive, tasty, and calorie-dense food.

Although the growth of television advertising is often thought of as the best example of using marketing tools—for good or ill—to shape consumer preferences and values, other industry advocacy practices also have shaped the landscape of the food system. Conventional food production companies have pursued growth through market segmentation and new product offerings for ever more selective tastes. Evidence also suggests that some companies have been able to find economic advantages from offering healthy options (Cardello and Wolfson, 2013).

Social movements are important drivers of food system changes. A wide range of social and political actors have sought to influence public policy and cultural values surrounding food. A tradition of critical food system journalism and literature goes back at least as far as Upton Sinclair, whose classic exposé of meat packing in Chicago led to dramatic reforms of labor law and public health regulations (Sinclair, 1906). This interest is exemplified by groups such as the Union of Concerned Scientists, the Center for Science in the Public Interest, and the Consumer Federation of America; organic producers; and food system critics like Michael Pollan and Mark Bittman. The organization of a consumer boycott and unionization of Californian farmworkers by Cesar Chavez in the 1960s dramatically changed the ability of farm employers in the fruit and vegetable industries to rely on poorly paid migrant workers to bring in their crops and stimulated changes in labor law, mechanization, and consumer awareness of the social costs of modern farm and food production (Holmes, 2010). The long history of academic research and writing also has contributed by raising concerns about the alignment of a market-driven food system with broader social interests, from the health, environmental, social, and economic concerns addressed in this report to issues such as stewardship of the oceans, climate, atmosphere, and other global "commons."

Many of these advocacy activities have made indelible marks on the food system. Information, private and public organizations, and social movements have contributed to many of the most significant changes in consumer food behaviors, public policy, industrial restructuring, and technological change over the past 100 years. Cooperatives, antitrust exemptions for producer groups, and farm/commodity programs are policy-based results of such forces.

Advocacy—by industry and its critics—has played and will continue to play a pivotal role in identifying food-related concerns, raising awareness of them, prompting research about them, and promoting debate about them. Some of these concerns ultimately prove to be marginal or misguided, but many of them reshape markets and technologies deployed in the food system or policies that regulate and guide it.

CONCLUDING REMARKS

By many measures, the U.S. food system is very successful. Productivity in agriculture is high due to mechanization, fertilizer and agrichemicals, genetic improvements, and improved information management practices. This has resulted in a food system that is able to nourish the majority of the population and provide food exports to much of the rest of the world. In terms of supporting farmers' incomes and wealth, from its inception in the Great Depression, farm policy has reduced volatility in farm income and food prices and raised the incomes and wealth of many farm households and landowners (Cochrane, 1993, 2003; Gardner, 2002; Pasour and Rucker, 2005). The food system contribution to the larger economy occurs off the farm, with more than 80 cents from each consumer dollar spent on food going to a wide range of input, output, and consumption services. The food system as a whole still provides about 10 percent of total U.S. employment.

Recognizing these benefits and attributes, this report describes some of the health, environmental, social, and economic effects (both positive and negative) of the U.S. food system and their interrelationships (see Chapters 3-5). Some of the most prominent issues relate to effects on human health, environment, climate change, food insecurity, and social and economic inequalities, which incur social and monetary costs. As demonstrated in this chapter, the effects of the U.S. food system reflect today's environmental and social/institutional contexts, each of which is constantly evolving in response to many drivers. With food demand globally projected to increase by 70 percent in the next 40 years, the food system will continue to evolve as it responds to new pressures and creates new issues. Although some of the health, environmental, social, and economic effects of this evolving food system will align with efficiency, others could entail added costs. This creates complex trade-offs that need to be teased out and understood as policy makers, consumers, and other actors make decisions. The analytical framework, discussed in Chapter 7, is aimed at providing tools to understand the effects, interactions, and trade-offs within the food system.

REFERENCES

Agriculture in the Classroom. 2014. *Growing a nation: The story of American agriculture. Historical timeline.* https://www.agclassroom.org/gan/timeline/index.htm (accessed November 24, 2014).

ARS (Agricultural Research Service). 2014. *ARS timeline. 144 years of ag research.* http://www.ars.usda.gov/is/timeline/chron.htm (accessed December 16, 2014).

Backstrand, J. R. 2002. The history and future of food fortification in the United States: A public health perspective. *Nutrition Reviews* 60(1):15-26.

Bell, D., and G. Valentine. 1997. *Consuming geographies: We are where we eat.* London: Routledge.

Benbrook, C. N. 2012. Impacts of genetically engineered crops on pesticide use in the U.S.—the first sixteen years. *Environmental Sciences Europe* 24(24):1-13.

Betson, D., M. Martinez-Schiferl, L. Giannarelli, and S. R. Zedlewski. 2011. *National- and state-level estimates of Women, Infants, and Children (WIC) eligibles and program reach, 2000-2009.* Washington, DC: U.S. Department of Agriculture, Food and Nutrition Service.

BLS (Bureau of Labor Statistics). 2014. *Labor force statistics from the Current Population Survey.* http://www.bls.gov/cps/cpsaat01.htm (accessed November 24, 2014).

Brownell, K. D., and K. B. Horgen. 2003. *Food fight: The inside story of the food industry: America's obesity crisis, and what we can do about it.* Columbus, OH: McGraw-Hill.

Buttel, F. H. 2003a. Continuities and disjunctures in the transformation of the U.S. agro-food system. In *Challenges for rural America in the twenty-first century*, edited by D. L. Brown and L. E. Swanson. University Park: The Pennsylvania State University Press.

Buttel, F. H. 2003b. Internalizing the societal costs of agricultural production. *Journal of Plant Physiology* 133(4):1656-1665.

Buzby, J. C., H. F. Wells, and T. G. Bentley. 2013. ERS's food loss data help inform the food waste discussion. USDA Economic Research Service. *Amber Waves.* Washington, DC: U.S. Department of Agriculture, Economic Research Service.

Buzby, J. C., H. F. Wells, and J. Hyman. 2014. *The estimated amount, value and calories of postharvest food losses at the retail and consumer levels in the United States.* Economic Information Bulletin, No. 121. Washington, DC: U.S. Department of Agriculture, Economic Research Service.

Calvin, L., and P. Martin. 2010. *The U.S. produce industry and labor: Facing the future in a global economy.* USDA-ERS Research Report 106. http://www.ers.usda.gov/publications/err-economic-research-report/err106.aspx (accessed November 25, 2014).

Canning, P. N. 2011. *A revised and expanded food dollar series. A better understanding of our food costs.* Economic Research Report, No. 114. Washington, DC: U.S. Department of Agriculture, Economic Research Service.

Cardello, H., and J. Wolfson. 2013. *Lower-calorie foods and beverages drive Healthy Weight Commitment Foundation companies' sales growth.* Interim report. Washington, DC: Hudson Institute.

Carson, R. 1962. *Silent spring*. New York: Houghton Mifflin.

CDC/NCHS (Centers for Disease Control and Prevention/National Center for Health Statistics). 2014. *Health, United States 2013. With special feature on prescription drugs*. Hyattsville, MD: NCHS. http://www.cdc.gov/nchs/hus.htm (accessed November 25, 2014).

Chandon, P., and B. Wansink. 2012. Does food marketing need to make us fat? A review and solutions. *Nutrition Reviews* 70(10):571-593.

Clay, J. 2004. *World agriculture and the environment: A commodity-by-commodity guide to impacts and practices*. Washington, DC: Island Press.

CNPP (Center for Nutrition Policy and Promotion). 2014. *Nutrient content of the U.S. food supply 1909-2010*. http://www.cnpp.usda.gov/USFoodSupply.htm (accessed November 25, 2014).

Cochrane, W. W. 1993. *The development of American agriculture: A historical analysis*. Minneapolis: University of Minnesota Press.

Cochrane, W. W. 2003. *The curse of American agricultural abundance*. Lincoln: University of Nebraska Press.

Cochrane, W. W., and C. F. Runge. 1992. *Reforming farm policy: Toward a national agenda*. 1st ed. Ames: Iowa State University Press.

Cronon, W. 1987. Revisiting the vanishing frontier: The legacy of Frederick Jackson Turner. *Western Historical Quarterly* 18(2):157-176.

Dutia, S. G. 2014. *AgTech: Challenges and opportunities for sustainable growth*. Kansas City, MO: Ewing Marion Kauffman Foundation.

EPA (U.S. Environmental Protection Agency). 2014a. *Agriculture. Overview*. http://water.epa.gov/polwaste/npdes/Agriculture.cfm (accessed November 24, 2014).

EPA. 2014b. *Sources of greenhouse gas emissions*. http://epa.gov/climatechange/ghgemissions/sources/agriculture.html (accessed November 24, 2014).

ERS (Economic Research Service). 2006. *Rural employment at a glance*. Economic Information Bulletin No. 21. Washington, DC: U.S. Department of Agriculture, Economic Research Service.

ERS. 2012. *County typology codes. Description and maps*. http://www.ers.usda.gov/data-products/county-typology-codes/descriptions-and-maps.aspx#.VD619RawSew (accessed November 25, 2014).

ERS. 2013a. *Food expenditure series*. http://ers.usda.gov/data-products/food-expenditures.aspx#.U71xNLEYePM (accessed November 25, 2014).

ERS. 2013b. *Foreign agricultural trade of the United States (FATUS): Value of U.S. agricultural trade, by calendar year*. http://www.ers.usda.gov/data-products/foreign-agricultural-trade-of-the-united-states-%28fatus%29/calendar-year.aspx#26444 (accessed November 7, 2014).

ERS. 2014a. *Ag and food sectors and the economy*. http://www.ers.usda.gov/data-products/ag-and-food-statistics-charting-the-essentials/ag-and-food-sectors-and-the-economy.aspx#.VD1ZXRawSAo (accessed November 25, 2014).

ERS. 2014b. *Food dollar series*. http://www.ers.usda.gov/data-products/food-dollar-series/documentation.aspx (accessed November 25, 2014).

ERS. 2014c. *Indicator table*. March 14. http://www.ers.usda.gov/amber-waves/2014-march/indicator-table.aspx#.VFjoypV0y71 (accessed November 4, 2014).

ERS. 2014d. *Manufacturing*. http://www.ers.usda.gov/topics/food-markets-prices/processing-marketing/manufacturing.aspx#.Uvowa_vwv3t (accessed November 24, 2014).

ERS. 2014e. *Organic market overview*. http://www.ers.usda.gov/topics/natural-resources-environment/organic-agriculture/organic-market-overview.aspx (accessed November 25, 2014).

ERS. 2014f. *Retail trends*. http://www.ers.usda.gov/topics/food-markets-prices/retailing-wholesaling/retail-trends.aspx#.Uu1RPCg7rj (accessed November 24, 2014).

FAO (Food and Agriculture Organization of the United Nations). 2014. *Biotechnology and food security fact sheet.* http://www.fao.org/worldfoodsummit/english/fsheets/biotech.pdf (accessed May 15, 2014).

FCWA (Food Chain Workers Alliance). 2012. *The hands that feed us: Challenges and opportunities for workers along the food chain.* http://foodchainworkers.org/wp-content/uploads/2012/06/Hands-That-Feed-Us-Report.pdf (accessed November 25, 2014).

FDA (U.S. Food and Drug Administration). 2007. Redbook 2000. *Guidance for industry and other stakeholders. Toxicological principles for the safety assessment of food ingredients.* http://www.fda.gov/Food/GuidanceRegulation/GuidanceDocumentsRegulatoryInformation/IngredientsAdditivesGRASPackaging/ucm2006826.htm#TOC (accessed November 24, 2014).

Fernandez-Cornejo, J., S. Wechsler, M. Livingston, and L. Mitchell. 2014. *Genetically engineered crops in the United States. Economic Research Report Number 162.* Washington, DC: Economic Research Service.

Fidelibus, M. W. 2014. Grapevine cultivars, trellis systems, and mechanization of the California Raisin Industry. *Journal of HortTechnology* 24(3):285-289.

Findeis, J. L., A. M. Vandeman, J. M. Larson, and J. L. Runyan. 2002. *The dynamics of hired farm labor: Constraints and community responses.* New York: CABI Publishing.

Flake, O., A. Jerardo, and D. Torgerson. 2013. *Outlook for U.S. agricultural trade: August 2013.* Washington, DC: U.S. Department of Agriculture, Economic Research Service and Foreign Agricultural Service.

FNS (Food and Nutrition Service). 2014. *Summary of annual data, FY 2009-2013.* http://www.fns.usda.gov/pd/overview (accessed November 25, 2014).

Food Institute. 2014. *The Food Institute report.* http://www.foodinstitute.com (accessed November 25, 2014).

Friedland, W., A. Barton, and R. Thomas. 1981. *Manufacturing green gold: Capital, labor, and technology in the lettuce industry.* Cambridge, UK: Cambridge University Press.

Fryer, C. D., and R. B. Ervin. 2013. Caloric intake from fast food among adults: United States, 2007-2010. *National Center for Health Statistics Data Brief* (114):1-8.

Fuglie, K., P. Heisey, J. King, and D. Schimmelfennig. 2012. Rising concentration in agricultural input industries influences new farm technologies. *Amber Waves* 10(4):1-6.

Garcia, M. A., and M. A. Altieri. 2005. Transgenic crops: Implications for biodiversity and sustainable agriculture. *Bulletin of Science, Technology & Society* 25(4):335-353.

Gardner, B. L. 2000. Economic growth and low incomes in agriculture. *American Journal of Agricultural Economics* 82(5):1059-1074.

Gardner, B. L. 2002. *American agriculture in the twentieth century: How it flourished and what it cost.* Cambridge, MA: Harvard University Press.

Golden, S. D., and J. A. Earp. 2012. Social ecological approaches to individuals and their contexts: Twenty years of health education & behavior health promotion interventions. *Journal of Health Education and Behavior* 39(3):364-372.

Gurian-Sherman, D. 2009. *Failure to yield. Evaluating the performance of genetically engineered crops.* Cambridge, MA: Union of Concerned Scientists.

Hendrickson, M., and W. Heffernan. 2007. *Concentration of agricultural markets.* Report prepared for National Farmers Union. http://www.nfu.org/media-galleries/document-library/heffernan-report/2007-Heffernan-Report (accessed November 25, 2014).

Holmes, T. 2010. The economic roots of Reaganism: Corporate conservatives, political economy, and the United Farm Workers movement, 1965-1970. *The Western Historical Quarterly* 41(1):55-80.

Hoppe, R. A., and D. E. Banker. 2010. *Structure and finances of U.S. farms.* EIB-66. Washington, DC: U.S. Department of Agriculture, Economic Research Service.

Hoppe, R. A., and J. MacDonald. 2013. *Updating the ERS farm typology.* Economic Information Bulletin No. 110. Washington, DC: U.S. Department of Agriculture, Economic Research Service.

Howard, P. H. 2009. Visualizing consolidation in the global seed industry: 1996-2008. *Sustainability* 1(4):1266-1287.

Howard, P. H. 2014. *Seed industry structure.* https://www.msu.edu/~howardp/seedindustry.html (accessed November 25, 2014).

IOM (Institute of Medicine). 2006. *Food marketing to children and youth: Threat or opportunity?* Washington, DC: The National Academies Press.

IPCC (Intergovernmental Panel on Climate Change). 2014. *Climate change 2014. Mitigation of climate change.* New York: Cambridge University Press. http://www.ipcc.ch/report/ar5/wg3 (accessed November 24, 2014).

IRI (Information Resources, Inc.). 2013. *Private label and national brands: Paving the path to growth together.* https://foodinstitute.com/images/media/iri/TTDec2013.pdf (accessed November 24, 2014).

Jakle, J. A., and K. A. Sculle. 1999. *Fast food: Roadside restaurants in the automobile age.* Baltimore, MD: Johns Hopkins University Press.

James, C. 2012. *Global status of commercialized biotech/GM Crops.* ISAAA Brief No. 44. Ithaca, NY: International Service for the Acquisition of Agri-Biotech Applications.

Josling, T., S. Tangermann, and T. K. Warley. 1996. *Agriculture in the GATT.* New York: St. Martin's Press.

Key, N. D., and W. McBride. 2007. *The changing economics of U.S. hog production.* Washington, DC: U.S. Department of Agriculture, Economic Research Service.

King, R. P., M. Anderson, G. DiGiacomo, D. Mulla, and D. Wallinga. 2012. *State level food system indicators, August 2012.* http://foodindustrycenter.umn.edu/Research/foodsystemindicators/index.htm (accessed November 24, 2014).

Kinsey, J. D. 2001. The new food economy: Consumers, farms, pharms, and science. *American Journal of Agricultural Economics* 83(5):1113-1130.

Kinsey, J. 2013. Expectations and realities of the food system. In *U.S. programs affecting food and agricultural marketing*, edited by W. J. Armbruster and R. Knutson. New York: Springer Science + Business Media. Pp. 11-42.

Liberty Beacon Staff. 2013. Genetically modified foods pose huge health risk. *The Liberty Beacon*, May 9, 2013. http://www.thelibertybeacon.com/2013/05/09/genetically-modified-foods-pose-huge-health-risk (accessed October 10, 2014).

Lin, B.-H., and J. Guthrie. 2012. *Nutritional quality of food prepared at home and away from home, 1977-2008.* Economic Information Bulletin, No. 105. Washington, DC: U.S. Department of Agriculture, Economic Research Service.

Lobao, L., and K. Meyer. 2001. The great agricultural transition: Crisis, change, and social consequences of twentieth century US farming. *Annual Review of Sociology* 27:103-124.

MacDonald, J. M., and W. D. McBride. 2009. *The transformation of U.S. livestock agriculture. Scale, efficiency and risks.* Economic Information Bulletin, No. 43. Washington, DC: U.S. Department of Agriculture, Economic Research Service.

Martin, P. 2009. *Importing poverty: Immigration and the changing face of rural America.* New Haven, CT: Yale University Press.

Martin, P. 2013. Immigration and farm labor: Policy options and consequences. *American Journal of Agricultural Economics* 95(2):470-475. http://ajae.oxfordjournals.org/content/95/2/470.full (accessed November 24, 2014).

Martin, P., and D. Jackson-Smith. 2013. An overview of farm labor in the United States. *Rural Connections* 8(1):21-24. http://wrdc.usu.edu/files/publications/publication/pub_2846540.pdf (accessed November 24, 2014).

Mintz, S. W., and C. M. Du Bois. 2002. The anthropology of food and eating. *Annual Review of Anthropology* 31:99-119.

NASS (National Agricultural Statistics Service). 2014a. *Farm labor*. http://usda.mannlib.cornell.edu/MannUsda/viewDocumentInfo.do?documentID=1063 (accessed November 25, 2014).

NASS. 2014b. *Quick stats*. http://quickstats.nass.usda.gov (accessed November 25, 2014).

NRC (National Research Council). 2000. *Genetically modified pest-protected plants: Science and regulation*. Washington, DC: National Academy Press.

NRC. 2002. *Environmental effects of transgenic plants: The scope and adequacy of regulation*. Washington, DC: The National Academies Press.

NRC. 2010. *Toward sustainable agricultural systems in the 21st century*. Washington, DC: The National Academies Press.

NRC and IOM. 2004. *Safety of genetically engineered food: Approaches to assessing unintended health effects*. Washington, DC: The National Academies Press.

Oskam, A., G. Backus, J. Kinsey, and L. Frewer. 2010. The new food economy. In *E.U. policy for agriculture, food and rural area*. Wageningen, The Netherlands: Wageningen Academic Publishers. Pp. 297-306.

Pardey, P. G., J. M. Alston, and C. Chan-Kang. 2013. *Public food and agricultural research in the United States: The rise and decline of public investments, and policies for renewal*. Washington, DC: AGree.

Pasour, E.C., Jr., and R. R. Rucker. 2005. *Plowshares and pork barrels: The political economy of agriculture*. Oakland, CA: The Independent Institute.

Pfeffer, M. J. 1983. Social origins of three systems of farm production in the United States. *Rural Sociology* 48:540-562.

Portnoy, S. 2013. *The U.S. role in a global food system—an agribusiness perspective*. Presentation to IOM Committee on a Framework for Assessing the Health, Environmental, and Social Effects of the Food System. Washington, DC, September 16.

Raney, T., and P. Pingali. 2007. Sowing a gene revolution. *Scientific American* 297(3):104-111.

Reinhardt, N., and P. Barlett. 1989. The persistence of family farms in the United States. *Sociologia Ruralis* 29(3/4):203-225.

Rosenbaum, D. 2013. *SNAP is effective and efficient*. Washington, DC: Center on Budget and Policy Priorities.

Runge, C. F., and B. Senauer. 2007. How biofuels could starve the poor. *Foreign Affairs* 86(3):41.

Schlosser, E. 2001. *Fast food nation: The dark side of the all-American meal*. Boston, MA: Houghton Mifflin.

Schnepf, R. 2013. *Farm-to-food price dynamics*. Congressional Research Service Report R40621. Washington, DC: Congressional Research Service.

Senauer, B., and L. Venturini. 2005. The globalization of food systems: A concept framework and empirical patterns. In *Food agriculture and the environment*, edited by E. Defrancesco, L. Galletto, and M. Thiene. Milan, Italy: FrancoAngeli. Pp. 197-224.

Sexton, R. J. 2013. Market power, misconceptions, and modern agricultural markets. *American Journal of Agricultural Economics* 95(2):209-219.

Sinclair, U. 1906. *The jungle*. New York: Doubleday, Page & Co.

St. Leger, L. 2001. Schools, health literacy and public health: Possibilities and challenges. *Health Promotion International* 16(2):197-205.

U.S. Census Bureau. 2014a. *Census of population and housing*. http://www.census.gov/prod/www/decennial.html (accessed November 25, 2014).

U.S. Census Bureau. 2014b. *Fast facts*. http://www.census.gov/history/www/through_the_decades/fast_facts (accessed November 25, 2014).

USDA (U.S. Department of Agriculture). 2003. *National range and pasture handbook. Revision 1.* Washington, DC: U.S. Department of Agriculture, Natural Resources Conservation Service.

USDA. 2009. *2007 Census volume 1, chapter 1: U.S. national level data.* Table 1. http://www.agcensus.usda.gov/Publications/2007/Full_Report/Volume_1,_Chapter_1_US (accessed February 10, 2014).

USDA. 2012. *Historical Census publications.* http://www.agcensus.usda.gov/Publications/Historical_Publications/index.php (accessed December 16, 2014).

USDA. 2014. *2012 Census of agriculture. United States.* http://www.agcensus.usda.gov/Publications/2012 (accessed November 25, 2014).

USDA and HHS (U.S. Department of Health and Human Services). 2010. *Dietary guidelines for Americans, 2010.* Washington, DC: USDA and HHS.

USDOJ (U.S. Department of Justice). 2012. *Competition and agriculture: Voices from the workshops on agriculture and antitrust enforcement in our 21st century economy and thoughts on the way forward.* http://www.justice.gov/atr/public/reports/283291.pdf (accessed October 27, 2014).

Vermeulen, S. J., B. M. Campbell, and J. S. I. Ingram. 2012. Climate change and food systems. *Annual Review of Environment and Resources* 37:195-222.

Ward, C. E., and T. C. Schroeder. 1994. Packer concentration and captive supplies. http://cals.arizona.edu/arec/wemc/cattlemarket/PckrConc.pdf (accessed December 16, 2014).

Wiebe, K. D. 2003. *Linking land quality, agricultural productivity, and food security.* Washington, DC: U.S. Department of Agriculture, Economic Research Service.

PART II

Effects of the U.S. Food System

Part II

Effects of the U.S. Food System

What does an ideal food system accomplish? In the committee's view, such a system should support human health; be nutritionally adequate and affordable and provide accessible food for all in a manner that provides a decent living for farmers and farm workers; and protect natural resources and animal welfare while minimizing environmental impacts. However, the activities that take place as we produce, process, consume, and dispose of food have positive and negative consequences in many realms of our physical and economic system, ranging from the more direct—providing nutrients needed for life—to the more indirect ones—contributing to changes in climate. Many individuals and organizations work on preventing or mitigating those negative consequences; on the other hand, some of the current challenges of the food system (see Chapter 2) may have resulted from making decisions based on siloed analyses, that is, analyses that explore effects only in one dimension and without considering the potential trade-offs. Better, informed decisions about interventions and possibly with fewer unintended consequences will be made if critical effects and trade-offs in various dimensions are first considered.

This report is intended to provide a framework for analyzing the health, environmental, social, and economic effects of the food system. To develop such a framework and illustrate issues it might need to address, the committee concluded that food system effects need to be examined in these varied domains. As described in Chapter 2, the food system is composed of many actors and processes; it is dynamic and circular (i.e., it is affected by interactions and loops) rather than linear; it affects populations in different ways; and the effects themselves can be acute and long term. There are interconnected markets that function (and result in impacts) at global, national, regional, and local levels. All of these features contribute to various challenges such as establishing boundaries, attributing cause and effect, and identifying mechanistic pathways of effects.

Part II is written as a background piece with brief descriptions of selected effects and complexities; for those selected, no systematic review of their potential associations with the food system was conducted. The chapter describes some complexities of the food system both conceptually and with examples. However, the connections to labor markets and social structures that have significant behavioral, social, and economic effects were not explored in detail. From this background piece, then, the reader should not imply any causality with the food system but, rather, potential associations. Also, although the committee recognizes that the U.S. food system has extensive and important connections to the global food system, the potential effects on other countries are not discussed. Finally, the chapters do not suggest (or even explore) alternative interventions to minimize any negative consequence or trade-off of current configurations.

In addition to highlighting some potential health (Chapter 3), environmental (Chapter 4), social (Chapter 5), and economic (Chapter 5) effects that arise as we produce, process, consume, and dispose of food, the chapters provide a brief summary of some methodologies that are used to identify and measure those effects. The introduction to each chapter aims to help the reader understand how the committee has categorized the effects in the health, environmental, social, and economic domains (e.g., food insecurity could be categorized as a health, social, or economic effect, but it has been included in Chapter 5 as a social and economic effect).

3

Health Effects of the U.S. Food System

This chapter describes health effects that are associated with the food system. It does not attempt to be comprehensive; rather, it reviews some of the most salient health effects affecting the U.S. population, their prevalence, and some potential causes. Important health effects resulting from exposure of the general population to environmental pollutants that are associated with food and agricultural operations also are included. Additionally, health effects of agriculture and food workers that are independent of food consumption are described in Chapter 5, where other health effects for this particular population are presented. Although the chapter focuses on health effects as primary outcomes, it also emphasizes that health effects are rarely independent of social and environmental effects; examples of trade-offs, interactions, and other complexities that are inherent in the current food system are briefly mentioned. Finally, the chapter points to important challenges encountered when measuring health outcomes and establishing associations with the food system. A list of selected data, metrics, and methodologies to measure health effects are in Tables B-1 through B-4 in Appendix B. The committee did not attempt to estimate non-market economic values for health effects.

THE FOOD SYSTEM AND HEALTH EFFECTS

The federal government invests resources to achieve certain public health goals. It monitors dietary patterns, nutrient intakes, and nutrition status indicators to promote human health and to prevent chronic disease.

It also encourages individuals to consume diets that promote health and prevent chronic disease by funding nutrition research and disseminating evidence-based nutrition information and guidelines, including the *Dietary Guidelines for Americans* (DGA) (USDA and HHS, 2010a) and the Dietary Reference Intakes (DRIs)[1] (IOM, 2014). Federal government resources also are invested in understanding acute disease associated with microbial or chemical foodborne illness. Regulations, warnings, and recommendations are issued to reduce the risks of foodborne illness and to protect the public's health.

Dietary practices in the United States are driven in part by consumer demands and preferences, influenced by culture, cost, taste, and convenience, and influenced by industry advertising and marketing practices (Hawkes, 2009; Popkin, 2011; Stuckler and Nestle, 2012). As Chapter 5 describes, the most profitable food production sectors are snack food producers, as opposed to producers of healthier alternatives. The unbalanced promotion of fewer nutritious products and their lower cost can influence dietary practices negatively (see below, e.g., on the association between marketing to children and obesity). Other drivers, such as policies, technology, and market forces, indirectly affect dietary practices by influencing food cost, preference formation, or accessibility (see Chapter 2). Market forces, including consumer demand, do not always support dietary practices that are consistent with public health nutrition recommendations, such as the DGA, and their associated public health goals (e.g., reducing chronic disease risk and micronutrient deficiencies). For example, current consumption of fruits and vegetables is well below recommended levels.

In some cases, interventions have been implemented to change food consumption patterns or alter the composition of consumed foods to achieve public health goals (see Box 3-1). These interventions include nutrient fortification regulations when common dietary practices fail to provide an adequate level of intake of a particular nutrient, and food assistance and nutrition-education programs that promote healthy diet planning and food preparation practices. In the absence of federal action, local governments have proposed policies to improve dietary practices by banning *trans* fats

[1] DRIs are nutrient intake standards for healthy individuals. The Estimated Average Requirement (EAR) is the average daily nutrient intake level estimated to meet the requirement of half of the healthy individuals in a particular life stage and gender group; the Recommended Dietary Allowance is the average daily nutrient intake level sufficient to meet the nutrient requirement of about 97-98 percent of the population in a particular life stage and gender group; the Upper Level is the highest level of daily nutrient intake for which there are no adverse health consequences in the population; and an Adequate Intake is established when insufficient data are available to establish an EAR, and it is based on observed or experimentally determined approximations of nutrient intake by a group of healthy people that are assumed to be adequate.

(Assaf, 2014), requiring menu labeling (Rutkow et al., 2008), or taxing or limiting the size of sugar-sweetened beverages (Mariner and Annas, 2013). Likewise, the federal government regulates food safety. Food safety is not considered a competitive advantage by the food industry in the United States. Thus, significant food safety advances are pioneered by industry as a whole and shared and adopted among companies.

Sometimes public health problems generated by market forces are not so easily corrected. This can occur when the relationships among causes and effects are not clear and therefore solutions are not easily identified. In other cases, potential interventions to promote health, such as proposed taxes on sugar-sweetened beverages or bans on advertising of low-nutrient foods on children's television programs, are rejected because the social, economic, or environmental impacts are not viewed favorably by key actors. In still other cases, feedback loops can reinforce a negative attribute of the food system. For example, the U.S. food system provides many low-cost, calorie-dense foods, which leads to an abundance of calories in the food supply but also to an increased likelihood of excessive calorie consumption, overweight, and obesity (Hawkes, 2009). This excessive consumption might be perceived as a need for higher production. At the same time, policies that subsidize a narrow number of commodities can increase calories in the food system at the expense of dietary diversity, leading to lower micronutrient intakes (Pingali, 2012).

Total alignment between market forces and public health goals for the general population, in fact, may not be possible. Population heterogeneity, including genetic, ethnic, life stage, and cultural groups, results in differing food preferences and needs among individuals within a population. Therefore, solutions increasingly may require targeted interventions and recommendations. Salient examples include susceptibility of individuals to food allergens or genetic and life-stage differences that affect nutrient requirements (Solis et al., 2008; Stover, 2006) (see folic acid fortification as an example below). Sometimes, consumer food preferences are not aligned with public health goals. For example, some groups within the population may have food beliefs that promote risky behavior, such as the consumption of raw milk despite the increased risk of foodborne illness. Unpasteurized dairy products were found to be 150 times more likely to cause illness than were pasteurized products based on the total volume of products sold in the U.S. marketplace (Langer et al., 2012). Cost, convenience, or taste can lead to dietary patterns that do not support public health goals (see also Chapter 5).

Trade-offs occur when a particular food source simultaneously promotes health (e.g., fish, which contains healthful omega-3 fatty acids) but carries health risks (e.g., fish also may contain harmful levels of methylmercury) (IOM, 2006b). Trade-offs also occur when beneficial public health

BOX 3-1
Examples of Public Health Interventions

Policies

- U.S. Department of Agriculture (USDA) nutrition assistance programs (e.g., Special Supplemental Nutrition Program for Women, Infants, and Children [WIC]; Supplemental Nutrition Assistance Program [SNAP]; the Food Emergency Program; National School Lunch Program; National School Breakfast Program)
- Food and Drug Administration (FDA) regulations requiring nutrient fortification of certain products
- USDA Pathogen Reduction and Hazard Analysis and Critical Control Points (HACCP) systems regulations, which requires meat and poultry processing plants to have safety plans to prevent contamination
- Food Safety Modernization Act, which mandates FDA to write policy to improve food safety management
- FDA Food Allergen Labeling and Consumer Protection Act, which informs consumers about allergens in foods
- FDA Food Code, a model of food safety regulations that state and local governments can adopt for the food retail and service industries
- FDA guidance with recommendations on the use of antimicrobials in foods (an attempt to voluntarily scale back the use of antibiotics in livestock) (FDA, 2013)
- FDA Nutrition Labeling and Education Act, which provides for the Nutrition Facts label to inform consumers about the nutrient content of packaged food products
- Competitive school foods rules as part of the Healthy, Hunger-Free Kids Act of 2010 (Public Law 111-296)

outcomes come at the expense of beneficial social, economic, or environmental outcomes. For example, meeting dietary omega-3 recommendations by consuming ocean fish has the potential to deplete fish stocks, a detrimental environmental outcome (Venegas-Caleron et al., 2010). Greenhouse gas emissions are similarly influenced by the architecture of the food system, including the balance between vegetable production and animal protein production (Macdiarmid et al., 2012). Achieving human health outcomes and reducing hunger may encourage labor and immigration policies that help maintain low food prices, which can be beneficial for the general population but carries social and economic inequalities. In other cases, social effects can create negative feedback loops across the dimensions of the food system, magnifying social and economic inequities, which in turn lead to health inequities. For example, some neighborhoods are character-

Voluntary Programs

- Industry-driven food safety initiatives (e.g., Global Food Safety Initiative, HACCP implementation before regulatory requirements, environmental monitoring for *Listeria monocytogenes* and other emerging pathogens)
- Food Allergy Research and Resource Program (industry-supported research and education)

Education Efforts

- Nutritional information on the front of the product package to inform consumers about salient benefits of the products
- Educational campaigns, such as the White House's Let's Move, which aims at improving the health of children and has nutrition as one of its core components
- Food safety education to consumers, such as the website foodsafety.com, established by the Centers for Disease Control and Prevention, FDA, and USDA
- Trade association food safety education on *Listeria* environmental monitoring and controls
- Nutrition education provided by USDA on the *Dietary Guidelines for Americans* (e.g., ChooseMyPlate.gov)
- State nutrition education standards, benchmarks, or expectations
- SNAP-Ed, administered by USDA with the goal of improving the food decisions of persons eligible for the SNAP program

ized by blight, crime, and disorder that can impede access to goods and services, including healthy food. The resulting negative health consequences of poor dietary practices may reinforce poverty and disadvantage among the affected populations (Bader et al., 2010).

Food system interventions are more likely to succeed if they are informed by an understanding of the intrinsic dynamics associated with public health, environmental, and social and economic outcomes, and an appreciation that their interactions are nonlinear and not always readily predicted. Maintaining alignment of the beneficial effects in all of these domains of the food system requires ongoing monitoring and evaluation of important health, environmental, social, and economic indicators, and implementation of interventions at key leverage points in the system that correct misalignments and limit the impact of trade-offs.

POTENTIAL SPECIFIC HEALTH EFFECTS OF THE FOOD SYSTEM

In the United States and in most Western countries, poor dietary patterns make the greatest contribution to the burden of noncommunicable disease (see Figure 3-1) (IHME, 2013).

The primary diet-related risks to disease of the current food system are related to food overconsumption, and contribute to the etiology of several leading causes of mortality and morbidity, including cardiovascular disease (CVD), type 2 diabetes, cancer, and osteoporosis (CDC, 2013b). Nutrient deficiencies and foodborne illness also contribute to diet-related disease.

	Australia	Austria	Belgium	Canada	Denmark	Finland	France	Germany	Greece	Ireland	Italy	Luxembourg	Netherlands	Norway	Portugal	Spain	Sweden	United Kingdom	United States
Dietary risks	1	1	1	1	2	1	1	1	1	1	1	1	2	1	1	1	1	1	1
Smoking	3	2	2	2	1	4	2	4	2	2	3	2	1	2	4	3	4	2	2
High body mass index	2	4	3	3	4	3	4	3	4	4	4	3	4	4	3	2	3	4	3
High blood pressure	4	3	4	4	3	2	3	2	3	3	2	4	3	3	2	4	2	3	4
High fasting plasma glucose	6	7	6	6	7	8	7	6	6	8	6	8	7	6	6	5	6	8	5
Physical inactivity	5	5	5	5	5	6	6	5	5	5	5	6	5	5	7	6	5	5	6
Alcohol use	8	6	7	8	6	5	5	8	9	6	9	5	6	8	5	7	8	6	7
High total cholesterol	7	8	8	7	8	7	8	7	7	7	7	7	8	7	8	8	7	7	8
Drug use	9	11	11	9	11	10	11	11	12	9	11	10	11	10	12	9	10	9	9
Ambient PM pollution	16	10	9	11	10	14	10	10	8	11	8	11	9	15	10	10	14	11	10
Occupational risks	10	9	10	10	9	9	9	9	10	10	10	9	10	9	9	11	9	10	11
Childhood sexual abuse	13	14	15	12	14	16	16	15	15	13	16	14	14	13	15	16	12	14	12
Intimate partner violence	14	13	14	13	13	12	13	14	14	14	14	12	12	12	14	14	13	15	13
Lead	11	15	12	16	15	13	14	13	11	12	13	17	15	17	11	12	16	12	14
Low bone mineral density	15	12	13	15	12	11	12	12	13	15	12	13	13	11	13	13	11	13	15
Radon	20	16	16	17	16	15	15	16	16	16	15	15	17	14	16	15	15	17	16
Ozone	23	18	18	18	18	19	18	18	17	18	17	18	18	18	18	17	19	18	17
Iron deficiency	12	17	17	14	17	17	17	17	19	17	18	16	16	16	17	18	17	16	18
Zinc deficiency	17	19	19	19	19	18	20	19	18	19	19	19	20	19	19	20	18	19	19
Unimproved water	22	23	23	22	23	23	23	23	23	23	21	23	23	23	23	23	23	23	20
Childhood underweight	18	20	20	20	20	20	21	20	20	20	20	20	19	20	21	19	20	20	21
Vitamin A deficiency	19	21	21	21	21	21	22	21	21	21	22	21	21	21	22	21	21	21	22
Sanitation	21	22	22	23	22	22	19	22	22	22	23	22	22	22	20	22	22	22	23

FIGURE 3-1 Heat map of the top risk factors that contribute to the burden of noncommunicable diseases in Western countries. The major dietary risks are low consumption of fruit, nuts, seeds, vegetables, and whole grains and elevated intakes of sodium, fat, processed meats, and trans fats. The colors and numbers designate the ranking based on number of risk factors, with red representing countries with a higher number of risk factors for a particular disease and therefore higher in the rank. A breakdown of dietary risks can be found at http://vizhub.healthdata.org/gbd-compare (accessed January 8, 2015).
NOTE: PM = particulate matter.
SOURCE: IHME, 2013. Reprinted with permission from the Institute for Health Metrics and Evaluation.

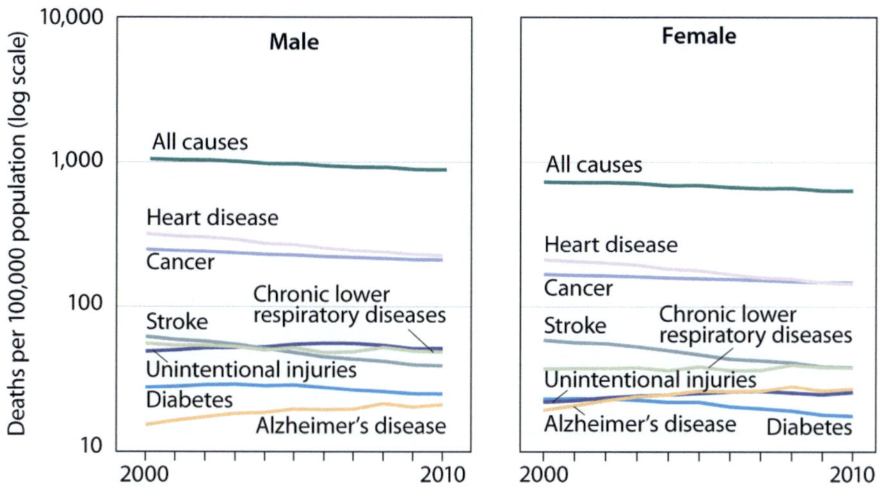

FIGURE 3-2 Age-adjusted death rates for selected causes of death for all ages, by gender: United States, 2000-2010.
NOTE: Cause of death is coded according to the 10th revision of the *International Statistical Classification of Diseases and Related Health Problems.*
SOURCE: CDC/NCHS, 2014a.

Figure 3-2 presents age-adjusted death rates for several chronic diseases[2] in the United States between 2000 and 2010 (CDC/NCHS, 2014a).

These diseases, together with their risk factors, including obesity, hypertension, and hypercholesterolemia, account for significant medical and productivity costs, and they exact a heavy toll on quality of life in the United States. The Centers for Disease Control and Prevention (CDC) estimates that 75 percent of our health care dollars are used to treat preventable chronic diseases and conditions. One estimate of the burden of cardiovascular disease in the United States is more than $300 billion each year, including the cost of health care services, medications, and lost productivity (Go et al., 2014). In 2012, the total burden of diabetes types 1 and 2 was estimated to be $245 billion, including hospital inpatient care, medications, and loss of productivity (ADA, 2013). In 2008, it was esti-

[2] Chronic disease, as defined by the U.S. National Center for Health Statistics, is a disease lasting 3 months or longer. About one-fourth of people with chronic conditions have one or more daily activity limitations, often understood as a hindrance or an inability to perform major activities in one's life.

mated that obesity cost the U.S. health care system around $147 billion (or 9.1 percent of annual medical spending) for treatment of obesity-related disorders, such as type 2 diabetes (Finkelstein et al., 2009).

A discussion of five broad categories of health outcomes of the food system follows, including (1) obesity; (2) chronic diseases (e.g., hypertension, CVD, and type 2 diabetes); (3) micronutrient deficiencies; (4) microbiological foodborne illness; and (5) chemical foodborne illness.

Obesity

The dynamics of the U.S. food system have created an abundant food supply, which has reduced hunger but also plays an important role in our current obesity epidemic. Obesity is classified as a disease by the American Medical Association, and it is also a risk factor for other common chronic diseases, such as CVD, type 2 diabetes, certain cancers, osteoarthritis, liver and gall bladder disease, and others (Dagenais et al., 2005; IOM, 2005; Malnick and Knobler, 2006). Obesity results from complex interactions among behavioral, genetic, and environmental factors (i.e., environments for physical activity, food and beverage, health care, work, and school) that influence what we eat throughout life. Ultimately, obesity is the result of habitually consuming more energy than is expended and the development of excess adipose tissue.

The National Health and Nutrition Examination Survey (NHANES; see section Methodologies to Measure Health Outcomes p. 109 and also Appendix B, Table B-3) tracks U.S. civilians in terms of health status and self-reported dietary intake. Data from NHANES show that in the period 2011-2012, 35.1 percent of U.S. adults were considered obese (body mass index [BMI] ≥30), while an additional 33.9 percent were considered overweight (BMI ≥25) (Fryar et al., 2014). The total prevalence of obesity among adults age 20 and older steadily increased from 1960-1962 to 2011-2012, from 10.7 to 33.9 percent for men and 15.8 to 36.6 percent for women (Fryar et al., 2014) (see Figure 3-3).

In 2009-2010, about 18 percent of children older than age 5 had obesity, a significant increase since 1976-1980, when the prevalence was about 5 percent (Fryar et al., 2012). Recent data from the Institute for Health Metrics and Evaluation (http://vizhub.healthdata.org/obesity [accessed January 8, 2015]) show that overweight and obesity among youth ages 10 to 14 in 2013 was 38 percent, and 18 percent in children ages 1 to 4 (see Figure 3-4), suggesting a flattening of the obesity rate for children. A recent article documented that this flattening of obesity growth is true for high-income categories but masks continued growth in obesity rates in lower income groups (Frederick et al., 2014).

Obesity prevalence varies by population and disproportionately affects

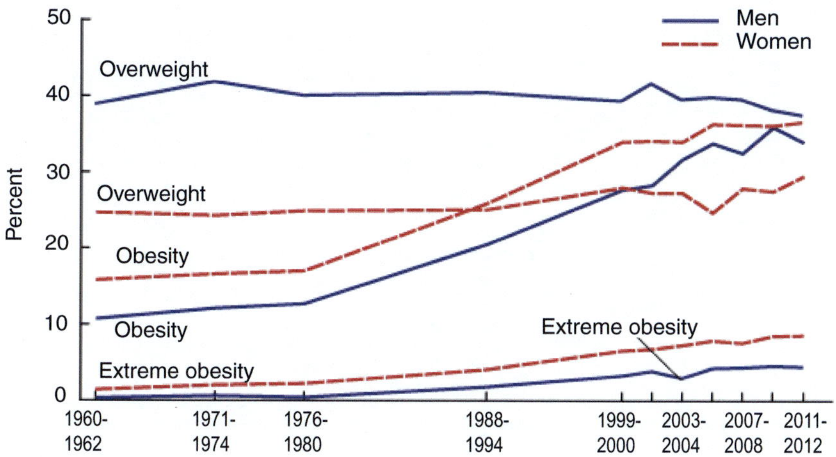

FIGURE 3-3 Trends in adult overweight, obesity, and extreme obesity among men and women ages 20-74: United States, selected years 1960-1962 through 2011-2012.
NOTES: Age-adjusted by the direct method to the year 2000 U.S. Census Bureau estimates using age groups 20-39, 40-59, and 60-74. Pregnant females were excluded. Overweight is body mass index (BMI) of 25 or greater but less than 30; obesity is BMI greater than or equal to 30; and extreme obesity is BMI greater than or equal to 40.
SOURCE: Fryar et al., 2014, with data from Centers for Disease Control and Prevention/National Center for Health Statistics, National Health Examination Survey 1960-1962; and National Health and Nutrition Examination Surveys 1971-1974, 1976-1980, 1988-1994, 1999-2000, 2001-2002, 2003-2004, 2005-2006, 2007-2008, 2009-2010, and 2011-2012.

certain race, ethnicity, and income groups. CDC reports that 49.5 percent of non-Hispanic blacks, 39.1 percent of Hispanics, and 34.3 percent of non-Hispanic whites had obesity (Flegal et al., 2012). From 2005 to 2008, the prevalence of obesity was 42 percent among women below the federal poverty level, compared to 32.9 percent among women above 130 percent of the poverty level.

Obesity: A Complex Etiology

The reasons for the marked increase in the rates of obesity in the U.S. population are complex and due to the interaction of many factors. Some evidence suggests that specific genes convey a higher risk for obesity if expressed (den Hoed et al., 2010; Dina et al., 2007; Frayling et al., 2007).

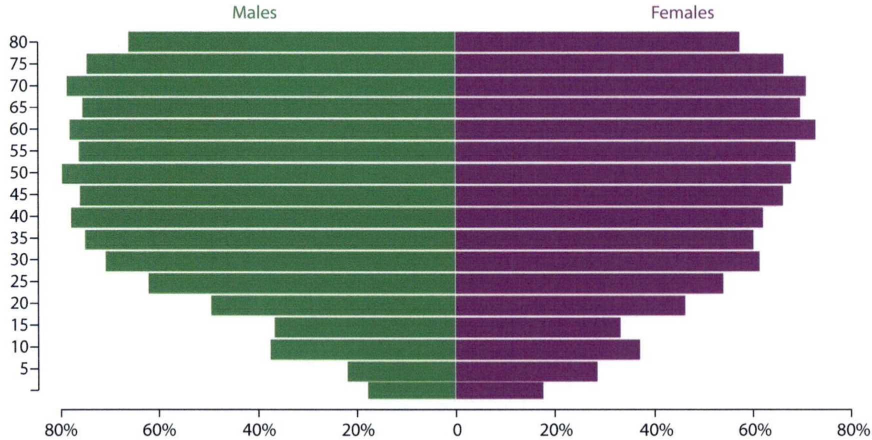

FIGURE 3-4 Percentage overweight and obesity (x-axis, body mass index greater than or equal to 25) by age (y-axis) and gender in the United States, 2013.
SOURCES: IHME, 2014; Ng et al., 2014. Reprinted with permission from the Institute for Health Metrics and Evaluation.

Leibel (2008) has argued that these genes act primarily on the central nervous system and affect both the conscious and the unconscious aspects of food intake and energy expenditure. He then postulated that no regulatory gene acting alone or with others can explain the risk of becoming obese, in part because its expression depends so much on the interaction with other genes as well as with the food environment. Although it is virtually impossible that a major genetic change has occurred in the U.S. population in the past 30 to 40 years, genes can sensitize individuals to obesity in obesity-promoting (obesogenic) environments. Therefore much attention has been given to the food environment in an effort to understand the dramatic rise in obesity.

Westerterp and Speakman (2008) have argued that Americans have not become less active during the period when obesity was rising at a rapid rate, but others have found otherwise (Archer et al., 2013; Church et al., 2011). There is no consensus at this time regarding the individual quantitative contributions of diet and physical activity to obesity in populations. Increases in the obesity rate in the United States since the 1980s, however, have coincided with substantial changes in the availability of food, food consumption, and the food environment. These changes, in turn, are driven by an evolution in technology, agricultural policies, marketing, and consumer life styles. The calories (not corrected for losses in processing and waste) available in the U.S. food supply remained relatively constant at about 3,300 calories per day from the early 1900s until the early 1980s. Available calories then rose to about 3,900 calories per day by the year 2000 (see Figure 3-5).

Researchers have suggested a number of potential pathways by which increased calorie levels in the food supply have translated into rising obesity rates. For example, individual studies and systematic analysis have found strong associations between eating an excess amount of sugar and weight gain (de Ruyter et al., 2012; Ebbeling et al., 2012; Malik et al., 2013; Perez-Morales et al., 2013; USDA and HHS, 2010b). In addition, the U.S.

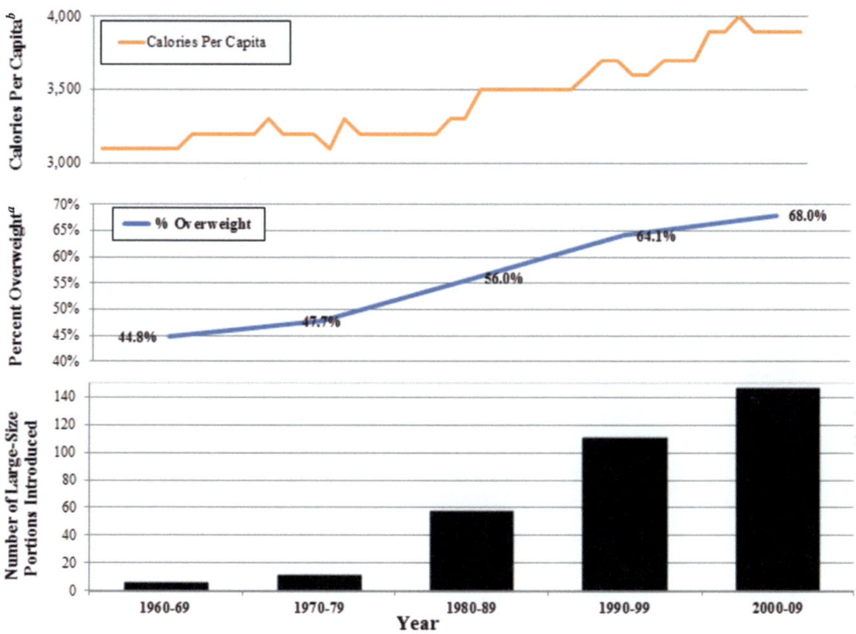

FIGURE 3-5 Available calories per capita per day, overweight, and number of large size portions introduced.
NOTES: The line for overweight includes both the percentage of overweight and obesity. Not corrected for losses in processing and waste.
[a] U.S. adults ages 20 years and above with BMI >25.
[b] Data from USDA food availability series.
SOURCE: Nestle and Nesheim, 2012. Reprinted with permission from the University of California Press.

Department of Agriculture's (USDA's) Economic Research Service has found evidence that eating one meal away from home each week, a growing trend, translates to an annual weight gain of 2 extra pounds each year, or 134 calories/day (Todd et al., 2010). Others have hypothesized that the trend to consume foods away from home, combined with the increases in portion sizes in food eaten away from home (Young and Nestle, 2007), is a potential reason for the parallel increase in average weight of the U.S. population.

A number of studies have explored how increased portion size increases caloric intake and food waste. In one study, participants consumed 30 percent more energy at lunch when offered the largest portion of food than when offered the smallest portion. This response to the variations in portion size was the same, regardless of who determined the amount of food on the plate, investigators or the subject (Rolls et al., 2002). Another study found that moviegoers ate more popcorn if randomly given a large container than a smaller one, even those subjects who reported not liking the popcorn (Wansink and Park, 2001). Further evidence of the influence of portion sizes on intake was found in a study of self-refilling soup bowls, in which participants unknowingly eating from self-refilling soup bowls ate 73 percent more soup than did those eating from normal bowls. The study authors suggest that, without visual cues, people are less able to self-monitor their intake (Wansink et al., 2005).

Price and preference formation also play an important role in household food purchasing, and thus in food consumption. Wilde et al. (2012) examined the relationship of food prices and the obesity epidemic and found support for the "food price hypothesis," which postulates that low prices of energy-dense foods relative to the price of less energy-dense foods leads to a higher risk of obesity. Evidence also suggests that marketing strategies to children contribute to an increased consumption of calorie-dense food. Based on evidence about industry's practices, mainly television advertising, and a systematic review of the relationship between those practices and health, the Institute of Medicine (IOM) report *Food Marketing to Children and Youth: Threat or Opportunity?* concluded that food and beverage marketing practices to children and youth are out of balance with healthful diets and contribute to food environments that put their health at risk (IOM, 2006a). Chandon and Wansink (2012) have proposed that food marketing has contributed to obesity by increasing the accessibility of bigger portions of inexpensive and calorie-dense food. They proposed that food marketers could continue to maintain profits by offering healthy foods to the consumer by altering marketing strategies. The evidence to support linkages among other aspects of food system dynamics and obesity is less clear. For example, the association between access to supermarkets and obesity is not entirely clear (Wilde et al., 2012).

Because of the complex etiology of obesity—that is, obesity is affected by many elements of the food system as well as other causes—reversing the rise in obesity in the United States does not have a simple solution. Several IOM reports that have analyzed the literature on evidence for contributors to obesity recommend a variety of strategies to make progress in obesity prevention, highlighting actions within the food and beverage environment as one salient strategy (IOM, 2005, 2012). One of these reports, *Accelerating Progress in Obesity Prevention: Solving the Weight of the Nation* (IOM, 2012), recommended a set of goals to deal with the rising prevalence of obesity in this country. These include interventions such as making physical activity a routine part of life, creating food and beverage environments in which healthy food and beverage options are the routine easy choice, and transforming messages about physical activity and nutrition, among others. These measures would have profound effects on the food system, the physical environment, and the socioeconomic aspects of life in the United States if they were fully implemented. The discourse about solutions is often dominated by arguments about choice, reflecting the often-contentious social and political environment surrounding food.

Chronic Diseases

Evidence supporting the relationships among diet and risk of chronic diseases has been graded and summarized in numerous reports and data resources (e.g., USDA's Nutrition Evidence Library [NEL, 2014a], World Cancer Research Fund/American Institute for Cancer Research Diet and Cancer Report [WCRF/AICR, 2007], American College of Cardiology and American Heart Association [Eckel et al., 2014; Jensen et al., 2014]). The conclusions presented here are from USDA's Nutrition Evidence Library, which grades the strength of evidence supporting an association among diet and health or disease as "strong" or "moderate" or "limited."

For CVD, strong and consistent evidence demonstrates that dietary patterns rich in fruits, vegetables, whole grains, nuts, legumes, low-fat dairy, fish, and unsaturated oils, and low in red and processed meat, saturated fat, sodium, and sugar-sweetened foods and drinks, are associated with decreased risk of fatal and nonfatal CVD (USDA, 2014). Consistent evidence also shows that vegetable and fruit intakes are inversely related to the incidence of myocardial infarction and stroke, with significantly larger positive effects when intakes are greater than five servings per day. Moderate evidence suggests that the intake of milk products and whole grains is inversely associated with CVD and that consumption of two servings per week of seafood containing omega-3 fatty acids is associated with lower cardiovascular mortality (NEL, 2014a).

Hypertension is a major risk factor for CVD and a condition that affects 29.1 percent of U.S. adults age 18 and older (Nwankwo et al.,

2013). Strong evidence among adults, and moderate evidence among children from birth to age 18, indicates that higher sodium intakes are associated with increased blood pressure. Conversely, considerable evidence shows that higher potassium intakes are associated with decreased blood pressure. Increased intakes of low-fat milk products and vegetable protein also are linked to lower blood pressure.

Strong evidence demonstrates that body fatness increases the risk of several cancers, including esophageal, pancreatic, colorectal, post-menopausal breast, endometrial, and renal. In addition, convincing evidence supports an increased risk of colorectal cancer with red and processed meat intakes and of liver cancer with aflatoxin intakes. Evidence also suggests that diets rich in dietary fiber, non-starchy vegetables, and fruits are protective for a number of cancers (NEL, 2014a).

Diet is a factor in type 2 diabetes, a major chronic disease that also is an independent risk factor for CVD. Strong evidence demonstrates that saturated fatty acid intakes are associated with increased insulin resistance and risk of type 2 diabetes, and that a substitution of just 5 percent of saturated fats with monounsaturated fatty acids or polyunsaturated fatty acids can improve insulin response. Furthermore, strong evidence shows that an improved lipid profile can be achieved with the substitution of monounsaturated or polyunsaturated fatty acids for saturated fatty acids. Moderate evidence indicates that milk and milk products are associated with a lower incidence of type 2 diabetes (NEL, 2014a). Limited evidence suggests that whole grain intakes also are associated with a reduced incidence of type 2 diabetes (NEL, 2014a).

Some races and ethnic populations and the poor are more likely to have chronic diseases, some of them related to food intake (Price et al., 2013). Type 2 diabetes risk varies by race and ethnicity and is more prevalent in non-Hispanic African Americans (19.0/100,000) than in Hispanic Americans (6.9 and 4.8/100,000 in males and females, respectively) and non-Hispanic whites (3.7/100,000). The disparities are likely related to multiple factors, including access to health insurance, poverty, food insecurity, and availability of healthy and affordable food. In 2013, CDC published a report on disparities in social and health indicators, *Health Disparities and Inequalities—United States, 2013* (CDC, 2013a). Despite limitations in the data, the report highlights the existence of inequalities that, in many cases, are increasing with time (see Table 3-1). For example, data from the 2009 National Vital Statistics System shows that blacks had higher age-adjusted rates of coronary heart disease (CHD) and stroke deaths than did other racial/ethnic groups.

Notably, dietary recommendations to control obesity, type 2 diabetes, CVD, hypertension, cancer, and osteoporosis are all remarkably similar (Krebs-Smith and Kris-Etherton, 2007; USDA and HHS, 2010a). For more

TABLE 3-1 Age-Adjusted Rates (number of cases/100,000) for Some Chronic Diseases Among Racial/Ethnic Groups; Data Sources and Years Vary

	Coronary Heart Disease and Stroke[a]	Obesity in Females[b]	Diabetes[c]	Hypertension[d]
American Indian/ Alaskan Native	92			
Asian/Pacific Islander	67.3			
Asian			7.9	
Black	141.3	51	11.3	41.3
Hispanic[e]	86.5		11.5	27.7
White	117.7	31	6.8	28.6
Mexican Americans		41		27.5
Total	116.1			29.6

[a] Data from 2009 National Vital Statistics Systems. Death rates per 100,000 U.S. standard population.
[b] Data from National Health and Nutrition Examination Survey (NHANES) 1999-2010. Prevalence per 100 population.
[c] Data from 2010 National Health Interview Survey; age-adjusted prevalence of diabetes of any duration per 100 population.
[d] Data from NHANES 2007-2010 prevalence of hypertension per 100 population.
[e] Persons of Hispanic ethnicity might be of any race.
SOURCE: CDC, 2013a.

than 30 years, federal dietary guidance has urged Americans to moderate their intakes of sodium and energy, especially from saturated fatty acids and simple carbohydrates. At the same time, they have encouraged relatively greater consumption of fruits, vegetables, and whole grains. The food supply is not aligned with these goals and, in spite of the recommendations, diets for most Americans have continued to be low in such foods and overabundant in refined grains, added sugars, saturated fats, and sodium.

Micronutrient Deficiencies

Clinical micronutrient deficiencies in the United States are uncommon, but risk of inadequacy occurs when the intake of a particular nutrient falls below reference values, referred to as DRIs (Trumbo et al., 2013). DRIs are nutrient intake standards for healthy individuals that are based on best available scientific evidence and are reviewed regularly. The specific measures and outcomes used to establish the Recommended Dietary Allowances (RDAs) vary by nutrient, but all relate to nutritional status or functional indicators that report on the level of nutrient intake required to prevent diseases associated with a particular micronutrient deficiency and/or to reduce chronic disease risk (Trumbo, 2008). Nutrient requirements can vary by population group, and the DRI process considers separate requirements for up to 22 distinct life stage and sex groups (Kennedy and Myers, 2005).

The micronutrient status of the U.S. population can be determined by comparing blood and urine measures of clinical cut-offs, accomplished primarily through NHANES (see p. 110 and Appendix B, Table B-3), or by national surveys that examine dietary intakes relative to the DRI reference values. The *Second National Report on Biochemical Indicators of Diet and Nutrition in the U.S. Population* (CDC, 2012) collected data on 58 biochemical indicators from specimens gathered during the period of 2003-2006 as part of NHANES. The data indicated that less than 10 percent of the general population had biochemical indicators below the clinical cut-off points. Vitamin B_6, iron, and vitamin D had the most prevalent low values (see Figure 3-6). Borderline indicators were found in young women for

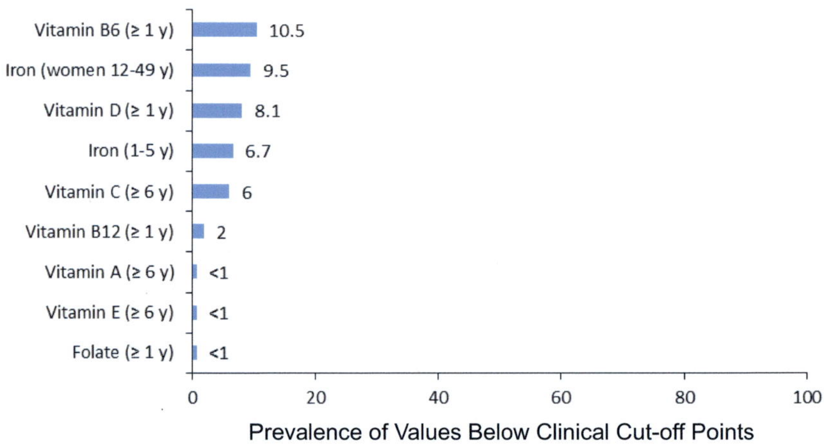

FIGURE 3-6 Prevalence estimates of nutrient deficiencies in U.S. persons, National Health and Nutrition Examination Survey, 2003-2006.
NOTES: Nutrition indicators were measured in different ages (e.g., age 1 year and older, age 6 years and older) and population groups (e.g., women ages 12-49 years, children ages 1-5 years). Cut-off values used to estimate prevalence are serum pyridoxal-5′-phosphate < 20 nmol/L, serum body iron < 0 mg/kg, serum 25-hydroxyvitamin D < 30 nmol/L, serum ascorbic acid < 114 µmol/L, serum cobalamin < 200 pg/mL, serum retinol < 20 µg/dL, serum alpha-tocopherol < 500 µg/dL, and red blood cell folate < 95 ng/mL.
SOURCE: CDC, 2012.

iodine, which is essential for normal growth and development of the fetus. Currently, most low micronutrient values in the United States are limited to particular population groups, and the rates vary by sex, age, and race/ethnicity. Non-Hispanic blacks and Mexican Americans are more likely to be low in vitamin D and folate (although rates of low values have decreased across all groups) compared to non-Hispanic whites. The prevalence of iron deficiency also varies by race and ethnicity. For children, the highest prevalence of deficiency is seen in Mexican Americans (10.9 versus 6.7 among all 1- to 5-year-old children) and, for adults, the highest prevalence deficiencies are seen in Mexican American (13.2 versus 9.5 among all women) and non-Hispanic black women (16.2 versus 9.5 among all women).

A report from USDA's Agricultural Research Service examined the usual intake levels of 24 nutrients from food in 8,940 individuals using 2001-2002 NHANES data and compared these to the Estimated Average Requirements (Moshfegh et al., 2005). The intakes of vitamins A, E, C, and magnesium were marginally low across all population groups, whereas group-specific low intakes were seen for vitamin B_6 and adult females, zinc for older adults, and phosphorus for young females. The latest data on phosphorus, magnesium, calcium, and vitamin D also found low intakes of those nutrients (Moshfegh et al., 2009). In contrast to using biomarker data, measuring micronutrient deficiency with intake data might be affected by reporting error.

The DRIs always have recognized that nutrient requirements differ by population groups, including age, sex, and life stage (e.g., pregnancy, lactation), but evidence is increasingly showing that requirements also are influenced by ethnicity and genetic variation (Solis et al., 2008) as well as obesity (Damms-Machado et al., 2012). Expanding knowledge of population heterogeneity (e.g., cultural, genetic, epigenetic, and BMI) and its impact on nutritional status have led to the idea of "individualized nutrition" (Ohlhorst et al., 2013). Individualized nutrition challenges intervention approaches at the population level because recommendations for one group within the population may be inappropriate for another group.

Microbiological Foodborne Illness

In the United States, foodborne disease surveillance is collected using both active and passive surveillance systems (see "Methodologies to Measure Health Outcomes" section on p. 109 and also Appendix B, Table B-3). The National Outbreak Reporting System (NORS) is a passive surveillance system that includes outbreaks (i.e., two or more people becoming ill from eating the same food) reported to CDC by state public health agencies. Data from NORS indicate that 831 foodborne illness outbreaks, 14,972 illnesses, 794 hospitalizations, and 23 deaths were reported in 2012 (CDC, 2014c).

Of the outbreaks with suspected or confirmed etiologies, 50 percent were associated with viruses, 42 percent with bacteria, 7 percent with chemicals and toxic agents, and 1 percent with parasites. The primary agents involved in confirmed illnesses were norovirus (50 percent) and *Salmonella* (28 percent). Of the hospitalizations, 61 percent of the cases involved *Salmonella,* 13 percent involved Shiga toxin-producing *Escherichia coli* (STEC), and 8 percent involved norovirus. Although the numbers of cases were not as high as those for other pathogens, severe disease is noted for *Clostridium botulinum* (21 illnesses, 1 death), *Listeria monocytogenes* (42 illnesses, 6 deaths), and mycotoxins (21 illnesses, 4 deaths). These data represent the "tip of the iceberg" in that underreporting of foodborne illness is significant (FoodNet data from 2000-2008 estimates 47.8 million illnesses annually).

The FoodNet (see next paragraph and Appendix B, Table B-3), an active surveillance program established in 1996 to monitor diarrheal foodborne illness attributed to eight bacterial pathogens and two parasites, provides better estimates than does NORS. Because data are normalized to the actual population size for participating sites, FoodNet data provide the basic metric to monitor trends from year to year. The incidence of foodborne illness associated with *Salmonella, Shigella,* STEC O157, *Listeria monocytogenes, Yersinia,* and *Cryptosporidium* in 2013 (CDC, 2014b) was not significantly different from a 2006-2008 baseline, while the incidence of *Campylobacter* and *Vibrio* increased 13 percent and 75 percent, respectively. The authors concluded that the lack of progress in recent years calls for more interventions and suggested possible causes. For example, the lack of progress in decreasing *Salmonella* infections since 2006-2008 could be due to a large outbreak associated with egg consumption in 2010, about the time when the Egg Safety Rule was being implemented. The increased incidence of *Vibrio* may be influenced by environmental and social factors. *Vibrio* spp. are naturally associated with a marine environment and seafood products. Increasingly warm coastal water temperatures provide a more favorable growth condition for *Vibrio*, thus increasing the risk of contamination. A majority of *Vibrio* foodborne illness outbreaks are associated with consumption of raw shellfish (Newton et al., 2012). Educational efforts to reduce consumption of these higher-risk products have not been effective (Newton et al., 2012).

FoodNet also is used as the basis for the current estimates of foodborne disease in the United States, which considers underreporting and the burden of disease related to unrecognized etiologies. For example, with data from 2000-2008, CDC estimates that 47.8 million illnesses, 127,839 hospitalizations, and 3,037 deaths related to foodborne illness occur every year in the United States, which translate into 1 in 6 Americans becoming ill every year from consuming contaminated food (Scallan et al., 2011a,b). Of these, known pathogens account for 9.4 million of these illnesses, 56,000 hospitalizations, and 1,400 deaths (Scallan et al., 2011a), illustrating that the burden from unknown agents is significant.

Foodborne illness estimates provided by FoodNet and NORS surveillance systems do not capture the true cost of foodborne disease. Some foodborne infectious diseases result in chronic sequelae, congenital disease, or death, which have an impact on productivity and quality of life. Quality-adjusted life year (QALY) estimates have been reported for 14 foodborne pathogens (Hoffman et al., 2012), which provide an estimate of economic and social costs of illness associated with major foodborne pathogens. The authors estimated that the annual cost of illness for the 14 pathogens ranged from $4.4 billion to $33 billion, and lost quality of life ranged from 19,000 to 145,000 QALYs. QALY calculations included factors for the estimated annual number of cases and the probability and duration of adverse health state. Non-typhoidal *Salmonella* spp., *Campylobacter* spp., *L. monocytogenes, Toxoplasma gondii*, and norovirus contributed to approximately 90 percent of the social and economic loss.

Chemical Foodborne Illness

Food risks are also related to chemicals, whether they are natural (e.g., allergens) or contaminants (e.g., they are not expected to be present in foods). Some contaminants have been known for many years while others are "emerging." Examples of chemical contaminants are polychlorinated biphenyls, polychlorinated dioxins/furans, methyl mercury, lead, arsenic, cadmium, aflatoxins, other mycotoxins, marine toxins, chromium VI, other metals, polybrominated diphenyl ethers, polyfluorinated carboxylates and sulfonates, and perchlorate.

Only 7 percent of foodborne outbreaks reported for 2012 (CDC, 2014b) with a confirmed or suspected etiologic agent were associated with a chemical or toxin hazard. This represented about 1 percent of the foodborne illnesses reported. Over the longer time frame of 1998-2010 (CDC, 2013c), seafood-related agents were the most common chemical food safety issue, with scombroid toxin/histamine (351 outbreaks), ciguatoxin (190 outbreaks), mycotoxins (18 outbreaks), and paralytic shellfish poison (13 outbreaks) identified as causing the majority of outbreaks. Heavy metals, cleaning agents, neurotoxic shellfish poison, plant/herbal toxins, pesticides, puffer fish tetrodotoxin, monosodium glutamate, and other chemicals and natural toxins also were listed as causing at least one outbreak.

The effects of long exposures to low levels of chemicals through food or other environmental routes related to food production are not routinely surveyed for the general population. The time lag makes the identification of associations difficult, so resources are typically prioritized to other surveillance activities that provide more accurate results. However, some studies have been conducted in specific populations that are exposed to higher levels of agrichemical residues through air or water, such as farmers, farm workers, or those in farming communities (see below for farming communities and Chapter 5 for health effects in farmers and farm workers).

A number of questions related to chemicals in foods are still unresolved. *State of the Science of Endocrine Disrupting Chemicals—2012* (WHO, 2013) points out that significant uncertainty exists regarding the potential risk of endocrine system disruption from many chemicals used in food. In humans, the contribution of these chemicals to risk of endocrine-related diseases and human exposure levels from food and nonfood sources are not clear at this time. However, the negative impact of persistent organic pollutants on certain wildlife populations has been demonstrated, leading to recommendations to ban certain chemicals to reduce exposure. For example, banning of the nonfood-system-related pesticides DDT and tributyltin (e.g., used in ships' paint) demonstrated positive effects on populations of birds and mollusks, respectively. Children and the developing fetus are more vulnerable to endocrine disruptors than are adults, again demonstrating that health outcomes related to the food supply can differ among human populations.

Environmental Pollutants

An important note is that in addition to food, some chemical exposures occur through air or water. For example, residents living near concentrated animal feeding operations[3] (CAFOs) are reported to have increased incidence of respiratory distress, digestive disorders, anxiety, depression, and sleep disorders. Children living on farms raising swine were reported to have a higher incidence of asthma, with increasing incidence as the size of the swine operation increased (Donham et al., 2007). A report from the Iowa Health Sciences Research Center (ISU/UI Study Group, 2002) concluded that the effects on residents of communities in the vicinity of CAFOs were less definitive than for workers in the facilities but suggested that residents had similar respiratory symptoms and a reduced quality of life. The Iowa group went on to conclude that CAFO air emissions constitute a public health hazard deserving of public health precautions. Others are less convinced that health effects in communities can be attributed to emissions from CAFOs. A review of existing studies funded by the National Soybean Board and the National Pork Board concluded that evidence of a

[3] CAFOs are agricultural enterprises where animals are confined on a small land area and feed is brought to the animals. The Environmental Protection Agency has delineated three categories of CAFOs, ordered in terms of capacity: large, medium, and small. The relevant animal unit for each category varies depending on species and capacity.

small increase in self-reported disease in people with allergies or familial history of allergies was inconsistent (O'Connor et al., 2010). The limitations in the quality and quantity of human health data related to CAFOs present challenges in assessing potential trade-offs associated with large-scale animal agriculture.

Likewise, ammonia (NH_3) pollution from agriculture has been cited recently as a major cause of health damage in the United States (Paulot and Jacob, 2014). Ammonia, which can enter the atmosphere from fertilizer and from animal urine and manure, reacts with other components of air to create particles that can affect the lungs and cause asthma attacks, bronchitis, and heart attacks. When ammonia reacts with oxides of nitrogen and sulfur, it can form particulate matter that is less than 2.5 microns wide, a size considered most dangerous. Long-term reductions in particulate matter in the atmosphere have been related to increased life expectancy (Pope et al., 2009) (see also "Environmental Contaminants and Pollutants" in Chapter 4).

COMPLEXITIES ASSOCIATED WITH HEALTH EFFECTS OF THE FOOD SYSTEM

Many decisions, whether made by individuals or by society, involve trade-offs between a specific benefit and certain risks. Comparisons are often challenging because adequate metrics do not exist or cannot be monetized into a single metric. Other complexities can occur when an effect implicates different populations or subgroups within populations. Although it has not been unusual to consider health and economic trade-offs in decision-making processes with health goals in mind, other dimensions (e.g., social, environmental) often have been overlooked. For example, Annex 1 in Chapter 7 includes a discussion on current advice for fish consumption (based on health benefits) that does not consider environmental risks. Below are some selected examples of trade-offs and other complexities that are inherent in the food system as it exists today.

Different Outcomes for Different Populations

Abundant Food Supply, Food Insecurity, and Obesity

Despite an abundant food supply, some regions and populations in the United States experience food insecurity, which ironically may contribute to obesity. Food insecurity, which in 2012 affected 15 percent of U.S. households (Coleman-Jensen et al., 2013), is categorized in this report as a social and economic effect (a more thorough exploration of the social and economic aspects of food insecurity can be found in Chapter 5). Food insecurity refers to those households that report lacking sufficient resources to acquire adequate food (Nord, 2013). Low-income, African American, and Latino households (Coleman-Jensen et al., 2013) are more likely to suffer food insecurity than are other population groups, and they are also at the highest risk for obesity and related illnesses such as type 2 diabetes, hypertension, and high cholesterol (Eisenmann et al., 2011; HER, 2010). Research also has shown that food insecurity affects children's mental health and well-being (Alaimo et al., 2001; Whitaker et al., 2006). Food insecurity can lead to hunger, which is associated with being sick more often and missing more school days and work days (Brown et al., 2007). Brown and colleagues estimated the total cost related to health consequences of hunger and food insecurity to be $67 billion per year in 2005 dollars. The authors considered the estimate to be conservative because indirect costs (i.e., non-medical costs incurred as a result of an illness, such as missed days of work) could not be included for all health outcomes. Thus, the true cost of hunger and food insecurity is likely much greater than reported.

Being food insecure may lead to weight gain because the most accessible food options for low-income households are typically not nutrient-rich but rather energy-dense foods (HER, 2010; Shier et al., 2012), and because food insecurity may increase an individual's need to depend on less nutritious foods that contain more calories but less nutritional value (Seligman and Schillinger, 2010). Bouts of both under- and overconsumption may lead to physiologic adaptation of increased body fat in response to episodic food shortages (CDC, 2003).

Residents of neighborhoods with higher concentrations of poverty and disadvantage often face multiple barriers to accessing healthy and affordable food (Lopez, 2007; Ver Ploeg et al., 2009). Moreover, households with limited resources tend to consume fewer healthful foods (e.g., fruits and vegetables) (Ludwig and Pollack, 2009) (see also Chapter 5). Higher socioeconomic status (SES) adults are more likely to come from households with better nutrition, fewer health risk behaviors, safer neighborhoods, and more economic resources (Crimmins et al., 2004). Therefore, consideration of the health effects of the food supply should consider the role of SES on morbidity and mortality (Marmot et al., 1991).

Different Nutritional Requirements for Different Populations: Folate

Folate is a B vitamin that is naturally present in many vegetables, nuts, beans, and fruits (Suitor and Bailey, 2000). Individuals require folate to make DNA and therefore produce and maintain new cells, particularly in tissues and cells that divide rapidly, such as blood cells (Beaudin and Stover, 2009). Folate nutrition is especially important for women of reproductive age. Clinical trials have established that folic acid intake before conception and throughout the first trimester can prevent up to 70 percent of neural tube defects, a common class of birth defects that include spina bifida and anencephaly (Crider et al., 2011).

Evidence suggests that the actual requirement for folate may vary among individuals by race and genotype. Individuals with a common polymorphism in the methylenetetrahydrofolate reductase gene (MTHFR 677 C→T) metabolize folate differently than those without it. They tend to exhibit lower red blood cell folate concentrations (Bagley and Selhub, 1998), and they are more susceptible to low folate status and deficiency. This genetic variant is nearly absent in individuals of African descent, but it does not protect against folate deficiency when folate dietary intake is insufficient. The gene variant is highly prevalent in Hispanic populations (Esfahani et al., 2003). Studies indicate that the current RDA is inadequate for Mexican American men with the MTHFR 677 TT genotype (Solis et al., 2008). Although uncommon in the general population, other population groups may be at risk for folate deficiency: persons with celiac disease, which decreases nutrient absorption; alcoholics; non-Hispanic blacks; and Mexican American adolescents (IOM, 2000; Kant and Graubard, 2012). Yet, an additional complexity is that although some groups in the population are achieving a benefit from fortification, it has been proposed, but not demonstrated, that others may accrue increased cancer risk (Mason, 2011). Although currently there is no known harm (including increased cancer risk) associated with current folic acid fortification levels, this remains an active area of research.

Interactions with Environmental, Social, or Economic Effects

Increase in Productivity Versus Exposure to Antibiotic Resistance Through Food and Environment

Health effects of the food system are the result of direct exposures to food through consumption; through exposure to other environmental media such as air, water, soil, or livestock; or through a combination of all of them during a lifetime. Attributing risk to a particular cause creates methodological challenges, but it is necessary when attempting to assess the effects of the food system and identifying solutions. Since the early 1930s, the use of antibiotics has intensified in human and veterinarian clinical settings, in agricultural production, and in household products, with many benefits to patients, producers, and consumers (Allen et al., 2013; Stanton, 2013). In animal production, antibiotics are used in disease treatment, disease prevention, and growth promotion (Allen et al., 2013). Although this implies the economic benefits, the widespread use of antibiotics also has led to the emergence of drug-resistant infections, a substantial cost to human and animal health. Many questions still remain about the causes of antibiotic resistance in agricultural applications and in the clinic, in part due to the lack of appropriate methods to study the complexities of resistance transference. Curtailing the spread of resistance in the absence of clear evidence or guidance from the scientific community can be difficult, while the incidence of antibiotic resistance has been increasing (Interagency Task Force on Antimicrobial Resistance, 2012), threatening human health and impacting animal agriculture. In 2013, the Food and Drug Administration (FDA) began implementing a voluntary plan with industry to phase out the use of certain antibiotics in food production (FDA, 2013). Antibiotic resistance is presented in Chapter 7 as an illustration of the application of the committee's framework.

Use of Pesticides to Increase Productivity Versus Potential Health Effects

The use of pesticides in agriculture, along with other technological improvements, has led to great achievements in agricultural productivity (Pretty, 2008). In 2010, it was estimated that 6,873,000 lbs of atrazine (the second most frequent herbicide used, after glysophate) was used in conventional corn in Iowa (NASS, 2011). Pesticides are of concern because they may cause both acute and long-term health and environmental effects. The use of pesticides serves as an example of a contentious trade-off because the benefits are easily identified and quantified, but the potential costs are elusive due to lack of methodologies to measure long-term effects of exposure to low levels of chemicals by consumers (however, in the case of exposure by farmers, there are documented effects; see Chapter 5). Our knowledge about the behavior of pesticides, both their life cycle in the environment and in human metabolism after exposure, is still evolving. Emerging questions today concern the extent to which the exposure to chemicals during fetal and childhood development contributes to health problems later in life, such as obesity, or the potential long-term endocrine-disrupting effects of atrazine (Vandenberg et al., 2012).

The use of pesticides in food crops is regulated by the U.S. Environmental Protection Agency (EPA), which uses risk assessment as a tool to help make decisions. Due to ethical considerations, the identification of human health consequences relies mainly on animal testing[4] and on human epide-

[4] (1) Animal testing includes acute testing (short-term exposure of a single exposure) for outcomes such as eye irritation, skin irritation, skin sensitization, and neurotoxicity; (2) subchronic testing (intermediate exposure; repeated exposure over a longer period of time) for outcomes such as neurotoxicity; and (3) chronic toxicity testing (long-term exposure; repeated exposure lasting for most of the test animal's life) for outcomes such as carcinogenicity (cancer). Developmental and reproductive functions,

miologic studies. The limitations of these experimental approaches add scientific uncertainties to the results and controversies related to limits needed to ensure safety of pesticides. The U.S. decision to approve use of atrazine is based on EPA's position that, based on current data, atrazine is not likely to cause cancer in humans. However, uncertainties in the data are recognized. The U.S. limits of atrazine levels in drinking water and foods are based on the reproductive effects of atrazine (EPA, 2013). Because of new research showing endocrine-disruptive activity at much lower levels of atrazine, the current limits are highly debated (Cragin et al., 2011; Hayes, 2004; Hayes et al., 2002; NRDC, 2010; Rohr and McCoy, 2010; Vandenberg et al., 2012). The monitoring frequency of water also is being challenged as there are times when atrazine concentrations have sometimes increased above the legal limits in some communities (EPA, 2013). The effects of atrazine on human health and the environment were due to be reviewed again in 2013 by EPA as part of the reregistration process. No updates were available at the time of this report's publication.

METHODOLOGIES TO MEASURE HEALTH OUTCOMES

Despite research gaps, uncertainties, or limitations in measurement and data collection, government policies are based on the best available scientific evidence, although other factors are considered, including feasibility, cost, impact on stakeholders, and legal considerations. Thus, the U.S. government, companies, and other stakeholders collect economic, social, demographic, lifestyle, as well as food, nutrition, and health data based on strategic plans and priorities. The types of data linking food systems to human health include indexes of food exposure (i.e., dietary intake), indicators of nutritional status, physiological functional indicators, and prevalence of disease. The two most common methods to quantify dietary intake of foods include the 24-hour dietary recall and the food frequency questionnaire (Tooze et al., 2012). The use and limitations of these methods, including measurement error, in health policy was recently reviewed (Hébert et al., 2014). Nutritional status indicators are typically direct or surrogate blood measurements that indicate whole-body tissue levels of a particular nutrient and require analytical methodologies for their assessment (Rohner et al., 2014). Physiological functional indicators of food or nutrient intake can include blood biomarkers of metabolic pathways or other functional indicators, including blood pressure, growth, cognitive function, and physical acuity and endurance (Rohner et al., 2014).

---

mutagenicity, and hormone disruption also are tested (http://www.epa.gov/pesticides/factsheets/riskassess.htm [accessed January 17, 2015]).

The most relevant health and nutrition survey is NHANES. Conducted annually from 1999 by the National Center for Health Statistics, NHANES covers a nationally representative sample of about 5,000 persons each year. NHANES includes an interview covering demographic, socioeconomic, dietary, and health-related questions and a physical examination that includes measurements of anthropometrics and key biomarkers of nutritional status (CDC/NCHS, 2014b). Among many other purposes, the data are used to assess the nutritional status of the U.S. population and to determine the prevalence of major diseases and their associated risk factors, including nutritional status. These data are available to the research community and are also used by the National Institutes of Health, FDA, and CDC to inform the implementation and evaluation of nutrition policies and initiatives.

Well-established methodologies to investigate foodborne illness have been developed (e.g., International Association for Food Protection, 2011) and are used to better understand the burden of foodborne disease in the United States. Previous publications provide a comprehensive discussion of datasets, metrics, and methodologies used in this area (e.g., IOM and NRC, 2003, 2010). As described earlier in this chapter, important surveillance methods used for foodborne illness are the passive surveillance NORS[5] and the active surveillance system FoodNet[6] (CDC, 2014a). NORS is used by state and local health departments to investigate foodborne illness on the local level. NORS summaries provide data on the number of illnesses, hospitalizations, and deaths attributed to unknown, suspected, and confirmed etiological agents (including bacteria, viruses, parasites, and chemicals) in food products. They also include information on settings where food was eaten, attribution to specific foods, factors contributing to contamination of the food, and settings where the food was prepared. FoodNet (CDC, 2014a) is an active surveillance system used by CDC to monitor illness, from the most common to the most severe foodborne causes of diarrheal disease and viral disease, respectively. In terms of chemical safety, no routine surveillance is conducted of exposures to chemicals through food or

[5] NORS is the primary source of information on agents involved in foodborne outbreaks. Annual summaries based on NORS data are published periodically, including the latest summarizing information for 2009-2010 (http://www.cdc.gov/foodsafety/fdoss/data/annual-summaries/index.html [accessed January 17, 2015]); http://www.cdc.gov/nors [accessed January 17, 2015]).

[6] FoodNet, launched in 1996, is a collaborative effort with 10 state health departments (Connecticut, Georgia, Maryland, Minnesota, New Mexico, Oregon, Tennessee, and certain counties in California, Colorado, and New York), FDA, and USDA's Food Safety and Inspection Service. The information collected is used to estimate the burden of illness caused by the bacteria *Campylobacter, Listeria, Salmonella,* Shiga toxin-producing *E. coli, Shigella, Vibrio,* and *Yersinia,* and the parasites *Cryptosporidium* and *Cyclospora.*

other environmental routes related to food production, although NHANES includes testing for some chemical contaminants that could be associated with food consumption. The Adverse Event Reporting System at FDA monitors post-marketing surveillance adverse events for FDA-regulated foods. FDA's Total Diet Study monitors levels of various contaminants at the retail level as an estimate of exposures to chemicals in foods. However, the sampling level is low (from about 280 foods).

These surveillance systems also are important because they are being used in health impact assessments (HIAs) of decisions affecting the food system. HIAs use a systematic approach to inform decision makers of the potential positive and negative health effects of policy proposals. Recommendations from HIAs aim to optimize beneficial health effects and minimize negative ones (NRC, 2011). HIAs have been used to identify the broad health effects of proposed changes to the Supplemental Nutrition Assistance Program, state-level legislation for farm-to-school and school garden programs, and USDA's proposed standards for snack and á la carte foods and beverages sold in schools (HIP, 2014). These HIAs have helped illuminate how each proposal could be modified in advance to better support optimal health.

Tables B-1 through B-4 in Appendix B include examples of data collected on a routine basis that relate to food safety, food and nutrient consumption, and health outcomes. The tables also include health metrics and analytical methodologies that are often used to answer questions regarding the health status of individuals and populations, including outcomes, contributing factors, and confounders, intended to identify potential interventions to address public health problems.

Challenges in Establishing Associations Between the Food System and Health Outcomes

Decision making in nutrition with respect to nutrition interventions (e.g., nutrient intake requirements) increasingly relies on systematic reviews of the available evidence using approaches similar to those used to evaluate medical diagnoses and treatments (Balk et al., 2007; Blumberg et al., 2010). The evidence-based approach is used to evaluate the nature and strength of scientific evidence obtained from human studies relative to a hierarchy of scientific evidence that best supports causality. Data derived from double-blinded, placebo-controlled, randomized controlled trials serve as the gold standard, followed by cohort studies, case-control studies, case series, case reports, and expert opinions. Other types of supporting information can also be considered, including ecological data and data from animal studies and in vitro systems. This approach was most recently applied in establishing the DRIs for vitamin D and calcium (IOM, 2010).

The process of systematic review involves a thorough examination and grading of published data within an analytic framework that permits relevant and answerable questions to be posited. The standards for this process continue to evolve, including those established by the Cochrane Collaboration (2014), the IOM (2011), and USDA's Nutrition Evidence Library. Central to these processes is a literature review that identifies relevant studies in a manner that is transparent and reproducible, comprehensive and unbiased, and takes into consideration the participants involved in the study, the nature of the intervention, the comparison groups, and the outcomes of interest. The strength of evidence is then evaluated relative to the consistency of findings, scientific quality, and absence of confounding factors. Similarly, limitations are evaluated, including inadequate design and/or controls, measurement error, insufficient or irrelevant data collection, and bias, including inclusion and exclusion criteria.

This general process for systematic reviews has been modified to incorporate the unique characteristics of nutrition research. Because no single standard exists to evaluate nutrition evidence, various groups have developed their own criteria and published reports. These groups include the Agency for Healthcare Research and Quality, the Academy of Nutrition and Dietetics, and the Dietary Guidelines for Americans Committee (DGAC). As an example, Table 3-2 shows the grading chart used by the 2010 DGAC to evaluate the strength of the body of evidence supporting the committee's conclusion statements. The criteria in the chart are adapted from the American Dietetic Association Evidence Analysis Library (NEL, 2014b). The process can be iterative depending on the available data and the need to refine or reframe the questions posited. The available evidence can be combined (e.g., a meta-analysis) and extrapolated, and uncertainties can be identified and used to inform policy making.

The application of the evidence-based approach to nutrition, especially in the context of food and food systems, presents unique challenges. For example, exposures to food and nutrients are chronic and required for life, thereby limiting the opportunity for true placebo treatments and therefore not practically or ethically amenable to randomized controlled trials (Maki et al., 2014). Other challenges include the long duration between an exposure and a chronic disease onset and the complex and variable composition of foods where multiple nutrient components can often affect the outcome of interest. As a result, many dietary recommendations are supported by the totality of evidence, with the majority of evidence being derived from observational data. Maki et al. (2014) describe limitations often inherent to observational data, including imprecise exposure quantification, collinearity among dietary exposures, displacement/substitution effects, healthy/unhealthy consumer bias, residual confounding, and effect modification.

As discussed above, the problem of rising obesity rates presents its own challenges due to its complex etiology. In contrast to other diseases that have declined as a result of 20th-century medical advances, the level of obesity in the United States has increased over the past several decades, perhaps due to its relationship with broad lifestyle and social and economic changes that have occurred simultaneously. In a review paper, Hammond (2009) found that obesity is a challenging problem to study due to several attributes: (1) the great breadth in levels of scale involved (e.g., genes, neurobiology, psychology, family structure and influences, social context and social norms, environment, markets, and public policy); (2) the substantial diversity of relevant actors; and (3) the multiplicity of mechanisms implicated. He proposed that these make the obesity problem a "complex adaptive system" and therefore, it can be studied using modeling techniques similar to those used by the field of complexity science (see also Chapter 6).

Challenges in Linking Foodborne Illness with Food

Although as mentioned above, methodologies to investigate foodborne illness are well established, identifying the specific agent responsible for foodborne illness is complicated (e.g., etiological agents also may come from nonfood sources, such as live animals, and the time between consumption of a contaminated food and the expression of symptoms can vary from minutes to weeks). Previous publications have commented extensively on the challenges of current datasets and attribution methods (e.g., IOM and NRC, 2003, 2010). For example, although the passive surveillance NORS is standardized, major limitations are the significant underreporting of foodborne disease, frequent lack of identification of causative agent, and exclusion of sporadic cases of illness (one individual becoming ill). To provide better national estimates of the burden of foodborne illness, CDC uses the active surveillance system FoodNet. Data from FoodNet provide the basic metrics used to monitor foodborne illness trends, to estimate the burden of disease, and to establish public health goals (e.g., in Healthy People 2020). Although data are representative of the population, a disadvantage of this surveillance system is that substantial percentages of illnesses, hospitalizations, and deaths are attributed to unspecified agents and they monitor only a fraction of the potential agents. CaliciNet is a national norovirus outbreak surveillance system used by CDC to link common sources of norovirus outbreaks. Because norovirus is easily transmitted person to person, many illnesses may not be foodborne.

PulseNet uses microbiological subtyping (e.g., DNA fingerprinting) of stool culture isolates in combination with epidemiological investigations and mathematical modeling to link sporadic cases or a cluster of cases to identify multistate outbreaks. A network of public health laboratories in the United States uses standardized methods to track isolates; matching strains

TABLE 3-2 Conclusion Grading Chart Used to Evaluate the Strength of the Body of Evidence Supporting Conclusion Statements by the Dietary Guidelines for Americans Committee

Elements	Strong	Moderate	Limited	Expert Opinion Only	Grade Not Assignable
Quality • Scientific rigor and validity • Study design and execution	Studies of strong design Free from design flaws, bias, and execution problems	Studies of strong design with minor methodological concerns OR only studies of weaker study design for question	Studies of weak design for answering the question OR inconclusive findings due to design flaws, bias, or execution problems	No studies available Conclusion based on usual practice, expert consensus, clinical experience, opinion, or extrapolation from basic research	No evidence that pertains to question being addressed
Consistency • Consistency of findings across studies	Findings generally consistent in direction and size of effect or degree of association, and statistical significance with very minor exceptions	Inconsistency among results of studies with strong design, OR consistency with minor exceptions across studies of weaker design	Unexplained inconsistency among results from different studies, OR single study unconfirmed by other studies	Conclusion supported solely by statements of informed nutrition or medical commentators	Not applicable
Quantity • Number of studies • Number of study participants	One large study with a diverse population or several good-quality studies Large number of subjects studied Studies with negative results have sufficiently large	Several studies by independent investigators Doubts about adequacy of sample size to avoid Type I and Type II error	Limited number of studies Low number of subjects studied and/or inadequate sample size within studies	Unsubstantiated by published research studies	Relevant studies have not been done

	sample size for adequate statistical power				
Impact • Importance of studied outcomes • Magnitude of effect	Studied outcome relates directly to the question Size of effect is clinically meaningful Significant (statistical) difference is large	Some doubt about the statistical or clinical significance of the effect	Studied outcome is an intermediate outcome or surrogate for the true outcome of interest OR size of effect is small or lacks statistical and/or clinical significance	Objective data unavailable	Indicates area for future research
Generalizability • Generalizability to population of interest	Studied population, intervention, and outcomes are free from serious doubts about generalizability	Minor doubts about generalizability	Serious doubts about generalizability due to narrow or different study population, intervention, or outcomes studied	Generalizability limited to scope of experience	Not applicable

SOURCE: USDA and HHS, 2010b.

are investigated further in an attempt to identify common sources. This methodology relies on culture isolates to generate the DNA fingerprint. As the health care system transitions to non-culture diagnostic methods, new "fingerprinting" techniques that do not depend on bacterial cultures will need to be developed. Risk assessment, the scientific element of a risk analysis framework, is an important methodology used to identify and attribute risk to foods and to food chemical and microbiological agents. Risk assessment is used by government agencies to guide the management of chemical and microbiological contaminants. Previous National Academy of Sciences reports provide a comprehensive description of the risk analysis framework (e.g., NRC, 2009). Formal risk assessment frameworks have evolved for both chemical and microbiological risks (see Table B-2). In-depth microbial risk assessments consider complexities associated with biological systems, such as variation in individual susceptibility, nonuniformity in the distribution of contamination, the ability of microbes to grow in food, and the potential for person-to-person spread for certain biological agents. Thus, microbial risk assessments can be resource intensive, presenting data gaps and uncertainties that must be articulated.

Chemical risk assessments also are resource intensive and traditionally use animal bioassays with extrapolation to humans. Due to the increasing number of chemicals to be tested, lower detection limits, and an urge to reduce animal testing, the merits of alternative approaches to prioritize and evaluate chemical safety are under discussion. For example, the use of risk assessment methodologies that could partly substitute in vitro testing for animal testing are evolving (e.g., computational and emerging in vitro methods such as in silico and high-throughput screening). This area of research faces numerous challenges, but it may decrease cost in the future (Bialk et al., 2013; Firestone et al., 2010; Kavlock and Dix, 2010; Krewski et al., 2010). In some cases, and when data are incomplete, the Threshold of Toxicological Concern approaches have been recommended when assessing the safety of chemicals in foods. Although less data intensive, applicability is limited to substances that meet specific criteria (Bialk et al., 2013; IFT, 2009).

SUMMARY

The U.S. food system supplies a wide variety of foods and sufficient calories at a low cost to meet the needs of the U.S. population. The major diet-related diseases and conditions of the current era in the United States are not related to nutrient inadequacy but mostly to inappropriate dietary patterns and overconsumption. Diet is a primary risk factor in the etiology of several leading causes of mortality and morbidity. However, despite the presence of this plentiful food supply, some segments of the U.S. population face issues of health, access, and food security.

Measuring those effects and identifying the mechanisms and pathways are challenging tasks presenting complexities at various levels. For example, government agencies have established dietary guidelines for healthy diets, but market forces (e.g., extensive advertising of unhealthy foods along with poor advertising of healthy foods) and consumer preferences do not always support recommended dietary practices. The etiology of many human health outcomes is multifactorial, with dietary practices being one of multiple interacting risk factors. Health outcomes related to the food system may vary among individuals and populations depending on their socioeconomic status or their individual physiology and genetics.

The diversity of the foods in the system provides resilience in maintaining a nutritious food supply without dependency on any single food or commodity. However, an appropriate variety of food is not equally accessible to all individuals in the population, which contributes to heterogeneity in health effects. For some foods and dietary patterns, there are both health benefits and risks associated with their consumption, illustrating the trade-offs that are inherent in the food system. Also, maximizing positive health effects may come at the expense of environmental, social, and economic effects.

Understanding the health effects of the food system and its trade-offs and interactions with the environment and social and economic domains is key to informing food system policies and interventions. Chapter 7 provides an analytical framework where all of these domains are considered.

REFERENCES

ADA (American Diabetes Association). 2013. Economic costs of diabetes in the U.S. in 2012. *Diabetes Care* 36(4):1033-1046.

Alaimo, K., C. M. Olson, and E. A. Frongillo, Jr. 2001. Food insufficiency and American school-aged children's cognitive, academic, and psychosocial development. *Pediatrics* 108(1):44-53.

Allen, H. K., U. Y. Levine, T. Looft, M. Bandrick, and T. A. Casey. 2013. Treatment, promotion, commotion: Antibiotic alternatives in food-producing animals. *Trends in Microbiology* 21(3):114-119.

Archer, E., R. P. Shook, D. M. Thomas, T. S. Church, P. T. Katzmarzyk, J. R. Hebert, K. L. McIver, G. A. Hand, C. J. Lavie, and S. N. Blair. 2013. 45-year trends in women's use of time and household management energy expenditure. *PLoS ONE* 8(2):e56620.

Assaf, R. R. 2014. Overview of local, state, and national government legislation restricting trans fats. *Clinical Therapeutics* 36(3):328-332.

Bader, M. D., M. Purciel, P. Yousefzadeh, and K. M. Neckerman. 2010. Disparities in neighborhood food environments: Implications of measurement strategies. *Economic Geography* 86(4):409-430.

Bagley, P. J., and J. Selhub. 1998. A common mutation in the methylenetetrahydrofolate reductase gene is associated with an accumulation of formylated tetrahydrofolates in red blood cells. *Proceedings of the National Academy of Sciences of the United States of America* 95(22):13217-13220.

Balk, E. M., T. A. Horsley, S. J. Newberry, A. H. Lichtenstein, E. A. Yetley, H. M. Schachter, D. Moher, C. H. MacLean, and J. Lau. 2007. A collaborative effort to apply the evidence-based review process to the field of nutrition: Challenges, benefits, and lessons learned. *American Journal of Clinical Nutrition* 85(6):1448-1456.

Beaudin, A. E., and P. J. Stover. 2009. Insights into metabolic mechanisms underlying folate-responsive neural tube defects: A minireview. *Birth Defects Research. Part A, Clinical and Molecular Teratology* 85(4):274-284.

Bialk, H., C. Llewellyn, A. Kretser, R. Canady, R. Lane, and J. Barach. 2013. Insights and perspectives on emerging inputs to weight of evidence determinations for food safety: Workshop proceedings. *International Journal of Toxicology* 32(6):405-414.

Blumberg, J., R. P. Heaney, M. Huncharek, T. Scholl, M. Stampfer, R. Vieth, C. M. Weaver, and S. H. Zeisel. 2010. Evidence-based criteria in the nutritional context. *Nutrition Reviews* 68(8):478-484.

Brown, J. L., D. Shepard, T. Martin, and J. Orwat. 2007. *The economic costs of domestic hunger.* Gaithersburg, MD: Sodexo Foundation.

CDC (Centers for Disease Control and Prevention). 2003. Self-reported concern about food security associated with obesity—Washington, 1995-1999. *Morbidity and Mortality Weekly Report* 52(35):840-842.

CDC. 2012. *Second national report on biochemical indicators of diet and nutrition in the U.S. population.* http://www.cdc.gov/nutritionreport/pdf/Nutrition_Book_complete508_final.pdf (accessed November 24, 2014).

CDC. 2013a. Health disparities and inequalities report—United States, 2013. *MMWR Supplement* 62(3):1-87.

CDC. 2013b. *Leading causes of death.* http://www.cdc.gov/nchs/fastats/leading-causes-of-death.htm (accessed November 24, 2014).

CDC. 2013c. Surveillance for foodborne disease outbreaks—United States, 2009-2010. *Morbidity and Mortality Weekly Report* 62(3):41-47.

CDC. 2014a. *CDC estimates of foodborne illness in the United States.* http://www.cdc.gov/foodborneburden/trends-in-foodborne-illness.html (accessed November 24, 2014).

CDC. 2014b. Incidence and trends of infection with pathogens transmitted commonly through food–foodborne diseases active surveillance network, 10 U.S. sites, 2006-2013. *Morbidity and Mortality Weekly Report* 63(15):328-332.

CDC. 2014c. *Surveillance for foodborne disease outbreaks, United States 2012, annual report.* Atlanta, GA: CDC.

CDC/NCHS (National Center for Health Statistics). 2014a. *Health, United States, 2013. With special feature on prescription drugs.* Hyattsville, MD: NCHS.

CDC/NCHS. 2014b. *National Health and Nutrition Examination Survey.* http://www.cdc.gov/nchs/nhanes.htm (accessed November 24, 2014).

Chandon, P., and B. Wansink. 2012. Does food marketing need to make us fat? A review and solutions. *Nutrition Reviews* 70(10):571-593.

Church, T. S., D. M. Thomas, C. Tudor-Locke, P. T. Katzmarzyk, C. P. Earnest, R. Q. Rodarte, C. K. Martin, S. N. Blair, and C. Bouchard. 2011. Trends over 5 decades in U.S. occupation-related physical activity and their associations with obesity. *PLoS ONE* 6(5):e19657.

Cochrane Collaboration. 2014. *Cochrane reviews.* http://www.cochrane.org/cochrane-reviews (accessed November 24, 2014).

Coleman-Jensen, A., M. Nord, and A. Singh. 2013. *Household food security in the United States in 2012.* Economic Research Report No. (ERR-155). Washington, DC: U.S. Department of Agriculture, Economic Research Service.

Cragin, L. A., J. S. Kesner, A. M. Bachand, D. B. Barr, J. W. Meadows, E. F. Krieg, and J. S. Reif. 2011. Menstrual cycle characteristics and reproductive hormone levels in women exposed to atrazine in drinking water. *Environmental Research* 111(8):1293-1301.

Crider, K. S., L. B. Bailey, and R. J. Berry. 2011. Folic acid food fortification—its history, effect, concerns, and future directions. *Nutrients* 3:370-384.

Crimmins, E.M., M. D. Hayward, and T. E. Seeman. 2004. Race/ethnicity, socioeconomic status, and health. In *Critical perspectives on racial and ethnic differences in health in late life*, edited by N. B. Anderson, R. A. Bulatao, and B. Cohen. Washington, DC: The National Academies Press.

Dagenais, G. R., Q. Yi, J. F. Mann, J. Bosch, J. Pogue, and S. Yusuf. 2005. Prognostic impact of body weight and abdominal obesity in women and men with cardiovascular disease. *American Heart Journal* 149(1):54-60.

Damms-Machado, A., G. Weser, and S. C. Bischoff. 2012. Micronutrient deficiency in obese subjects undergoing low calorie diet. *Nutrition Journal* 11:34.

de Ruyter, J. C., M. R. Olthof, J. C. Seidell, and M. B. Katan. 2012. A trial of sugar-free or sugar-sweetened beverages and body weight in children. *New England Journal of Medicine* 367(15):1397-1406.

den Hoed, M., U. Ekelund, S. Brage, A. Grontved, J. H. Zhao, S. J. Sharp, K. K. Ong, N. J. Wareham, and R. J. Loos. 2010. Genetic susceptibility to obesity and related traits in childhood and adolescence: Influence of loci identified by genome-wide association studies. *Diabetes* 59(11):2980-2988.

Dina, C., D. Meyre, C. Samson, J. Tichet, M. Marre, B. Jouret, M. A. Charles, B. Balkau, and P. Froguel. 2007. Comment on "a common genetic variant is associated with adult and childhood obesity." *Science* 315(5809):187.

Donham, K. J., S. Wing, D. Osterberg, J. L. Flora, C. Hodne, K. M. Thu, and P. S. Thorne. 2007. Community health and socioeconomic issues surrounding concentrated animal feeding operations. *Environmental Health Perspectives* 115(2):317-320.

Ebbeling, C. B., H. A. Feldman, V. R. Chomitz, T. A. Antonelli, S. L. Gortmaker, S. K. Osganian, and D. S. Ludwig. 2012. A randomized trial of sugar-sweetened beverages and adolescent body weight. *New England Journal of Medicine* 367(15):1407-1416.

Eckel, R. H., J. M. Jakicic, J. D. Ard, J. M. de Jesus, N. Houston Miller, V. S. Hubbard, I. M. Lee, A. H. Lichtenstein, C. M. Loria, B. E. Millen, C. A. Nonas, F. M. Sacks, S. C. Smith, Jr., L. P. Svetkey, T. A. Wadden, and S. Z. Yanovski. 2014. 2013 AHA/ACC guideline on lifestyle management to reduce cardiovascular risk: A report of the American College of Cardiology/American Heart Association task force on practice guidelines. *Journal of the American College of Cardiology* 63(25 Pt B):2960-2984.

Eisenmann, J. C., C. Gundersen, B. J. Lohman, S. Garasky, and S. D. Stewart. 2011. Is food insecurity related to overweight and obesity in children and adolescents? A summary of studies, 1995-2009. *Obesity Reviews* 12(5):e73-e83.

EPA (U.S. Environmental Protection Agency). 2013. *Atrazine updates.* http://www.epa.gov/oppsrrd1/reregistration/atrazine/atrazine_update.htm (accessed November 24, 2014).

Esfahani, S. T., E. A. Cogger, and M. A. Caudill. 2003. Heterogeneity in the prevalence of methylenetetrahydrofolate reductase gene polymorphisms in women of different ethnic groups. *Journal of the American Dietetic Association* 103(2):200-207.

FDA (U.S. Food and Drug Administration). 2013. *Phasing out certain antibiotic use in farm animals.* http://www.fda.gov/forconsumers/consumerupdates/ucm378100.htm (accessed November 24, 2014).

Finkelstein, E. A., J. G. Trogdon, J. W. Cohen, and W. Dietz. 2009. Annual medical spending attributable to obesity: Payer- and service-specific estimates. *Health Affairs (Millwood)* 28(5):w822-w831.

Firestone, M., R. Kavlock, H. Zenick, and M. Kramer. 2010. The U.S. Environmental Protection Agency strategic plan for evaluating the toxicity of chemicals. *Journal of Toxicology and Environmental Health. Part B Critical Reviews* 13(2-4):139-162.

Flegal, K. M., M. D. Carroll, B. K. Kit, and C. L. Ogden. 2012. Prevalence of obesity and trends in the distribution of body mass index among US adults, 1999-2010. *Journal of the American Medical Association* 307(5):491-497.

Frayling, T. M., N. J. Timpson, M. N. Weedon, E. Zeggini, et al. 2007. A common variant in the *FTO* gene is associated with body mass index and predisposes to childhood and adult obesity. *Science* 316(5826):889-894.

Frederick, C. B., K. Snellman, and R. D. Putnam. 2014. Increasing socioeconomic disparities in adolescent obesity. *Proceedings of the National Academy of Sciences of the United States of America* 111(4):1338-1342.

Fryar, C. D., M. D. Carroll, and C. L. Ogden. 2012. *NCHS Health E-Stat: Prevalence of obesity among children and adolescents: United States, trends 1963-1965 through 2009-2010.* http://www.cdc.gov/nchs/data/hestat/obesity_child_09_10/obesity_child_09_10.htm (accessed November 24, 2014).

Fryar, C. D., M. D. Carroll, and C. L. Ogden. 2014. *NCHS E-Stat: Prevalence of overweight, obesity, and extreme obesity among adults: United States, 1960-1962 through 2011-2012.* http://www.cdc.gov/nchs/data/hestat/obesity_adult_11_12/obesity_adult_11_12.htm (accessed November 24, 2014).

Go, A. S., D. Mozaffarian, V. L. Roger, E. J. Benjamin, J. D. Berry, et al. 2014. Heart disease and stroke statistics—2014 update: A report from the American Heart Association. *Circulation* 129(3):E28-E292.

Hammond, R. A. 2009. Complex systems modeling for obesity research. *Preventing Chronic Disease* 6(3):A97.

Hawkes, C. 2009. Sales promotions and food consumption. *Nutrition Reviews* 67(6):333-342.

Hayes, T. B. 2004. There is no denying this: Defusing the confusion about atrazine. *BioScience* 54(12):1138-1149.

Hayes, T. B., A. Collins, M. Lee, M. Mendoza, N. Noriega, A. A. Stuart, and A. Vonk. 2002. Hermaphroditic, demasculinized frogs after exposure to the herbicide atrazine at low ecologically relevant doses. *Proceedings of the National Academy of Sciences of the United States of America* 99(8):5476-5480.

Hébert, J. R., T. G. Hurley, S. E. Steck, D. R. Miller, F. K. Tabung, K. E. Peterson, L. H. Kushi, and E. A. Frongillo. 2014. Considering the value of dietary assessment data in informing nutrition-related health policy. *Advances in Nutrition* 5(4):447-455.

HER (Healthy Eating Research). 2010. *Food insecurity and risk for obesity among children and families: Is there a relationship?* http://www.rwjf.org/content/dam/farm/reports/reports/2010/rwjf58903 (accessed November 24, 2014).

HIP (Health Impact Project). 2014. *The Health Impact Project.* http://www.healthimpactproject.org (accessed November 24, 2014).

Hoffmann, S., M. B. Batz, and J. G. Morris, Jr. 2012. Annual cost of illness and quality-adjusted life year losses in the United States due to 14 foodborne pathogens. *Journal of Food Protection* 75(7):1292-1302.

IFT (Institute of Food Technologists). 2009. Making decisions about the risks of chemicals in foods with limited scientific information. An IFT Expert Report funded by the IFT Foundation. *Comprehensive Reviews in Food Science and Food Safety* 8:269-303.

IHME (Institute for Health Metrics and Evaluation). 2013. *GBD 2010 heat map.* http://vizhub.healthdata.org/irank/heat.php (accessed June 14, 2014).

IHME. 2014. *Overweight and obesity patterns (BMI≥25) for both sexes adults (20+).* http://vizhub.healthdata.org/obesity (accessed June 16, 2014).

Interagency Task Force on Antimicrobial Resistance. 2012. *A public health action plan to combat antibiotic resistance.* http://www.cdc.gov/drugresistance/actionplan/aractionplan.pdf (accessed November 24, 2014).

International Association for Food Protection. 2011. *Procedures to investigate foodborne illness*, 6th ed. New York: Springer.

IOM (Institute of Medicine). 2000. *Dietary reference intakes for thiamin, riboflavin, niacin, vitamin B6, folate, vitamin B12, pantothenic acid, biotin, and choline.* Washington, DC: National Academy Press.

IOM. 2005. *Preventing childhood obesity. Health in the balance.* Washington, DC: The National Academies Press.

IOM. 2006a. *Food marketing to children and youth: Threat or opportunity?* Washington, DC: The National Academies Press.

IOM. 2006b. *Seafood choices: Balancing benefits and risks.* Washington, DC: The National Academies Press.

IOM. 2010. *Dietary reference intakes for calcium and vitamin D.* Washington, DC: The National Academies Press.

IOM. 2011. *Finding what works in health care: Standards for systematic reviews.* Washington, DC: The National Academies Press.

IOM. 2012. *Accelerating progress in obesity prevention: Solving the weight of the nation.* Washington, DC: The National Academies Press.

IOM. 2014. *Dietary reference intakes tables and application.* http://www.iom.edu/Activities/Nutrition/SummaryDRIs/DRI-Tables.aspx (accessed November 24, 2014).

IOM and NRC (National Research Council). 2003. *Scientific criteria to ensure safe food.* Washington, DC: The National Academies Press.

IOM and NRC. 2010. *Enhancing food safety. The role of the Food and Drug Administration.* Washington, DC: The National Academies Press.

ISU/UI Study Group (Environmental Health Sciences Research Center CAFO Air Quality Study Iowa State University/University of Iowa Study Group). 2002. *Iowa Concentrated Animal Feeding Operations Air Quality Study.* http://www.public-health.uiowa.edu/ehsrc/pubs/cafo-aqs.html (accessed November 24, 2014).

Jensen, M. D., D. H. Ryan, C. M. Apovian, J. D. Ard, A. G. Comuzzie, K. A. Donato, F. B. Hu, V. S. Hubbard, J. M. Jakicic, R. F. Kushner, C. M. Loria, B. E. Millen, C. A. Nonas, F. X. Pi-Sunyer, J. Stevens, V. J. Stevens, T. A. Wadden, B. M. Wolfe, and S. Z. Yanovski. 2014. *2013 AHA/ACC/TOS guideline for the management of overweight and obesity in adults: A report of the American College of Cardiology/American Heart Association Task Force on Practice Guidelines and The Obesity Society. Circulation* 129(25 Suppl 2):S102-S138.

Kant, A. K., and B. I. Graubard. 2012. Race–ethnic, family income, and education differentials in nutritional and lipid biomarkers in US children and adolescents: NHANES 2003-2006. *American Journal of Clinical Nutrition* 96(3):601-612.

Kavlock, R., and D. Dix. 2010. Computational toxicology as implemented by the US EPA: Providing high throughput decision support tools for screening and assessing chemical exposure, hazard and risk. *Journal of Toxicology and Environmental Health. Part B, Critical Reviews* 13(2-4):197-217.

Kennedy, E., and L. Meyers. 2005. Dietary reference intakes: Development and uses for assessment of micronutrient status of women—a global perspective. *American Journal of Clinical Nutrition* 81(5):1194S-1197S.

Krebs-Smith, S. M., and P. Kris-Etherton. 2007. How does MyPyramid compare to other population-based recommendations for controlling chronic disease? *Journal of the American Dietetic Association* 107(5):830-837.

Krewski, D., D. Acosta, Jr., M. Andersen, H. Anderson, J. C. Bailar III, K. Boekelheide, R. Brent, G. Charnley, V. G. Cheung, S. Green, Jr., K. T. Kelsey, N. I. Kerkvliet, A. A. Li, L. McCray, O. Meyer, R. D. Patterson, W. Pennie, R. A. Scala, G. M. Solomon, M. Stephens, J. Yager, and L. Zeise. 2010. Toxicity testing in the 21st century: A vision and a strategy. *Journal of Toxicology and Environmental Health, Part B, Critical Reviews* 13(2-4):51-138.

Langer, A. J., T. Ayers, J. Grass, M. Lynch, F. J. Angulo, and B. E. Mahon. 2012. Nonpasteurized dairy products, disease outbreaks, and state laws—United States, 1993-2006. *Emerging Infectious Diseases* 18(3):385-391.

Leibel, R. L. 2008. Energy in, energy out, and the effects of obesity-related genes. *New England Journal of Medicine* 359(24):2603-2604.

Lopez, R. P. 2007. Neighborhood risk factors for obesity. *Obesity (Silver Spring)* 15(8):2111-2119.

Ludwig, D. S., and H. A. Pollack. 2009. Obesity and the economy: From crisis to opportunity. *Journal of the American Medical Association* 301(5):533-535.

Macdiarmid, J. I., J. Kyle, G. W. Horgan, J. Loe, C. Fyfe, A. Johnstone, and G. McNeill. 2012. Sustainable diets for the future: Can we contribute to reducing greenhouse gas emissions by eating a healthy diet? *American Journal of Clinical Nutrition* 96(3):632-639.

Maki, K. C., J. L. Slavin, T. M. Rains, and P. M. Kris-Etherton. 2014. Limitations of observational evidence: Implications for evidence-based dietary recommendations. *Advances in Nutrition* 5(1):7-15.

Malik, V. S., A. Pan, W. C. Willett, and F. B. Hu. 2013. Sugar-sweetened beverages and weight gain in children and adults: A systematic review and meta-analysis. *American Journal of Clinical Nutrition* 98(4):1084-1102.

Malnick, S. D., and H. Knobler. 2006. The medical complications of obesity. *QJM* 99(9):565-579.

Mariner, W. K., and G. J. Annas. 2013. Limiting "sugary drinks" to reduce obesity—who decides? *New England Journal of Medicine* 368(19):1763-1765.

Marmot, M. G., G. D. Smith, S. Stansfeld, C. Patel, F. North, J. Head, I. White, E. Brunner, and A. Feeney. 1991. Health inequalities among British civil-servants—the Whitehall II study. *Lancet* 337(8754):1387-1393.

Mason, J. B. 2011. Unraveling the complex relationship between folate and cancer risk. *Biofactors* 37(4):253-260.

Moshfegh, A., J. Goldman, and L. Cleveland. 2005. *What we eat in America, NHANES 2001-2002: Usual nutrient intakes from food compared to dietary reference intakes.* http://www.ars.usda.gov/main/site_main.htm?modecode=80-40-05-30 (accessed November 24, 2014).

Moshfegh, A., J. Goldman, J. Ahuja, D. Rhodes, and R. LaComb. 2009. *What we eat in America, NHANES 2005-2006: Usual nutrient intakes from food and water compared to 1997 dietary reference intakes for vitamin D, calcium, phosphorus, and magnesium.* http://www.ars.usda.gov/main/site_main.htm?modecode=80-40-05-30 (accessed November 24, 2014).

NASS (National Agricultural Statistics Service). 2011. *2011 Iowa agricultural statistics: USDA National Agricultural Statistics Service, Iowa Field Office and Iowa Farm Bureau.* http://www.nass.usda.gov/Statistics_by_State/Iowa/Publications/Annual_Statistical_Bulletin/index.asp (accessed November 21, 2014).

NEL (Nutrition Evidence Library). 2014a. *Nutrition evidence library.* http://www.nel.gov (accessed November 24, 2014).

NEL. 2014b. *Conclusion grading chart (2010 DGAC).* http://www.nel.gov/topic.cfm?cat=3210 (accessed November 24, 2014).

Nestle, M., and M. Nesheim. 2012. *Why calories count: From science to politics*. Berkeley, CA: University of California Press.

Newton, A., M. Kendall, D. J. Vugia, O. L. Henao, and B. E. Mahon. 2012. Increasing rates of vibriosis in the United States, 1996-2010: Review of surveillance data from 2 systems. *Clinical Infectious Diseases* 54(Suppl 5):S391-S395.

Ng, M., T. Fleming, M. Robinson, B. Thomson, N. Graetz, C. Margono, E. C. Mullany, S. Biryukov, C. Abbafati, S. F. Abera, J. P. Abraham, N. M. Abu-Rmeileh, et al. 2014. Global, regional, and national prevalence of overweight and obesity in children and adults during 1980-2013: A systematic analysis for the Global Burden of Disease Study 2013. *Lancet* 384(9945):766-781.

Nord, M. 2013. Food insecurity in U.S. households rarely persists over many years. *Amber Waves*. Washington, DC: U.S. Department of Agriculture, Economic Research Service.

NRC (National Research Council). 2009. *Science and decisions: Advancing risk assessment*. Washington, DC: The National Academies Press.

NRC. 2011. *Improving health in the United States: The role of health impact assessment*. Washington, DC: The National Academies Press.

NRDC (Natural Resources Defense Council). 2010. *Still poisoning the well. Atrazine continues to contaminate surface water and drinking water in the United States*. http://www.nrdc.org/health/atrazine/files/atrazine10.pdf (accessed November 24, 2014).

Nwankwo, T., S. S. Yoon, V. Burt, and Q. Gu. 2013. Hypertension among adults in the United States: National Health and Nutrition Examination Survey, 2011-2012. *NCHS Data Brief* (133):1-8.

O'Connor, A. M., B. Auvermann, D. Bickett-Weddle, S. Kirkhorn, J. M. Sargeant, A. Ramirez, and S. G. Von Essen. 2010. The association between proximity to animal feeding operations and community health: A systematic review. *PLoS ONE* 5(3):e9530.

Ohlhorst, S. D., R. Russell, D. Bier, D. M. Klurfeld, Z. Li, J. R. Mein, J. Milner, A. C. Ross, P. Stover, and E. Konopka. 2013. Nutrition research to affect food and a healthy life span. *American Journal of Clinical Nutrition* 98(2):620-625.

Paulot, F., and D. J. Jacob. 2014. Hidden cost of U.S. agricultural exports: Particulate matter from ammonia emissions. *Environmental Science & Technology* 48(2):903-908.

Perez-Morales, E., M. Bacardi-Gascon, and A. Jimenez-Cruz. 2013. Sugar-sweetened beverage intake before 6 years of age and weight or BMI status among older children; systematic review of prospective studies. *Nutrición hospitalaria* 28(1):47-51.

Pingali, P. L. 2012. Green revolution: Impacts, limits, and the path ahead. *Proceedings of the National Academy of Sciences of the United States of America* 109(31):12302-12308.

Pope, C. A., M. Ezzati, and D. W. Dockery. 2009. Fine-particulate air pollution and life expectancy in the United States. *New England Journal of Medicine* 360(4):376-386.

Popkin, B. M. 2011. Agricultural policies, food and public health. *EMBO Reports* 12(1):11-18.

Pretty, J. 2008. Agricultural sustainability: Concepts, principles and evidence. *Philosophical Transactions of the Royal Society of London, Series B, Biological Sciences* 363(1491):447-465.

Price, J. H., J. Khubchandani, M. McKinney, and R. Braun. 2013. Racial/ethnic disparities in chronic diseases of youths and access to health care in the United States. *BioMed Research International* 2013:1-12.

Rohner, F., M. Zimmermann, P. Jooste, C. Pandav, K. Caldwell, R. Raghavan, and D. J. Raiten. 2014. Biomarkers of nutrition for development—iodine review. *Journal of Nutrition* 144(8):1322S-1342S.

Rohr, J. R., and K. A. McCoy. 2010. A qualitative meta-analysis reveals consistent effects of atrazine on freshwater fish and amphibians. *Environmental Health Perspectives* 118(1):20-32.

Rolls, B. J., E. L. Morris, and L. S. Roe. 2002. Portion size of food affects energy intake in normal-weight and overweight men and women. *American Journal of Clinical Nutrition* 76(6):1207-1213.

Rutkow, L., J. S. Vernick, J. G. Hodge, Jr., and S. P. Teret. 2008. Preemption and the obesity epidemic: State and local menu labeling laws and the Nutrition Labeling and Education Act. *Journal of Law, Medicine and Ethics* 36(4):772-789.

Scallan, E., R. M. Hoekstra, F. J. Angulo, R. V. Tauxe, M. A. Widdowson, S. L. Roy, J. L. Jones, and P. M. Griffin. 2011a. Foodborne illness acquired in the United States—major pathogens. *Emerging Infectious Diseases* 17(1):7-15.

Scallan, E., P. M. Griffin, F. J. Angulo, R. V. Tauxe, and R. M. Hoekstra. 2011b. Foodborne illness acquired in the United States—unspecified agents. *Emerging Infectious Diseases* 17(1):16-22.

Seligman, H. K., and D. Schillinger. 2010. Hunger and socioeconomic disparities in chronic disease. *New England Journal of Medicine* 363(1):6-9.

Shier, V., R. An, and R. Sturm. 2012. Is there a robust relationship between neighbourhood food environment and childhood obesity in the USA? *Public Health* 126(9):723-730.

Solis, C., K. Veenema, A. A. Ivanov, S. Tran, R. Li, W. Wang, D. J. Moriarty, C. V. Maletz, and M. A. Caudill. 2008. Folate intake at RDA levels is inadequate for Mexican American men with the methylenetetrahydrofolate reductase 677tt genotype. *Journal of Nutrition* 138(1):67-72.

Stanton, T. B. 2013. A call for antibiotic alternatives research. *Trends in Microbiology* 21(3):111-113.

Stover, P. J. 2006. Influence of human genetic variation on nutritional requirements. *American Journal of Clinical Nutrition* 83(2):436S-442S.

Stuckler, D., and M. Nestle. 2012. Big food, food systems, and global health. *PLoS Medicine* 9(6):e1001242.

Suitor, C. W., and L. B. Bailey. 2000. Dietary folate equivalents: Interpretation and application. *Journal of the American Dietetic Association* 100(1):88-94.

Todd, J. E., L. Mancino, and B.-H. Lin. 2010. *The impact of food away from home on adult diet quality*. Washington, DC: U.S. Department of Agriculture, Economic Research Service.

Tooze, J. A., S. M. Krebs-Smith, R. P. Troiano, and A. F. Subar. 2012. The accuracy of the Goldberg method for classifying misreporters of energy intake on a food frequency questionnaire and 24-h recalls: Comparison with doubly labeled water. *European Journal of Clinical Nutrition* 66(5):569-576.

Trumbo, P. R. 2008. Challenges with using chronic disease endpoints in setting dietary reference intakes. *Nutrition Reviews* 66(8):459-464.

Trumbo, P. R., S. I. Barr, S. P. Murphy, and A. A. Yates. 2013. Dietary reference intakes: Cases of appropriate and inappropriate uses. *Nutrition Reviews* 71(10):657-664.

USDA (U.S. Department of Agriculture). 2014. *A series of systematic reviews on the relationship between dietary patterns and health outcomes*. Alexandria, VA: USDA/Center for Nutrition Policy and Promotion. http://www.nel.gov/vault/2440/web/files/Nutrition%20Education%20Systematic%20Review%20Report%20-%20CHAP%201-5_FINAL.pdf (accessed November 24, 2014).

USDA and HHS (U.S. Department of Health and Human Services). 2010a. *Nutrition and your health: Dietary guidelines for Americans, 2010*, 7th ed. Washington, DC: USDA.

USDA and HHS. 2010b. *Report of the Dietary Guidelines Advisory Committee on the Dietary Guidelines for Americans, 2010, to the Secretary of Agriculture and the Secretary of Health and Human Services*. Washington, DC: USDA.

Vandenberg, L. N., T. Colborn, T. B. Hayes, J. J. Heindel, D. R. Jacobs, Jr., D. H. Lee, T. Shioda, A. M. Soto, F. S. vom Saal, W. V. Welshons, R. T. Zoeller, and J. P. Myers. 2012. Hormones and endocrine-disrupting chemicals: Low-dose effects and nonmonotonic dose responses. *Endocrine Reviews* 33(3):378-455.

Venegas-Caleron, M., O. Sayanova, and J. A. Napier. 2010. An alternative to fish oils: Metabolic engineering of oil-seed crops to produce omega-3 long chain polyunsaturated fatty acids. *Progress in Lipid Research* 49(2):108-119.

Ver Ploeg, M., V. Breneman, T. Farrigan, K. Hamrick, D. Hopkins, P. Kaufman, B-H. Lin, M. Nord, T.A. Smith, R. Williams, K. Kinnison, C. Olander, A. Singh, and E. Tuckermanty. 2009. *Access to affordable and nutritious food measuring and understanding food deserts and their consequences: Report to Congress.* Washington, DC: U.S. Department of Agriculture, Economic Research Service.

Wansink, B., and S. B. Park. 2001. At the movies: How external cues and perceived taste impact consumption volume. *Food Quality and Preference* 12(1):69-74.

Wansink, B., J. E. Painter, and J. North. 2005. Bottomless bowls: Why visual cues of portion size may influence intake. *Obesity Research* 13(1):93-100.

WCRF/AICR (World Cancer Research Fund/American Institute for Cancer Research). 2007. *Food, nutrition, physical activity, and the prevention of cancer: A global perspective.* Washington, DC: AICR.

Westerterp, K. R., and J. R. Speakman. 2008. Physical activity energy expenditure has not declined since the 1980s and matches energy expenditures of wild mammals. *International Journal of Obesity* 32(8):1256-1263.

Whitaker, R. C., S. M. Phillips, and S. M. Orzol. 2006. Food insecurity and the risks of depression and anxiety in mothers and behavior problems in their preschool-aged children. *Pediatrics* 118(3):e859-e868.

WHO (World Health Organization). 2013. *State of the science of endocrine disrupting chemicals—2012: An assessment of the state of the science of endocrine disruptors prepared by a group of experts for the United Nations Environment Programme (UNEP) and WHO.* Edited by A. Bergman, J. J. Heindel, S. Jobling, K. A. Kidd, and R. Thomas Zoeller. Geneva, Switzerland: WHO/United Nations Environment Programme.

Wilde, P., J. Llobrera, and N. Valpiani. 2012. Household food expenditures and obesity risk. *Current Obesity Reports* 1(3):123-133.

Young, L. R., and M. Nestle. 2007. Portion sizes and obesity: Responses of fast-food companies. *Journal of Public Health Policy* 28(2):238-248.

4

Environmental Effects of the U.S. Food System

The U.S. food system (described in Chapter 2) is widely recognized to have direct and indirect effects on the environment. The degree to which each sector of the food system affects the environment depends on a variety of natural and human-driven processes. For example, increased use of mineral fertilizers is responsible for much of the growth in productivity in U.S. agriculture over the past 50 years, but it also has led to negative impacts on the environment, such as greater greenhouse gas (GHG) emissions and deterioration of water quality. GHG emissions also can result from the burning of fossil fuels in the food manufacturing process and during food distribution.

The ongoing intensification of agricultural production[1] has had particularly notable effects on the environment. According to the 2012 Agricultural Census, 2.1 million farms and ranches operate in the United States, of which two-thirds sell less than $25,000 worth of livestock or crops. In contrast, large farms (about 80,000 of them) represent only 4 percent of the total farm population but are responsible for two-thirds of the agricultural production in the United States today (USDA, 2014b). Intensive agricultural production has become highly efficient, which reduces costs per unit of product (thus, likely reducing costs to consumers) and can alter environmental impacts per unit of product. For example, Capper et al. (2009) showed historic advances in dairy production, where 2007 cows produced

[1] There are a variety of definitions of agricultural intensification but they all refer to increasing agricultural inputs to improve productivity or yields of a fixed land area rather than expanding land under cultivation.

43 percent less methane and 56 percent less nitrous oxide per 1 billion kilograms of milk than did 1944 cows. Similar trends have been described for the beef sector (Capper, 2011), where the number of cattle was reduced by 40 percent over this time span, but the total amount of beef produced remained the same (USDA, 2014b). On the other hand, large concentrations of livestock (concentrated animal feeding operations,[2] or CAFOs) can lead to regional air and water quality issues if the animal waste is not properly managed. CAFOs can cause nuisance and health issues for neighboring communities—including dust, odors, flies, and gaseous emissions—and therefore often face public scrutiny. In addition, runoff from CAFOs can create food safety problems by contaminating water or downstream agriculture fields with pathogens. Increasingly, livestock CAFOs attempt to counteract these challenges by collecting manure from the animal housing and placing it into treatment facilities like composters or anaerobic digesters, which can convert waste to energy.

The impact of contaminated surface or groundwater from excessive nitrogen fertilizer applications, in both inorganic and organic forms, may affect a local community over a short period of time, or decades later, sometimes miles from the initial nutrient inputs. The impact within a community also may be disparate, as disadvantaged portions of the community may not have the resources to ensure a safe drinking water source. (Health effects related to environmental contaminants and their differential effects on the general population are discussed in Chapters 3 and 5, respectively.)

Although the U.S. food system's impacts on the environment are often undesirable, the current system can provide environmental benefits as well (see Figure 4-1 for examples). Benefits such as carbon sequestration, biodiversity conservation, aesthetically pleasing landscapes, and sustained food and fiber production can all be realized, particularly when an ecological approach is used by agricultural producers (Robertson and Swinton, 2005; Swinton et al., 2007; Zhang et al., 2007). An ecological approach requires actors to recognize not only how management choices affect the environment, both temporally and spatially but also how managing the system for multiple ecosystem services[3] can often result in significant mitigation of these impacts, acknowledging also that trade-offs are inevitable (Robertson and Swinton, 2005).

Agricultural producers are chiefly in business to produce food, fiber, and fuel products for sale, but most also place a high value on ecosys-

[2] CAFOs are agricultural enterprises where animals are raised in a confined, small land area and feed is brought to the animals. The Environmental Protection Agency has delineated three categories of CAFOs, ordered in terms of capacity: large, medium, and small. The relevant animal unit for each category varies depending on species and capacity.

[3] Ecosystem services are any positive benefit that wildlife or ecosystems provides to people. The benefits can be direct or indirect, small or large.

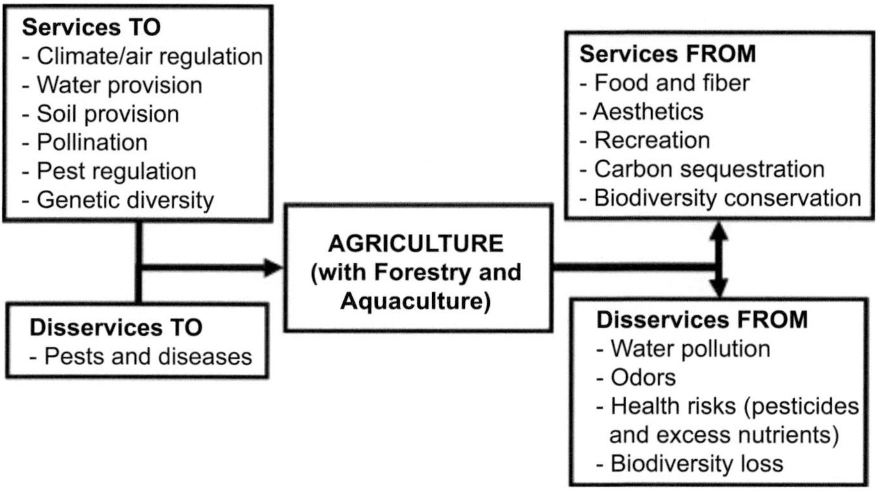

FIGURE 4-1 Examples of ecosystem services to and from agriculture.
SOURCE: Swinton et al., 2007. Reprinted with permission.

tem services from their farms, especially those that offer private benefits (e.g., enhanced soil fertility and organic matter). However, many producers believe ecosystem services that offer distant benefits (e.g., climate or water quality regulation) are costly to provide without financial incentives and technical resources (Ma et al., 2012; Smith and Sullivan, 2014). Understanding how actors in the food system make decisions is important when assessing the environmental impacts of the system.

Broadly, the U.S. food system's environmental effects can be grouped into three categories: (1) environmental contaminants/pollutants, (2) depletion and replenishment of natural resources, and (3) population and community disruption. In this chapter, each of these broad effects categories is described briefly, highlighting the major environmental features and mechanisms of each category. The chapter further discusses the dynamic nature of environmental effects, including the importance of understanding how human behavior influences direct and indirect, and positive and negative, impacts on the environment. The chapter concludes with a basic overview of the various approaches used to quantify the performance of a dynamic environmental system, including direct measurement, the use of indicators, and simulation modeling. A comprehensive list of environmental data sources, metrics, and models commonly employed to quantify environmental impacts is included in Tables B-1 through B-4 of Appendix B.

CATEGORIES OF POTENTIAL ENVIRONMENTAL EFFECTS AND ASSOCIATED MECHANISMS

Environmental Contaminants and Pollutants

The U.S. food system has seen a substantial increase in product output over the past 50 years. Although more food is produced than ever, the current system also leads to unintended environmental consequences depicted in the pollution life cycle shown in Figure 4-2. Contaminants are emitted into the environment, are transported and/or transformed, and eventually are deposited in a location where they may negatively affect human and ecosystem health. These negative effects on human and ecosystem health are most often dealt with through the implementation of regulations to reduce or eliminate emissions of the contaminant.

A considerable amount of effort by the scientific community has gone into determining the identity, fate, and transport paths of environmental contaminants associated with the various components of the U.S. food and agriculture system. These contaminants include nutrients (i.e., nitrogen and phosphorus), pesticides, pharmaceuticals, pathogens, gases and inhalants (i.e., ammonia, nitrogen oxide, methane, odors, and fine particulate matter, or PM), and soil sediment (including the chemicals and organisms it may contain). When a contaminant reaches pollutant levels, it leads to the

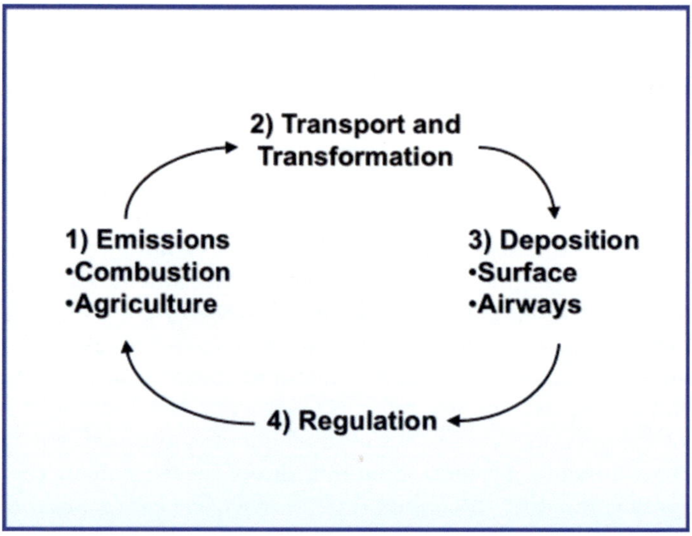

FIGURE 4-2 The pollution life cycle. Regulations at various levels (federal, state, and local) address negative impacts to human and ecosystem health.

degradation of water, soil, air, or habitat and to potential consequences on human health. For example, nutrient-laden runoff can lead to eutrophication[4] of downstream waters (EPA, 2011), excessive GHG emissions can contribute to global warming (EPA, 2013), and pesticides transported in runoff or in groundwater recharge can result in toxicity to humans, aquatic life, and wildlife (Gilliom et al., 2006). The extent to which these contaminants result in environmental degradation depends on a number of factors, including but not limited to contaminant concentration, timing of exposure, extent of biodegradation and bioaccumulation, and the frequency of exposure. The following discussion focuses on the major classes of contaminants (nutrients, pesticides, sediment, and pathogens) and the mechanisms leading to environmental contamination. An extensive discussion of nitrogen as a nutrient contaminant and pollutant in agricultural production can be found in Annex 4 of Chapter 7.

Agricultural activities in the United States contribute significantly to the release of numerous air quality and climate change-related emissions, especially those of ammonia (agriculture contributes to ~90 percent of total U.S. emissions), reduced sulfur (unquantified), $PM_{2.5}$[5] (~16 percent), PM_{10} (~18 percent), methane (~29 percent), and nitrous oxide (72 percent) (Aneja et al., 2009). Once these materials are released into the air, they can undergo various transformational steps (Aneja et al., 2001). For example, a large percentage of ammonia is deposited near its source. However, ammonia can readily transform into ammonium, which can be transported over greater distances from the source. As the most prevalent base found in the atmosphere, ammonia can also readily react with acidic nitrogen and sulfur species, forming fine particulate matter (i.e., $PM_{2.5}$). Carbon molecules also can transform from one form to another. For example, volatile organic compounds[6] (VOCs), which are produced during fermentation and decomposition of organic materials as well as during combustion of fossil fuels, contribute to ozone formation when combined with oxides of nitrogen (NOx) and sunlight (Shaw et al., 2007). Ozone can form smog, which constitutes one of the most pressing air quality issues in parts of the United States, such as California. Some VOCs also cause health effects such as eye, nose, and throat irritation (EPA, 2014).

Figure 4-3 shows an example of how primary (e.g., ammonia) and secondary (e.g., fine particulate matter, $PM_{2.5}$) air emissions are most often transported by wind and eventually undergo dry or wet deposition. These

---

[4] Eutrophicaton is excessive plant and algal growth due to the increased availability of one or more limiting growth factors needed for photosynthesis, such as sunlight, carbon dioxide, and nutrient fertilizers.

[5] $PM_{2.5}$ refers to particulate matter less than 2.5 μm in diameter.

[6] Volatile organic compounds are gases from certain solids or liquids that include a variety of chemicals, some of which may have short- and long-term adverse health effects.

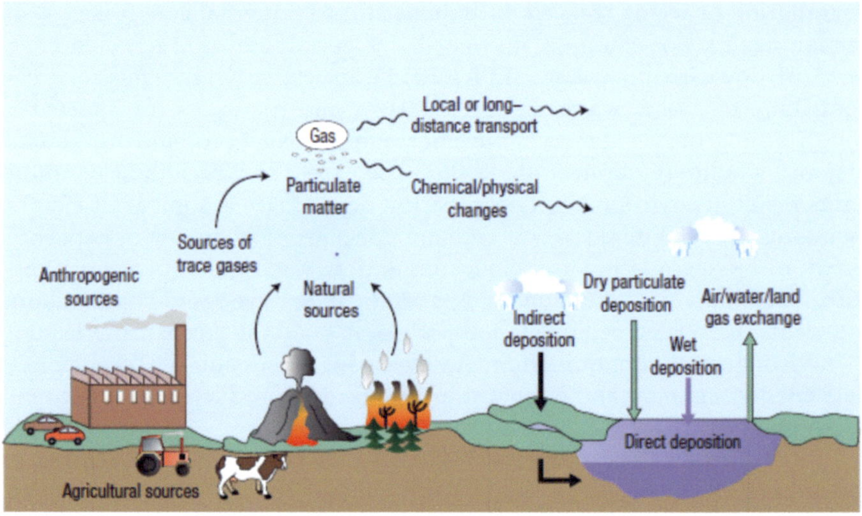

FIGURE 4-3 Atmospheric emissions, transport/transformation, and deposition.
SOURCE: Reprinted by permission from Macmillan Publishers Ltd.: Aneja, V. P., W. H. Schlesinger, and J. W. Erisman. 2008. Farming pollution. *Nature Geoscience* 1(7):409-411.

can affect both ecosystem (e.g., eutrophication, acidification) and human health (e.g., respiratory conditions).

Water pollution occurs when pollutants are leached through the soil and the unsaturated zone above the water table into the aquifer (groundwater), or when surface water quality is impaired due to runoff or drainage discharge from agricultural land. Major issues related to water quality in agricultural production focus on nitrogen, phosphorus, salinity, and pathogen occurrence. Nitrogen and phosphorus are the principal nutrient pollutants of major concern regarding water quality. Ammonia from manure or other nitrogen forms contained in chemical fertilizers undergoes nitrification in the soil leading to nitrate formation. Nitrate is readily taken up by crops, but if applications are beyond the need of the plant (i.e., agronomic rates), excess will leach into the groundwater (see also Chapter 7, Annex 4). Phosphorus, on the other hand, generally binds to soil particles, and most pollution to water bodies occurs due to soil erosion and direct runoff of soluble reactive phosphate from fields.

Pathogens

Even though the United States has one of the safest food supplies globally, millions of cases of human foodborne illnesses still occur (see Chapter 3). Animal agriculture is a considerable source of microorganisms, some of which are pathogens, including bacteria such as *Salmonella, Escherichia coli* O157:H7, and *Campylobacter*. Other pathogens of major importance are Norovirus, *Clostridia*, and *Staphylococcus*. Concentrated animal feeding operations, grazing lands, and lands receiving animal waste are all potential sources of pathogens to waterways and agricultural products. Pathogen contamination of manure can lead to foodborne diseases in people when waste is applied as fertilizers to crops and the produce is not washed appropriately before consumption. For example, a large *E. coli* O157:H7 outbreak in 2006 was associated with contaminated spinach. Similarly, manure has the potential to contaminate meat at the packing plant, which can potentially lead to foodborne illnesses in people, particularly if meat is undercooked.

Pesticides

The advent of synthetic pesticides, much like the rise of synthetic fertilizer use, led to significant increases in crop yields through the protection of crops from destructive pests. Pesticides are predominately used to protect crops from yield reductions resulting from insect damage and competition from weeds. The annual amount of pesticide active ingredients used by the agricultural sector from 1988 to 2007 (shown in Figure 4-4) has remained relatively unchanged except for minor increases and decreases in the specific use of certain pesticide types.

Although agricultural pesticide use has allowed for increased production of food and fiber at a lower cost, widespread use of pesticides in a variety of crops increases the likelihood of negative impacts on the environment.

Pesticides and associated breakdown products are readily mobilized through air, water, and sediment pathways, resulting in the potential exposure of non-target organisms, including humans, to acute and/or chronic toxicity conditions. Depending on a pesticide's properties, the environmental conditions during and after application, and the management practices used by a farmer, a pesticide or its breakdown products can be: carried in drift during application, in dust created by wind or tillage activities, in surface runoff during irrigation or rainfall, or in sediment carried by runoff; leached through the soil into groundwater; or volatized into the air and deposited onto surfaces near or a considerable distance from the application site. A 2007 U.S. Geological Survey (USGS) assessment reported

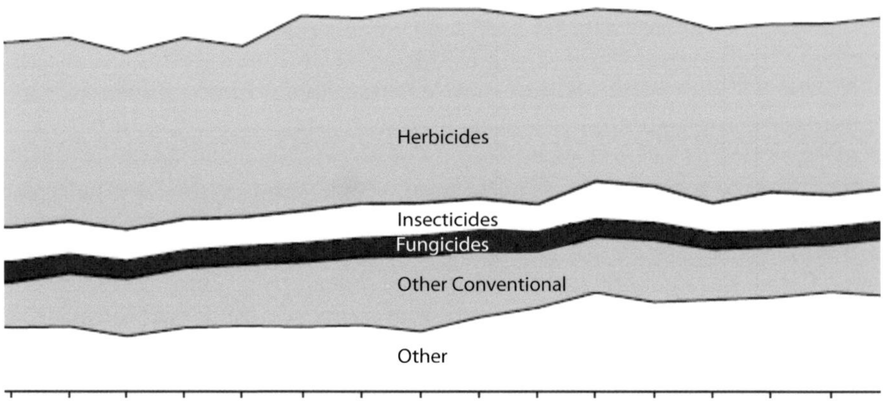

FIGURE 4-4 Annual amount of pesticide active ingredient used in the United States by pesticide type, 1988-2007 Estimates Agricultural Market Sector.
SOURCE: Grube et al., 2011.

the detection of pesticide compounds in streams of developed watersheds more than 90 percent of the time (Gilliom, 2007). In agricultural areas of the United States where sampling was conducted, pesticides were detected in 97 percent of samples in streams and 61 percent of samples in shallow groundwater areas. Additionally, organochlorine compounds, the majority of which are no longer used and which are considered "legacy" pesticides, were detected in 92 percent of fish tissue samples and 57 percent of aquatic bed sediment samples.

Because ecosystems are generally exposed to mixtures of pesticide compounds and their degradation products at varying concentrations, assessing environmental toxicity can be difficult, especially if only a single pesticide is evaluated (Gilliom, 2007). The issue is further complicated by toxicity arising from the use of currently registered pesticides and those used historically but with long half-lives, such as organochlorines. In addition, as a result of the lack of a comprehensive pesticide use database, except in certain states such as California, studies evaluating pesticide risk to the environment and human health are limited. Researchers in California studying pesticide risk in almond production were able to overcome this limitation by using the Pesticide Use Reporting (PUR) database and a Pesticide Use Risk Evaluation (PURE) indicator to assess the risks of pesticide use to air, water, and soil (Zhan and Zhang, 2012, 2014). The spatial and temporal data contained within PUR combined with the use of the PURE indicator demonstrated a shift to more environmentally friendly insect control measures, such as the use of oils and *Bacillus thuringiensis* (Bt) instead of less water-quality-friendly organophosphate compounds, while also revealing an increasing use of herbicides possibly linked to herbicide resistance (Zhan and Zhang, 2014).

The type and the amount of pesticides used by the U.S. food system are driven by a number of different forces. These forces include food marketing standards and consumer demands, varying pest pressure, real and perceived human health issues through both worker and consumer exposure, detection of pesticide or breakdown compounds in various environmental media (especially water), and increased use of crops with both natural and engineered (i.e., transgenic) resistance to pests. For example, aquatic toxicity and human health concerns attributed to chlorpyrifos and diazinon resulted in a shift away from these organophosphate insecticides to pyrethroid insecticides, which are less water soluble and have lower mammalian toxicity characteristics (Anderson et al., 2003; Bradman et al., 2011; Fenske et al., 2005; Hunt et al., 2003; Loewenherz et al., 1997). See Chapter 5 for a discussion on exposure effects on farmers and farm workers. Although this shift has reduced the impact of organophosphates on water quality and human health toxicity, a significant body of literature now exists demonstrating increased detections and aquatic toxicity of pyrethroids in the sediment downstream of agricultural lands, including in marine receiving waters (Amweg et al., 2005; Anderson et al., 2014; Ding et al., 2010; Domagalski et al., 2010; Weston et al., 2013). Pesticide use in response to pest outbreaks is always variable due to shifting environmental conditions, presence of host plants, and population of natural predators, but use may be more significant in response to invasive pests, especially where existing natural biological control organisms are inadequate or unable to control the pest. The detection of the soybean aphid, Aphis glycines Matsumura, in the United States in 2000 is an example of an outbreak of an invasive pest on an economically important crop that resulted in a significant increase in pesticide use where previously little pesticide was required. Chemical treatment for soybean aphid consists of foliar applications of pyrethroids and organophosphates as well as seed treatments with neonicotinoids (Ragsdale et al., 2011). Figure 4-5 illustrates the increase in the use of the neonicotinoids compounds imidacloprid and thiamethoxam as seed treatments as well as the increase in the use of pyrethroid compound lambda-cyhalothrin as a foliar treatment for controlling soybean aphid.

Depletion and Replenishment of Natural Resources

The U.S. food and agriculture system relies on vast quantities of natural resources, especially arable land and water. The availability and quality of these natural resources is influenced not only by human decisions (e.g., contamination of aquifers with pesticides and fertilizers or excessive erosion

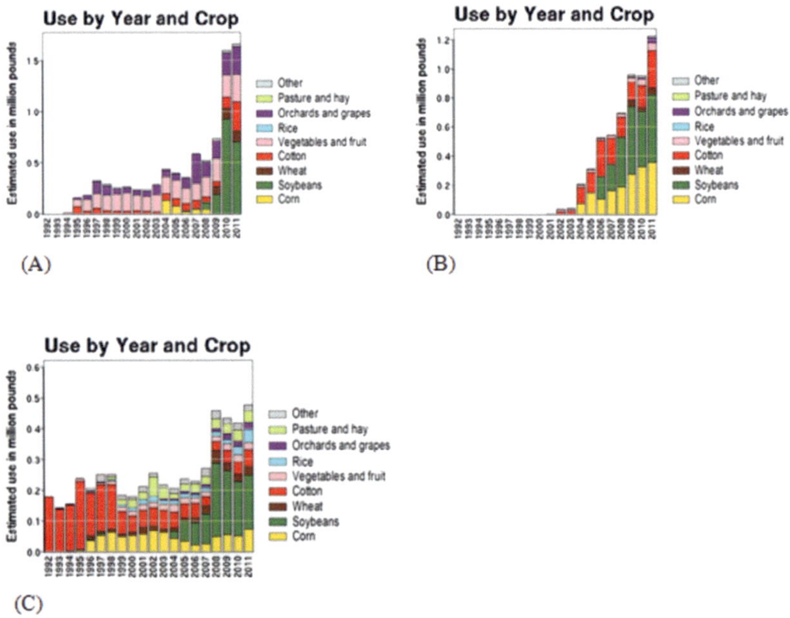

FIGURE 4-5 Estimated agricultural use for imidacloprid (A), thiamethoxam (B), and lambda-cyhalothrin (C), 2011.
SOURCE: Adapted from the Pesticide National Synthesis Project, U.S. Geological Survey. https://water.usgs.gov/nawqa/pnsp/usage/maps/index.php (accessed January 8, 2015).

due to improper tillage practices) but also by factors outside human control (e.g., floods and droughts). In some cases, rates of resource depletion can be matched by rates of replenishment or regeneration: for example, rates of water use in irrigation are matched by recharge of surface and groundwaters by snow melt or rainfall. Alternatively, rates of resource depletion can exceed rates of recharge, leading to slow or rapid degradation of the resource base on which agricultural production depends.

The recognition of the need to better manage soil and water resources on farms, on grazing lands, and in forests began formally in the United States with the formation of the U.S. Department of Agriculture (USDA) Soil Conservation Service in 1935, renamed the Natural Resources Conservation Service (NRCS) in 1994. Financial and technical support provided by NRCS continues to help landowners implement natural resource conservation strategies that address soil erosion, water quality, water conservation, and wildlife habitat. However, climate change and weather extremes, such as intense rainfall events or drought, as well as the need to produce more food on the same or less arable land, will require a renewed commitment to further research and extension capacity into the development and implementation of economically feasible conservation strategies that minimize imbalances in the stocks and flows of natural resources.

Soil Resources

Disruption of the balance between soil erosion and soil formation illustrates how agriculture can have a profound effect on the environment through net resource depletion. Erosion is a natural process that occurs on nearly all soils, though rates depend on multiple site-specific factors that include climate conditions and topography. The process occurs in two stages: detachment of soil particles from the soil surface and their subsequent transport and deposition. Erosion by water can occur in sheets,[7] rills,[8] and gullies[9] when rainfall rates exceed a soil's infiltration capacity; erosion by wind can occur when soil is dry and loose, the surface is bare and smooth, and the landscape has few physical barriers to block the movement of air (Magdoff and van Es, 2009).

Erosion is perhaps the most important land degradation process associated with agriculture (Cruse et al., 2013). Direct comparisons of soil erosion rates under different forms of land management have shown 1.3- to 1,000-fold differences, with mean erosion rates of 0.05 mm year^{-1} for sites under native vegetation and 3.94 mm year^{-1} for agricultural sites managed conventionally (Montgomery, 2007). Soil disturbance and exposure due to tillage and cropping practices are the prime culprits for accelerated rates of erosion on land under agricultural management (Magdoff and van Es, 2009; Montgomery, 2007). Erosion of agricultural soils tends to deplete soil organic matter, fertility, and water holding capacity (Magdoff and van Es, 2009) and, consequently, can cause significant reductions in crop yields (den Biggelaar et al., 2004; Fenton et al., 2005).

Soil formation is the result of the weathering of parent rock materials and additions and transformations of organic matter derived from plants, animals, and microbes. It is a geological process that is slow in comparison to the time span of a human generation and to rates of erosion incurred on agricultural land. In an investigation of 18 watersheds worldwide,

[7] Sheet erosion is removal of soil in thin layers by raindrop impact and shallow surface flow. It results in loss of the finest soil particles that contain most of the available nutrients and organic matter in the soil.

[8] Rills are shallow drainage lines that develop when surface water concentrates in paddock depressions, eroding the soil.

[9] Gullies are channels deeper than 30 cm that occur when smaller water flows concentrate, cutting a channel through the soil.

Alexander (1988) found soil formation rates ranged from 0.002 to 0.09 mm $year^{-1}$, with a mean value of 0.04 mm $year^{-1}$.

Wakatsuki and Rasyidin (1992) also studied soil dynamics at multiple sites worldwide and estimated the mean rate of soil formation to be 0.06 mm $year^{-1}$. Cruse et al. (2013) reported a mean rate of soil formation of 0.11 mm $year^{-1}$ for four soil series used intensively for crop production in Iowa.

The mean rate of sheet and rill erosion on U.S. cropland in 2010 was estimated by the USDA (NRCS, 2013) at 6.1 megagrams (Mg) ha^{-1} $year^{-1}$; the mean rate of wind erosion that year was estimated at 4.6 Mg ha^{-1} $year^{-1}$. Erosion due to water in ephemeral gullies can also be an important form of soil loss (Cruse et al., 2013; Gordon et al., 2008), but it is not assessed in widely used soil erosion assessment tools such as the Revised Universal Soil Loss Equation 2 (USDA, 2008) and the Water Erosion Prediction Project model (USDA, 2012). Nonetheless, by combining values for sheet, rill, and wind erosion, the minimum mean value for erosion on U.S. cropland is 10.7 Mg ha^{-1} $year^{-1}$ (see Figure 4-6). Assuming a soil bulk density of 1.3 Mg m^{-3}, that rate is equivalent to the loss of 0.82 mm of soil per $year^{-1}$.

Though erosion of soil from cropland at a rate of 0.82 mm $year^{-1}$ may seem insignificant, it is at least an order of magnitude greater than the rates of soil formation cited earlier. Consequences of this imbalance can be seen in an evaluation of soil dynamics in Iowa, which contains some of the most productive rain-fed croplands in the United States. Based on the mean rate of soil formation reported by Cruse et al. (2013) for four Iowa soil series (0.11 mm $year^{-1}$) and the mean rate of erosion due to sheet, rill, and wind losses on Iowa cropland (0.98 mm $year^{-1}$) reported by the USDA (NRCS, 2013), net loss of soil would be 0.87 mm $year^{-1}$. Viewed in a more historical context, net loss of soil would be 87 mm per century.

Despite the loss of considerable amounts of topsoil from U.S. croplands due to erosion, crop yields have generally increased over the past century, largely because technological advances, including more intensive use of fertilizers, have been able to mask the potential effects of soil degradation. However, as noted by Cruse et al. (2013), to make use of technological advances in the next century, especially those related to plant genetics, soil quality must be maintained or improved, especially soil's capacity to supply increasing amounts of water and nutrients. In this regard, changes in tillage and cropping practices that retard erosion will be critical, especially increased adoption of minimum tillage and zero tillage techniques, greater use of cover crops, and more widespread use of perennial, sod-forming crops (Magdoff and van Es, 2009; Montgomery, 2007).

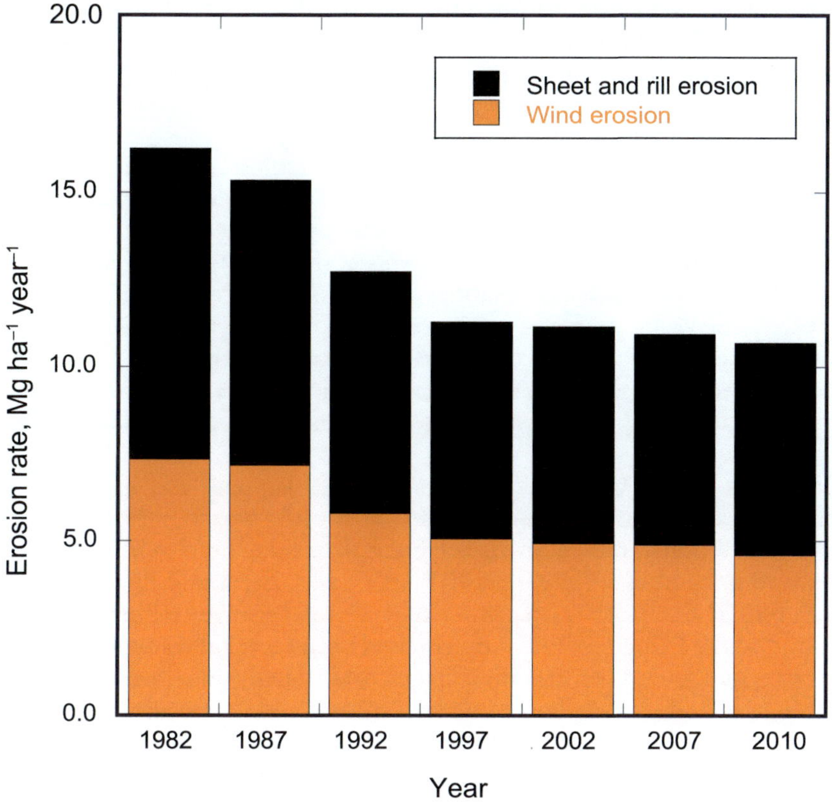

FIGURE 4-6 Estimated mean sheet, rill, and wind erosion on U.S. cropland, measured in megagrams per hectare per year (Mg ha^{-1} year^{-1}), 1982-2010.
SOURCE: NRCS, 2013.

Water Supply

Though irrigation is used on only 15 to 20 percent of total U.S. cropland, it is used on about 70 percent of land used for vegetable production, about 80 percent of land used for orchard crops, and essentially 100 percent of land used for rice production (Schaible and Aillery, 2012). Changes in irrigation technology, competition for water between urban and agricultural users, spatial and temporal patterns of drought, biofuel production from irrigated crops such as corn, and shifts in domestic and international markets for crops with different water use efficiencies and profit characteristics now intersect with the need to balance between water resource use and water resource replenishment. In general, rates of groundwater withdrawal are increasing throughout the United States relative to rates of replenishment (Konikow, 2013). In some cases, such as for croplands drawing on the Ogallala (High Plains) Aquifer, the imbalance between water withdrawal and recharge may prove too costly or impractical to maintain current levels of crop production (Konikow, 2013).

Relatively inefficient irrigation systems are still used for much of the U.S. irrigated cropland (Schaible and Aillery, 2012). The authors noted that long-term sustainability of irrigated agriculture will depend on adopting innovative, more efficient irrigation systems at the farm level. Some of these innovations include soil- and plant-moisture–sensing devices, commercial irrigation-scheduling services, and simulation models that help producers with irrigation decisions, among others. Another approach, currently being assessed in the Central Valley of California, is the artificial recharge of groundwater using excess surface water in non-drought years (Scanlon et al., 2012).

In areas of the United States where water supplies are limited and groundwater is susceptible to overdraft (most often due to periodic severe drought conditions), reused water is increasingly being used to irrigate both edible and nonedible crops. The 2007 Ag Census, Farm and Ranch Irrigation Survey (USDA, 2009) reported that more than 1.8 million acres of farmland in the United States were irrigated with recycled water, defined as water previously used for irrigating crops. Additionally, more than 700,000 acres of farmland used reclaimed wastewater treated for non-potable reuse (USDA, 2009). USDA, in recognition of the increasing frequency and severity of droughts in many parts of the United States where food and fiber are grown, identified water reuse as one of six broad areas on which to focus research, education, and extension efforts to ensure agriculture water security by 2025 (Dobrowolski and O'Neill, 2005). Water reuse provides significant opportunities to reduce groundwater depletion, but it is not without its challenges. These include matching supply and demand, the risk of contamination of stored water with pathogens from wildlife, negative impacts on crop yields due to increased salinity, health concerns related to emerging contaminants, and the public's perception of its use on edible crops (Dobrowolski et al., 2008). USGS provides a tremendous amount of information on agricultural impacts on water quality (see also Appendix B on selected metrics, methods, data, and models for USGS data sources).

Population and Community Disruption

Population and community dynamics among species within ecosystems can be affected by contaminants released into the environment at pollutant levels and by shifts in the availability of natural resources. The degree of ecosystem impact at each stage of the food and agriculture system depends on management decisions and the resulting response of the environment to the stressors created by those decisions.

For example, a broad-spectrum pesticide applied to a crop to control a pest during production may have significant adverse impacts on non-target pollinating insects in both farmed and non-farmed areas of the ecosystem. The loss of pollinators, by pesticide exposure and a variety of other drivers, affects both wild plant population and community diversity as well as yields of insect-pollinated crops, especially fruits and nuts. A current review of the decline in pollinators on a global scale advocates for investment in both a better understanding and implementation of "agri-environment schemes" to protect pollination services (Potts et al., 2010).

The Sacramento-San Joaquin Delta provides another example of how the balance of an ecosystem can be affected by management decisions. Vast acres of farmland in the southern Central Valley of California depend on water withdrawals from the Delta, as do two-thirds of the state's households. At the same time, the Delta provides critical habitat to a number of native fish, birds, mammals, and reptiles. For example, the Yolo Bypass floodplain is a fertile setting both for salmon reproduction and crop production (Garnache and Howitt, 2011). The high demands on water supply by agriculture as well as the general population, especially during drought years, significantly affect the population and community dynamics of the Delta. Lund et al. (2008) noted the importance of planning efforts to balance the water supply with the Delta's ecosystem needs. Keeping this idea at the forefront of any decision making would improve the likelihood of providing benefits to agriculture and the environment. The report identified an "ecosystem solution" that includes strategies such as coordinating planning efforts, minimizing the entry of toxicants and invasive species into the Delta, creating wildlife-friendly agriculture, and restoring habitat diversity. These two examples demonstrate how management decisions can have intended and unintended consequences on ecosystem health, emphasizing the importance of a more thorough understanding of the interconnectedness of agriculture and the environment as well as a recognition of the complex nature of these connections.

COMPLEXITIES ASSOCIATED WITH ENVIRONMENTAL EFFECTS

As should be clear from Chapter 2 and the previous discussion in this chapter, the U.S. food and agriculture system constitutes a prominent example of a coupled social–ecological system, in which people are inextricably linked with key components of the environment, including soil, water, air, sunlight, and a diverse biota (Rivera-Ferre et al., 2013). Natural resources are used to produce food, feed, fuel, and fiber for residents of the United States and other countries, thereby supporting a considerable portion of the U.S. economy. However, in recent years, societal demands on the food and agriculture system have expanded beyond production and profitability to include better stewardship of natural resources and improved protection of environmental quality.

Unlike most other ecosystems, agroecosystems explicitly reflect human knowledge, technology, labor, attitudes, and intentions, which in turn are affected by broader socioeconomic factors like markets, regulations, and education. Farmers, policy makers, businesspeople, and consumers repeatedly make decisions that affect the components and performance of agroecosystems. Consequently, agroecosystems are dynamic and can change quickly in response to social, economic, physical, biological, and technical factors.

Because the U.S. food and agriculture system has many interrelated components and processes, decisions about ways to adjust or refine one portion of the system can have significant consequences for other portions. Optimizing system performance in relation to productivity and environmental goals depends on several sets of tasks and types of information. These include identifying the multiple interacting and interdependent parts of the system; understanding how these parts are related; quantifying the status of system components; monitoring fluxes of materials and energy into, within, and out of the system; and determining key decision points affecting system dynamics. In some cases, empirical experiments can be designed, implemented, and monitored to compare the performance of contrasting systems of agricultural production, processing, and distribution. In other cases, empirical data derived from a range of sources can be used to develop models with which to compare system performance characteristics. For both approaches, it is important to recognize the dynamic characteristics of relevant environmental effects.

Characteristics of Environmental Effects

Interactions among food, agriculture, and the environment are of major importance in the United States for three reasons: the large land area the system occupies, the large quantities of resources it consumes, and the strong connections that can exist between agricultural and nonagricultural ecosystems. Of the 9.16 million square kilometers of total land in the United States, 18 percent is used for cropland and 27 percent is used for pasture and rangeland; within the continental United States, agriculture occupies 54 percent of total land area (Nickerson et al., 2011). Water use exemplifies the disproportionate impact of the U.S. food and agriculture system on natural resources. Food and agriculture, principally irrigation, account for about 80 percent of the nation's total consumption of freshwater stocks (ERS, 2013).

Exports (i.e., outflows) of nutrients, pesticides, and other materials from agroecosystems into nonagricultural ecosystems (i.e., inflows) can be substantial. For example, Alexander et al. (2008) estimated that nearly 1 million metric tons of nitrogen are delivered annually into the Gulf of Mexico from agricultural lands lying upstream in the Mississippi River Basin, leading to formation of a coastal hypoxic zone. Of the 34,000 metric tons of the herbicide atrazine that are applied each year to U.S. cropland (Grube et al., 2011), about 1 percent moves into associated streams, creating conditions that can exceed thresholds for safeguarding aquatic organisms and human health (Gilliom et al., 2006; Larson et al., 1999). Heathcote et al. (2013) studied trends in sedimentation for 32 lakes in Iowa and found that agricultural intensification over the past 50 years had led to accelerating increases in soil sediment deposition in the lakes due to erosion, despite soil conservation efforts. Fluxes between farms and the atmosphere also are important. Agricultural practices, principally fertilizer use and manure management, are responsible for about 74 percent of U.S. emissions of the greenhouse gas nitrous oxide and 84 percent of the nation's emissions of ammonia and other NH_x-nitrogen compounds (EPA, 2011, 2013).

As these examples illustrate, environmental effects of the U.S. food and agriculture system reveal traits of a complex system. In particular, they can involve spatial displacement, with large distances possible between sites of pollutant discharge and sites of their ultimate impacts. The system's environmental effects also may be characterized by temporal lags, with effects remaining largely invisible or unrecognized for months or years. For example, following the introduction of chlorinated hydrocarbon insecticides, such as DDT and dieldrin, in the 1940s and 1950s, declines in bird populations were not recognized as being related to use of these chemicals for a number of years. Because their toxic effects included reduced reproductive efficiency, rather than just direct mortality, and because concentrations did not reach critical levels until "biomagnifications" had occurred with movement of the pesticides through the food web (Mineau, 2002), cause-and-effect relationships were initially difficult to discern. By the 1970s, when understanding of the large effects of this class of pesticides on non-target organisms increased, most of the chemicals were banned or severely restricted in many developed countries. Currently, there is concern over the ecological impacts of neonicotinoid insecticides, which were introduced in the 1990s due to their lower mammalian toxicity relative to organophosphate and carbamate compounds and are now widely used throughout U.S. agriculture. Emerging data indicate these compounds may be primary factors in the decline of honeybee populations through chronic effects on behavior, health, and immunity, and increased susceptibility to pathogens and parasites (Di Prisco et al., 2013; Henry et al., 2012; Pettis et al., 2012).

Temporal lags in agroecosystems also may present positive, desirable effects, such as the increase in soil nitrogen fertility and reduced requirement for mineral fertilizer that occur when nitrogen-fixing crops like alfalfa are followed in rotation sequences by cereals and other crops that do not fix atmospheric nitrogen (Peoples et al., 1995).

Environmental effects of the food and agriculture system can be indirect. Indirect effects may occur through loops and webs of interconnected species so that the impact on one species of a change in management practices or system composition and configuration is mitigated by other species. The effects of neonicotinoid insecticides on honeybees by way of pathogens and parasites illustrate this concept. It is also exemplified by the phenomenon known as "target pest resurgence" whereby an insect pest population increases rapidly following application of a chemical intended to control it, often to a level higher than existed before the control measure was applied (Dutcher, 2007). Although an insecticide may destroy more than 99 percent of a target pest population, it rarely eliminates all of the pests; frequently, however, it kills a large portion of the pest's natural enemies and disrupts food webs that would otherwise promote natural enemy persistence and efficacy (Bottrell, 1979; NRC, 1996). With many fewer natural enemies present, surviving pest populations increase rapidly, posing an enhanced threat to crop production. Alternatively, biological control of crop pests by natural enemies may be enhanced by maintaining natural and seminatural vegetation in agricultural landscapes, thereby allowing natural enemies to move among habitats that provide them with refugia and resources that may be scarce in crop fields (Power, 2010). Losey and Vaughan (2006) estimated that insect predators and parasitoids acting as natural enemies of crop pests save $4.5 billion in the United States each year by reducing crop losses to insect damage and lowering expenditures on insecticides. Thus, ignoring or failing to appropriately manage indirect effects in the U.S. food and agriculture system may have serious economic implications.

Nonlinear effects are common in complex systems like food and agriculture, with small changes in management or system composition or configuration giving little or no response or a disproportionately large response. The latter class of effects can be particularly important for both physical and biological processes in agroecosystems. For example, in a field experiment comparing contrasting patterns of land use in watersheds used for corn and soybean production, Helmers et al. (2012) observed that conversion of 10 percent of the cropland area to filter strips composed of reconstructed prairie vegetation resulted in a 96 percent reduction in the export of soil sediment from the watersheds. Pesticides that disrupt the endocrine system of non-target animals can also exhibit nonlinear, nonproportional effects, with exposure to low or intermediate concentrations causing equal or larger changes in hormone levels relative to changes elicited by high concentrations. Endocrine-disrupting agricultural pesticides have been found to alter rates of growth and development, immune system function, and other health parameters (Rohr and McCoy, 2010; Vandenberg et al., 2012). Exposure to them at low, ecologically relevant concentrations has been suggested as contributing to population declines of amphibian species (Hayes et al., 2002, 2010).

Though the food and agriculture system exerts substantial pressure on the environment, environmental factors also can have strong effects on various aspects of the food and agriculture system, especially crop and livestock productivity. Environmental stressors, especially droughts, floods, exceptionally high and low temperatures, and pest infestations, are notable for their lack of predictability in both space and time. Consequently, a key system characteristic is the degree of resilience the environment manifests when stressed by physical and biotic factors. Resilient systems resist change due to stressors and rebound quickly after perturbation; non-resilient systems are strongly altered by stressors and recover more slowly, if ever. Pimentel et al. (2005) noted differences in resilience in a long-term cropping systems experiment that included a conventionally managed corn–soybean rotation and two organically managed, more diverse rotations. During 5 drought years when growing season precipitation was less than 70 percent of average levels, corn yields were 28 to 34 percent higher in the more diverse organic systems. This effect was attributed to higher levels of soil organic matter, with concomitant increases in soil water storage and plant-available water. Resilience also can be evident with regard to the effects of crop diversity on pest management. Blackshaw (1994) found that the mean density and year-to-year variance of population densities of the grass weed Bromus tectorum were markedly higher in fields in which wheat was grown continuously compared with wheat grown in rotation with canola. In general, diversified crop rotation systems offer important opportunities for minimizing threats of weed infestation while reducing requirements for herbicide inputs (Nazarko et al., 2005), a consideration that is especially relevant to addressing growing problems associated with the management of herbicide-resistant weeds (Beckie, 2006).

Because the food and agriculture system covers a broad geographic area and intersects with numerous organisms and multiple portions of the economy, changes in the configuration of the system can incur consequences that may be difficult to anticipate without careful analysis. For example, biofuel production from crop materials has been championed as a means of reducing fossil fuel use and limiting GHG emissions, but some analysts have concluded that it can be responsible for environmentally undesirable indirect land-use change effects,[10] whereby shifts from food and feed production to biofuel production in one region may lead to the conversion of grasslands and forest lands to croplands in others, with concomitant increases in net carbon dioxide (CO_2) emissions, soil erosion, and nutrient emissions to water (Fargione et al., 2008; Searchinger et al., 2008; Secchi et al., 2010). The evolution of pesticide resistance in target pests also exemplifies how agricultural management practices can elicit unwanted effects that might be avoided by analysis of alternative management systems. Since the mid-1990s introduction of transgenic crops resistant to the herbicide glyphosate, glyphosate use in the United States has increased 10-fold (USGS, 2014), making it the most heavily used pesticide in U.S. agriculture and a strong selection force acting on weed population genetics. Concomitantly, glyphosate-resistant weeds have become increasingly prevalent and problematic (Heap, 2014). In an analysis of ways to address this problem, Mortensen and colleagues (2012) concluded that simply stacking new genes for resistance to additional herbicides in crop genomes was unlikely to prevent further cases of herbicide resistance in weeds, and that a more efficacious approach would be to develop and implement integrated weed management systems that employ a diverse set of tactics, such as crop rotation, cover cropping, planting of competitive crop cultivars, and appropriate use of tillage and herbicides application.

The multiple dimensions of the food and agriculture system can provide multiple pathways toward solutions to complex problems. For example, increasing food production is not the only pathway to increase food availability to a growing human population. This is fortunate, because increased food production tends to either require more land (through the conversion of more forests and grasslands to arable crop production) or the intensification of fertilizer and pesticide use on existing arable land, with attendant environmental problems such as elevated GHG emissions, loss of biodiversity, water contamination, and soil erosion. Food availability also can be increased by reducing food waste and shifting dietary patterns toward a greater proportion of plant-based foods (Foley et al., 2011). In 2010, an estimated 31 percent of the 195 billion kilograms of food available in the United States at retail and consumer levels was not eaten (Buzby et al., 2013). In an analysis of the consequences of a radical shift in global dietary patterns, Cassidy et al. (2013) concluded that growing food exclusively for direct human consumption rather than animal feed and biofuels could increase available food calories by as much as 70 percent, enough to feed an additional 4 billion people. Such a shift would be particularly profound

[10] Indirect land use change effects refers to the effects that increasing biofuel production in one location will have on expanded cultivation of land in other locations.

in the United States, where corn, the nation's largest crop, is chiefly destined for animal feed and biofuel production (ERS, 2014; Foley, 2013).

DRIVERS OF HUMAN BEHAVIOR AFFECTING THE ENVIRONMENT

It seems paradoxical that humans would undermine the quality of their habitat by depleting, contaminating, and unbalancing the natural environment. But maintaining the natural environment is one among many human goals. Human behavior makes more sense when different kinds of people and different group sizes are examined in their specific socioeconomic and biophysical contexts. Like the environment as a dynamic system, human behavior also displays spatial displacement, temporal lags, and nonlinear feedbacks—all peppered with random effects.

Human decisions are made in the context of desires, incentives, constrained resources, imperfect information, and bounded rationality. Human institutions, like laws and markets, shape incentives for decision makers (Schmid, 2004). Of particular importance for behavior related to the natural environment are property rights—what and how people are allowed to own things. For environmental impacts, two cases of property rights are especially important. When one decision maker's actions influence the welfare of another person, an economic externality exists. The term comes from the fact that the affected person's welfare is external to the decision. The externality may be positive (e.g., acquiring honey bees that also pollinate a neighbor's trees) (Meade, 1952) or negative (e.g., pesticide runoff into a river with swimmers downstream). But the key factor is that the external person lacks the property right to protect himself or herself from the external effect without taking special measures. Hence, the decision maker takes into account some, but not all, of the costs and benefits experienced by the public. What is optimal from a private perspective may not be so from a public one.

The second case of property rights that affect environmental behavior is that of common property resources that are shared (like a grazing commons or the atmosphere) (Blaikie and Brookfield, 1987). In both cases, no one has the right to exclude others from using the resource, creating an incentive for depletion or misuse. Consequently, what is optimal for the individual is not so in the aggregate because the resource gets overexploited.

Because many important environmental impacts of the food system occur during agricultural production, the following sections first examine farmer decision processes and then explore decisions by other food system actors, such as processors, distributors, and consumers.

Private Producer Perspective

Most food is produced by farmers who rely on agriculture for their livelihood. Although evidence abounds that farmers care about environmental stewardship, surveys repeatedly show that profitability is an overriding concern (Ma et al., 2012). Farmers in the United States hold property rights that give broad latitude over how to manage their land so long as they do not cause harm in direct and measurable ways (Norris et al., 2008). However, their actions may cause economic externalities through air, water, or biotic changes that are indirect and often hard to measure.

The profit-maximizing approach to nitrogen fertilizer application on corn illustrates a rational process where an economic externality can lead to environmental degradation. To begin, note that fertilizer, land, and corn are private goods that belong to the farmer. But the aquifer under the farm, the streams nearby, and the atmosphere have no owners—they are common property resources. Corn yield typically increases with increasing applications of nitrogen, but yield increases at a decreasing rate and ultimately reaches a plateau due to genetic yield potential or shortages of other inputs. For a corn producer who is deciding how much nitrogen fertilizer to apply to a corn crop, the standard rule for profit maximization is to apply more fertilizer up to the point where the pay-off from adding more fertilizer just equals the cost of acquiring and spreading that fertilizer. Up to that point, each added unit of fertilizer will fetch greater value of marketable corn. As fertilizer application rises and corn yield tails off, a rising share of fertilizer applied is not taken up by the corn plant. Instead, it converts to nitrate and is carried by water into streams that may contribute to marine hypoxia (Alexander et al., 2008); it may also convert into nitrous oxide and move into the atmosphere as a GHG (McSwiney and Robertson, 2005; Shcherbak et al., 2014). Because no one owns the waterways or the air, the costs to other people of using those environmental media as waste recipients are external to the farmer's decision. Similar external costs can accrue from other privately rational decisions by farmers. Examples include specializing in highly profitable crops at the expense of biodiverse natural areas that provide habitat for beneficial species, such as songbirds, pollinators, and the natural enemies of certain agricultural pests.

The common property dynamic contributes importantly to depletion of shared resources like the Ogallala (High Plains) Aquifer. In the century since farmers learned that the semiarid High Plains region was underlain by this vast aquifer, irrigation has dramatically expanded crop production. However, due to low rainfall in the current era, the aquifer's recharge rate is dwarfed by water withdrawals, resulting in a 30 percent depletion of the groundwater supply today in western Kansas, with continuing depletion expected despite rising private costs of withdrawing water from greater depths (Steward et al., 2013). Because no one owns the groundwater, there is no assurance that if one person conserves, that person will have more of the resource available later.

Societal Perspective and Environmental Policy

Although environmental problems in agriculture are driven by a certain logic, solutions that can protect the public interest are possible. The fact that one decision maker holds the right to take actions that affect others does not mean those actions are inevitable. As Ronald Coase (1960) famously observed, it simply means the affected parties must pay for the right to prevent harm. A variety of regulatory and voluntary approaches to mitigating the impacts of the U.S. food system on the environment have been taken by regulatory agencies, environmental conservation groups, and actors within each of the food system sectors (see Box 4-1).

Because U.S. farmers have broad property rights to manage their land as they see fit, U.S. agricultural environmental protection policy focuses on paying farmers for environmental services. A variety of federal programs under the historic series of farm bills since 1985 (most recently the Agricultural Act of 2014) (USDA, 2014a) pay farmers for environmental services through sharing the cost of environmental stewardship practices (e.g., under the Environmental Quality Incentives Program), renting farmland that offers conservation benefits (e.g., Conservation Reserve Program), or paying for environmental services from working lands (e.g., Conservation Stewardship Program). In the private sector, efforts are expanding to establish markets for ecosystem services, such as the provision of clean water or of wildlife habitat. Although such markets are currently small, their emergence has raised a set of important questions about how to ensure that environmental stewardship practices truly add to environmental quality ("additionality") and whether it makes sense to pay separately for different services that arise from the same stewardship practice ("stacking" ecosystem services) (Cooley and Olander, 2012; Hanley et al., 2012; Woodward, 2011).

Another approach to protect the public interest is regulation that directly mandates actions or sets limits on pollutants. In this instance, the public holds the right, for example, to clean water and air, so polluters must incur the cost of meeting clean standards. A prime example of this is the multipronged effort to curb the unintended consequences of unwanted nutrient flows and resultant pollutants into air and water using regulations and voluntary programs at the national, regional, and state levels. Often these regulatory approaches mandate emission mitigation to avoid not only ecosystem impacts but also the impacts these emissions have on human health.

BOX 4-1
Examples of Environmental Mitigation Interventions

Laws/Regulations

- The Clean Water Act
- The Clean Air Act
- Federal Insecticide, Fungicide, and Rodenticide Act
- Endangered Species Act
- Coastal Zone Act Reauthorization Amendments of 1990
- Safe Drinking Water Act
- Resource Conservation and Recovery Act
- Food Quality Protection Act
- Toxic Substances Control Act
- National Ambient Air Quality Standards
- Conservation compliance linked to crop insurance subsidies (Sodsaver Program)

Voluntary (Incentive Programs)

- Agricultural Management Assistance (AMA)
- Conservation Reserve Program (CRP)
- Conservation Stewardship Program (CSP)
- Environmental Quality Incentives Program (EQIP)
- Agricultural Conservation Easement Program
- Healthy Forests Reserve Program (HFRP)

Education/Technical Assistance

- The U.S. Department of Agriculture (USDA) Natural Resources Conservation Service Conservation Technical Assistance Program
- USDA state and locally funded Cooperative Extension offices

The Clean Air Act mandated the Environmental Protection Agency (EPA) to set air quality standards for six pollutants, namely, carbon monoxide, lead, nitrogen dioxide, PM less than 10 μm in diameter (PM_{10}), PM less than 2.5 μm in diameter ($PM_{2.5}$), ozone, and sulfur dioxide (EPA, 2009a). Primary standards address public health concerns and secondary standards protect general public welfare (e.g., visibility and environmental effects) (EPA, 2008; Pope et al., 2009). The major agricultural air pollutants are PM, ammonia, and VOCs, as well as hydrogen sulfite. Currently, no federal standards regulate agricultural ammonia and VOC atmospheric emissions directly, but ammonia can contribute to PM formation (Pinder et al., 2007) and VOCs contribute to ozone formation (EPA, 2008).

The anthropogenic GHGs of greatest concern are carbon dioxide, methane, and nitrous oxide. These gases have different potentials for trapping heat in the Earth's atmosphere, known as global warming potential.[11] Currently, the United States neither requires mandatory reporting nor regulates total GHG emissions. At the state level, California became the first state to regulate and mandate reporting of GHG emissions with Assembly Bill 32 (California Global Warming Solutions Act of 2006). This bill does not exempt GHG emissions from the agriculture sector.

The Clean Water Act (CWA), passed in 1972 and significantly amended in 1977 and 1987, provides the basis for EPA to regulate point sources of pollution to surface waters using the National Pollutant Discharge Elimination System (NPDES) permitting system. Except for certain agricultural facilities, such as large animal feedlots, agricultural discharges are classified as non-point sources and therefore exempt from the point source NPDES permitting system. The 1987 amendments to the CWA recognized non-point source pollution (NPS) as a significant impairment to U.S. surface waters and in response created, under section 319, the Nonpoint Source Management Program. This program provides grant money to support the development and implementation of technologies, educational programs, and—most importantly—funds for water quality monitoring to determine the effectiveness of non-point implementation projects. Non-point source pollutants arising from agricultural production and addressed by this program include nutrients, sediment, pathogens, and pesticides.

Agricultural NPS continues to be a significant impairment to surface water quality, as stated in the 2004 National Water Quality Inventory Report to Congress (EPA, 2009b), where it was identified as the leading source of water quality impacts to rivers and lakes. California has implemented additional water quality regulations to address non-point sources from agriculture. The Irrigated Lands Regulatory Program, administered by the California State Water Resources Control Board (SWRCB), issues growers either waste discharge requirements (WDRs) or conditional waivers of WDRs in order to regulate discharges from irrigated agricultural lands. The program allows for irrigated discharges to occur, but under a condition of monitoring the water quality of receiving waters and the implementation of management practices to correct any impairments. In 2014, the SWRCB reported approximately 6 million acres and 40,000 growers had been enrolled in the program.

Apart from payments for environmental services and regulations to

[11] Global warming potential is a relative measure of how much heat a GHG traps in the atmosphere.

control pollutants, several other approaches encourage improved environmental stewardship. These incentive-based methods include certifications of good environmental performance. Certifications may serve to inform the consumer about invisible production process traits or to protect the farmer against lawsuits for alleged poor stewardship. The USDA organic label is the best known of these, but a wide variety of certifications of general agro-environmental stewardship and specific practices exist, such as pesticide safety or groundwater protection (Greene, 2001; Segerson, 2013; Waldman and Kerr, 2014).

METHODOLOGIES TO QUANTIFYING SYSTEM PERFORMANCE

This section identifies some relevant measurement and modeling methods used to capture environmental effects. It describes general methods used to assess environmental effects with the understanding of the difficulty in establishing clear cause-and-effect relationships without using a combination of methods. Assessing environmental effects begins with determining how large they are. Some environmental effects can be measured directly. Others are diffuse or hard to observe, so they are measured indirectly, using indicators, or they are simulated, using mathematical models. Life cycle assessments (LCAs) are typically used to account for environmental effects over the life of a product.

Datasets covering environmental effects are available from EPA, USDA, USGS, and private-sector sources (see Appendix B, Table B-3). U.S. surface water quality is tracked by the USGS National Water Information System. Air quality and chemical toxins are tracked by EPA's Air Quality System and ECOTOX databases. The environmental effects of farming practices are tracked by USDA's Agricultural Resource Management Survey and NRCS databases, while pesticide residues on food are covered by the USDA Pesticide Data Program.

Apart from the size of a direct environmental effect, it can be equally important to measure feedbacks and repercussions elsewhere in the food system. Such feedbacks are generally simulated using models.

Direct Measurement

The direct measurement approach seeks to directly quantify causal relationships between key ecosystem attributes and the entities selected for measurement (Lindenmayer and Likens, 2011). An advantage of the direct measurement approach is that it can result in the development of effective monitoring programs and successful implementation of management practices as long as the entities directly measured are selected based on answering carefully designed questions about the system being studied. For example, if a question is about whether surface runoff from dairy production in a particular watershed is a source of *Giardia* or *Cryptosporidium* detected in a local drinking water supply, then measurement of *Giardia* or *Cryptosporidium* at various locations within the watershed would be the most direct and efficient method to answer the question. Direct measurements under situations such as this are used to answer specific environmental questions as long as adequate resources are available.

Although the direct measurement approach has its advantages, significant disadvantages and/or limitations exist with its use in quantifying environmental effects. It is often costly and both labor and time intensive. Moreover, it is frequently impossible to measure and evaluate all the environmental processes and factors needed to thoroughly quantify the system of interest (Bockstaller and Girardin, 2003; Lindenmayer and Likens, 2011). Even with continued advances in technology allowing for easier and more economical analyses of organisms and chemicals (e.g., pathogens, pesticides, nutrients), some ecosystem evaluations, such as soil biodiversity, require the use of alternative measurements that are easier and more cost-effective to conduct (Eckschmitt et al., 2003). Chemical and biological toxicity testing are commonly used to identify the pollutant(s) responsible for water quality impairments, but only after less expensive biosurvey techniques, such as EPA's Rapid Bioassessment Protocols, detect a potential impairment (Barbour et al., 1999).

Indicators

Indicators are used to detect and evaluate changes in environmental conditions in response to environmental stressors. Environmental and ecological indicators measure a variety of environmental parameters, including plant health (water stress, nutrient content, and pest damage), biodiversity, ecosystem services, aquatic toxicity, soil erosion, emissions, and water quality. The advantage of the indicator approach over direct measurement is that indicators are generally more cost-effective, require less time to obtain results, and respond predictably to environmental stressors across space and time. Table 4-1 provides a sampling of the types of indicators used to measure environmental conditions affected by the U.S. food system. Box 4-2 describes *Daphnia* as a biological indicator.

Remote sensing, geographic information systems (GISs), and global positioning systems technology deserve special attention as they allow for the assessment of environmental conditions on both a site-specific and a global scale through the frequent and reliable measurement of a variety of environmental indicators. Atzberger's (2013) review of advances in remote sensing of agriculture highlights the potential role the technology could provide in reducing the environmental impacts of the U.S. food system.

TABLE 4-1 Example Indicators and the Associated Environmental Condition Monitored

Indicator	Condition of the Environment Monitored
Sun-induced chlorophyll fluorescence (SIF)	Agricultural productivity, crop photosynthesis
Aquatic macroinvertebrates	Biological health of streams and rivers, pollution, water quality
Heat shock proteins in fish	Thermal pollution of streams and rivers
Lichens and mosses	Air pollution
Visual and acoustic remote sensing of birds	Biodiversity
Fecal indicators (such as *E. coli*)	Water quality
Soil organic matter, pH, bulk density	Soil health

BOX 4-2
Daphnia, A Biological Indicator of Environmental Status

Indicator species are frequently employed to evaluate ecosystem integrity in response to environmental stressors. Properly selected indicator species are sensitive to stressors and allow for the integrity of the ecosystem to be examined in a timely and cost-effective manner (Carignan and Villard, 2002). Some of the most common indicator species are those used to examine the impacts of agricultural and nonagricultural activities on aquatic environments.

Daphnia, a genus of small freshwater crustaceans, is commonly used in water quality monitoring due to its sensitivity to physical and chemical changes in the aquatic environment, its important role in the aquatic food web, and its ease to cultivate under laboratory conditions. Its wide use as an indicator species in freshwater systems also has created an extensive database of acute and subacute responses to numerous environmental stressors, such as pesticides, heavy metals, and sedimentation.

Simulation Modeling

Simulation models are used to estimate the size or probability of environmental effects that are hard to observe. Simulation models that link multiple components of the food system can also predict indirect effects, and dynamic models can capture feedbacks that lead to delayed, indirect repercussions. When simulation models can be run in concert with random variables, like weather data, they also can capture important environmental impacts that occur only under special conditions when a threshold is exceeded. An applicable example to use such a model is in predicting the impact of algal blooms. Harmful algal blooms are rare, but when heavy rains washed agricultural phosphorus into the Maumee River and temperatures warmed up rapidly in the summer of 2011, devastating consequences ensued for Lake Erie fisheries and beaches (Michalak et al., 2013). The general uses of simulation models are described in Chapter 7, but this section will survey important simulation modeling approaches used for environmental impacts.

For environmental assessments, the two broad classes of simulation modeling are biophysical and socioeconomic. There are ecosystem service models, such as InVEST developed by the Natural Capital Project, that attempt to link biophysical and socioeconomic components in a GIS context, which can be useful for evaluating alternative land-use and land-management scenarios.

Biophysical Models

Biophysical models vary widely according to the environmental media on which they focus (soil, plants, animals, water, biodiversity, air, climate). They also vary in spatial scale (field, watershed, airshed, globe) (see examples in Appendix B, Table B-4).

Most water and air pollutants are either intermediate or by-products of several basic biochemical or geochemical reactions, namely, decomposition, ammonification, nitrification, denitrification, ammonium-ammonia equilibrium, ammonia volatilization, fermentation, etc. Incorporating the basic reactions in the modeling framework is essential. Biogeochemical models like DNDC (Denitrification/Decomposition) (Li et al., 2012) have been developed to simulate those reactions for soil, livestock, and crop environmental emissions. Models like DNDC predict water and air emissions under both aerobic and anaerobic conditions using theoretical concepts (e.g., water and gas formation and transfer) along with empirical measured parameters that drive these.

One important group of biogeochemical models predicts crop growth and associated environmental consequences (EPIC, CENTURY/DAYCENT) (Gassman et al., 2005; Hanks and Ritchie, 1991; Parton et al., 1987). These models draw parameters from a particular location on soils and weather, and combine these parameters with data on plant genetics and management methods to predict crop growth and yields and the associated movement of key elements (especially carbon, nitrogen, phosphorus) into the plant and in the surrounding soil. They are often linked to erosion models (e.g., RUSLE2 [Revised Universal Soil Loss Equation 2] or WEPP [Water Erosion Prediction Project]) or to hydrological flow models that predict where water carries eroded soil sediments and dissolved nutrients (e.g., SWAT [Soil and Water Assessment Tool] or GLEAMS [Groundwater Loading

Effects of Agricultural Management Systems]) (Arnold et al., 1998), allowing aggregation of geochemical movements at the groundwater or surface watershed level.

Another important class of physical models simulates and predicts climate changes. At the planetary level, general circulation models predict global climate changes at a decadal time step. Such models are widely used both to test policy and technological scenarios to mitigate climate change and to simulate conditions to which humans will need to adapt. Global climate forecasts from the Intergovernmental Panel on Climate Change are frequently used to generate parameters for agricultural models (such as those mentioned above) to simulate how to adapt food production to projected climate change (IPCC, 2013).

Socioeconomic Models

For environmental assessments, socioeconomic models aim to simulate human behavior and how it affects the environment. The main economic models used in environmental assessments focus on producers and markets. At local and regional scales, producer models tend to assume that farmers maximize profits, taking prices as given (Weersink et al., 2002). However, large-scale changes in producer or consumer behavior will trigger changes in prices, which are captured in computable general equilibrium (CGE) models (discussed in Chapter 7). Major CGE models used in agricultural environmental impact assessments include FASOM (Forest and Agricultural Sector Optimization Model) and GTAP (Global Trade Analysis Project), both of which have been used to estimate the effects of agricultural policies in the face of climate change (Hertel et al., 2010; Schneider, 2007). The linking of economic and environmental models is discussed further in Chapter 5 in the context of modeling complex feedbacks.

Life Cycle Assessment

LCA is a methodology that describes environmental assessment of a product or service (e.g., a kilogram of beef or lettuce) over its life cycle. Used for biochemical and energy flows, it is based on inventory data of a product and the emissions to the environment at each stage of the life cycle. The data on resources and emissions are measured and aggregated over the whole life cycle and classified into specific environmental impact categories (e.g., climate change, acidification, eutrophication). LCA arrives at values for each impact category and the results are expressed per unit of the studied product (i.e., functional unit), which is often expressed as mass of the product of a certain quality (e.g., carbon emissions per kg of fat and per protein in milk). LCA is overwhelmingly applied to energy use and GHG emissions; for example, GHG emissions have been closely studied in the dairy sector (Rotz et al., 2010). It is noteworthy that until recently, hardly any consistency was observed for LCAs conducted even within one sector of food production. For example, 21 peer-reviewed LCAs have been conducted for the U.S. beef sector with a wide divergence of methodologies, making comparisons of findings impossible. The most comprehensive cradle-to-grave LCA for the U.S. beef sector was recently conducted by Battagliese et al. (2013). However, the lack of harmonization across global LCA methodologies, especially for the livestock sector, has led the United Nations' Food and Agriculture Organization to conduct a 3-year project titled LEAP (Livestock Environmental Assessment and Performance Partnership), which aims to develop one global ISO (International Organization for Standardization) standard-compliant LCA methodology to ensure that environmental assessments of the livestock sector follow a scientifically consistent method and not individual bias. It is hoped that the resulting LEAP guidelines will be applicable to other sectors of the food system to allow for a complete and fair environmental assessment of current production processes and potential effects of mitigation.

SUMMARY

The U.S. food system depends heavily on the climate, soil, and water resources that allow a highly productive and varied agriculture to flourish. The environmental effects of the current agricultural system in the United States are positive and negative as well as intended and unintended. Any assessment of the current system must recognize that agricultural production systems may in many instances deplete natural resources of land and water, disturb ecosystem balance, involve the use of environmental contaminants such as pesticides and nitrogen that pollute the natural environment, and present challenges to human health. At the same time, many of these effects can be mitigated by management practices that promote soil and water conservation, minimize nutrient and pesticide emissions, foster sequestration of carbon, and allow appropriate manure disposal from animal feeding operations.

This chapter reviews the environmental effects of food production systems and discusses their salient characteristics, along with drivers of human behavior that influence the environmental impact of food systems, including both the perspectives of private producers and broader societal goals.

Assessments of the environmental effects of food systems are often difficult to conduct because there may be long distances between sites of pollutant discharge and the resulting changes in the abundance and health of non-target areas or species. Nitrogen runoff and effects on distant water ecosystems represent an example of such effects. Similarly, long delays may occur before the effects of some pollutant discharges become evident, with nitrate impacts on groundwater as an example. Webs of interconnectivity among species that are affected by pesticide use also may occur but not be readily apparent. Ignoring indirect effects of agricultural practices that are expressed through multiple species may have serious long-term implications.

The pathways by which a food system leads to environmental effects display characteristics of complex systems, in that they are dynamic and adaptive, are subject to lags and feedbacks, and include many interdependent actors. As this chapter makes clear, the environmental effects of food systems are intertwined with health, social, and economic domains. Measuring interdependencies within and among these domains presents analytical and modeling challenges that require special methods. Chapter 6 elaborates on the characteristics of complex adaptive systems, and Chapter 7 describes analytical methods that are appropriate for assessing the environmental effects of food systems.

REFERENCES

Alexander, E. B. 1988. Rates of soil formation: Implications for soil-loss tolerance. *Soil Science* 145:37-45.

Alexander, R. B., R. A. Smith, G. E. Schwarz, E. W. Boyer, J. V. Nolan, and J. W. Brakebill. 2008. Differences in phosphorus and nitrogen delivery to the Gulf of Mexico from the Mississippi river basin. *Environmental Science and Technology* 42(3):822-830.

Amweg, E. L., D. P. Weston, and N. M. Ureda. 2005. Use and toxicity of pyrethroid pesticides in the Central Valley, California, USA. *Environmental Toxicology and Chemistry* 24(4):966-972.

Anderson, B., J. W. Hunt, B. M. Phillips, P. A. Nicely, K. D. Gilbert, V. de Vlaming, V. Connor, N. Richard, and R. S. Tjeerdema. 2003. Ecotoxicologic impacts of agricultural drain water in the Salinas River, California, USA. *Environmental Toxicology and Chemistry* 22:2375-2384.

Anderson, B., B. Phillips, J. Hunt, K. Siegler, J. Voorhees, K. Smalling, K. Kuivila, M. Hamilton, J. A. Ranasinghe, and R. Tjeerdema. 2014. Impacts of pesticides in a Central California estuary. *Environmental Monitoring and Assessment* 186(3):1801-1814.

Aneja, V. P., P. A. Roelle, G. C. Murray, J. Southerland, J. W. Erisman, D. Fowler, W. A. H. Asman, and N. Patni. 2001. Atmospheric nitrogen compounds II: Emissions, transport, transformation, deposition and assessment. *Atmospheric Environment* 35:1903-1911.

Aneja, V. P., W. H. Schlesinger, and J. W. Erisman. 2008. Farming pollution. *Nature Geoscience* 1(7):409-411.

Aneja, V. P., W. H. Schlesinger, and J. W. Erisman. 2009. Effects of agriculture upon the air quality and climate: Research, policy, and regulations. *Environmental Science and Technology* 43(12):4234-4240.

Arnold, J. G., R. Srinivasan, R. S. Muttiah, and J. R. Williams. 1998. Large area hydrologic modeling and assessment—Part I, model development. *Journal of the American Water Resources Association* 34(1):73-89.

Atzberger, C. 2013. Advances in remote sensing of agriculture: Context description, existing operational monitoring systems and major information needs. *Remote Sensing* 5:949-981.

Barbour, M. T., J. Gerritsen, B. D. Snyder, and J. B. Stribling. 1999. *Rapid bioassessment protocols for use in streams and wadeable rivers: Periphyton, benthic macroinvertebrates and fish*, 2nd ed. EPA 841-B-99-002. Washington, DC: U.S. Environmental Protection Agency, Office of Water.

Battagliese, T., J. Andrade, I. Schulze, B. Uhlman, and C. Barcan. 2013. *More sustainable beef optimization project: Phase 1 final report*. Florham Park, NJ: BASF Corporation.

Beckie, H. J. 2006. Herbicide-resistant weeds: Management tactics and practices. *Weed Technology* 20:793-814.

Blackshaw, R. E. 1994. Rotation affects downy brome (*Bromus tectorum*) in winter wheat (*Triticum aestivum*). *Weed Technology* 8:728-732.

Blaikie, P., and H. Brookfield. 1987. The degradation of common property resources. In *Land degradation and society*, edited by P. Blaikie and H. Brookfield. London, UK: Methuen. Pp. 186-207.

Bockstaller, C., and P. Girardin. 2003. How to validate environmental indicators. *Agricultural Systems* 76:639-653.

Bottrell, D. R. 1979. *Integrated pest management*. Washington, DC: Council on Environmental Quality.

Bradman, A., R. Castorina, D. Boyd Barr, J. Chevrier, M. E. Harnly, E. A. Eisen, T. E. McKone, K. Harley, N. Holland, and B. Eskenazi. 2011. Determinants of organophosphorus pesticide urinary metabolite levels in young children living in an agricultural community. *International Journal of Environmental Research and Public Health* 8(4):1061-1083.

Buzby, J. C., H. F. Wells, and J. Bentley. 2013. ERS's food loss data help inform the food waste discussion. *Amber Waves* June 2013. http://www.ers.usda.gov/amber-waves/2013-june/ers-food-loss-data-help-inform-the-food-waste-discussion.aspx#.U1lc2sfqIzE (accessed November 25, 2014).

Capper, J. L. 2011. The environmental impact of beef production in the United States: 1977 compared with 2007. *Journal of Animal Science* 89(12):4249-4261.

Capper, J. L., R. A. Cady, and D. E. Bauman. 2009. The environmental impact of dairy production: 1944 compared with 2007. *Journal of Animal Science* 87(6):2160-2167.

Carignan, V., and M. A. Villard. 2002. Selecting indicator species to monitor ecological integrity: A review. *Environmental Monitoring and Assessment* 78:45-61.

Cassidy, E. S., P. C. West, J. S. Gerber, and J. A. Foley. 2013. Redefining agricultural yields: From tonnes to people nourished per hectare. *Environmental Research Letters* 8(3):1-8.

Coase, R. 1960. On the problems of social cost. *Journal of Law and Economics* 3:1-44.

Cooley, D., and L. Olander. 2012. Stacking ecosystem services payments: Risks and solutions. *Environmental Law Reporter* 42(2):10150-10165.

Cruse, R. M., S. Lee, T. E. Fenton, E. Wang, and J. Laflen. 2013. Soil renewal and sustainability. In *Principles of sustainable soil management in agroecosystems*, edited by R. Lal and B. A. Stewart. Boca Raton, FL: CRC Press. Pp. 477-500.

den Biggelaar, C., R. Lal, R. K. Wiebe, H. Eswaran, V. Breneman, and P. Reich. 2004. The global impact of soil erosion on productivity. Effects on crop yields and production over time. *Advances in Agronomy* 81:49-95.

Di Prisco, G., V. Cavaliere, D. Annoscia, P. Varricchio, E. Caprio, F. Nazzi, G. Gargiulo, and F. Pennacchio. 2013. Neonicotinoid clothianidin adversely affects insect immunity and promotes replication of a viral pathogen in honeybees. *Proceedings of the National Academy of Sciences of the United States of America* (46):18466-18471.

Ding, Y., A. D. Harwood, H. M. Foslund, and M. J. Lydy. 2010. Distribution and toxicity of sediment-associated pesticides in urban and agricultural waterways from Illinois, USA. *Environmental Toxicology and Chemistry* 99(1):149-157.

Dobrowolski, J. P., and M. P. O'Neill. 2005. *Agricultural water security listening session final report*. Washington, DC: U.S. Department of Agriculture Research Education and Economics.

Dobrowolski, J., M. O'Neill, L. Duriancik, and J. Throwe. 2008. *Opportunities and challenges in agricultural water reuse: Final report*. Washington, DC: U.S. Department of Agriculture Cooperative State Research, Education, and Extension Service.

Domagalski, J. L., D. P. Weston, M. Zhang, and M. Hladik. 2010. Pyrethroid insecticide concentrations and toxicity in streambed sediments and loads in surface waters of the San Joaquin Valley, California, USA. *Environmental Toxicology and Chemistry* 29(4):813-823.

Dutcher, J. D. 2007. A review of resurgence and replacement causing pest outbreaks in IPM. In *General concepts in integrated pest and disease management*, edited by A. Ciancio and K.G. Mukerji. Dordrecht, The Netherlands: Springer. Pp. 27-43.

Eckschmitt, K., T. Stierhof, J. Dauber, K. Kreimes, and V. Wolters. 2003. On the quality of soil biodiversity indicators: Abiotic and biotic parameters as predictors of soil faunal richness at different spatial scales. *Agriculture Ecosystems and Environment* 98:273-283.

EPA (U.S. Environmental Protection Agency). 2008. *National air quality: Status and trends through 2007*. Washington, DC: EPA. http://www.epa.gov/air/airtrends/2008/report/TrendsReportfull.pdf (accessed March 1, 2014).

EPA. 2009a. *National ambient air quality standards (NAAQS)*. Washington, DC: EPA. http://epa.gov/air/criteria.html (accessed March 1, 2014).

EPA. 2009b. *National water quality inventory: Report to Congress. 2004 Reporting cycle*. EPA 841-R-08-001. Washington, DC: EPA.

EPA. 2011. *Reactive nitrogen in the United States–an analysis of inputs, flows, consequences, and management options*. EPA-SAB-11-013. Washington, DC: EPA. http://yosemite.epa.gov/sab/sabproduct.nsf/WebBOARD/INCSupplemental?OpenDocument (accessed November 25, 2014).

EPA. 2013. *Inventory of U.S. greenhouse gas emissions and sinks: 1990-2011*. EPA 430-R-13-001. Washington, DC: EPA. http://www.epa.gov/climatechange/Downloads/ghgemissions/US-GHG-Inventory-2013-Main-Text.pdf (accessed November 25, 2014).

EPA. 2014. *An introduction to indoor air quality. Volatile organic compounds (VOCs)*. http://www.epa.gov/iaq/voc.html#Health_Effects (accessed November 25, 2014).

ERS (Economic Research Service). 2013. *Irrigation and water use*. Washington, DC: U.S. Department of Agriculture Economic Research Service. http://www.ers.usda.gov/topics/farm-practices-management/irrigation-water-use.aspx#.Us8MH_a6X2A (accessed November 25, 2014).

ERS. 2014. *Corn*. Washington, DC: U.S. Department of Agriculture, Economic Research Service. http://www.ers.usda.gov/topics/crops/corn/background.aspx#.U1liscfqIzF (accessed November 25, 2014).

Fargione, J., J. Hill, D. Tilman, S. Polasky, and P. Hawthorne. 2008. Land clearing and the biofuel carbon debt. *Science* 319:1235-1238.

Fenske, R. A., C. Lu, C. L. Curl, J. H. Shirai, and J. C. Kissel. 2005. Biologic monitoring to characterize organophosphate pesticide exposure among children and workers: An analysis of recent studies in Washington State. *Environmental Health Perspectives* 113(11):1651-1657.

Fenton, T. E., M. Kazemi, and M. A. Lauterbach-Barrett. 2005. Erosional impact on organic matter content and productivity of selected Iowa soils. *Soil and Tillage Research* 81:163-171.

Foley, J. A. 2013. It's time to rethink America's corn system. *Scientific American* March 2013. http://www.scientificamerican.com/article.cfm?id=time-to-rethink-corn (accessed November 25, 2014).

Foley, J. A., N. Ramankutty, K. A. Brauman, E. S. Cassidy, J. S. Gerber, M. Johnston, N. D. Mueller, C. O'Connell, D. K. Ray, P. C. West, C. Balzer, E. M. Bennett, S. R. Carpenter, J. Hill, C. Monfreda, S. Polasky, J. Rockstrom, J. Sheehan, S. Siebert, D. Tilman, and D. P. M. Zaks. 2011. Solutions for a cultivated planet. *Nature* 478:337-342.

Garnache, C., and R. Howitt. 2011. *Species conservation on a working landscape: The joint production of wildlife and crops in the Yolo Bypass floodplain.* Selected paper, annual meeting of the Agricultural and Applied Economics Association, Pittsburgh, PA, July 24-26. http://purl.umn.edu/103973 (accessed November 25, 2014).

Gassman, P. W., J. R. Williams, V. W. Benson, R. C. Izaurralde, L. M. Hauck, C. A. Jones, J. D. Atwood, J. R. Kiniry, and J. D. Flowers. 2005. *Historical development and applications of the EPIC and APEX models.* Working Paper 05-WP 397. Ames: Center for Agriculture and Rural Development, Iowa State University.

Gilliom, R. J. 2007. Pesticides in U.S. streams and groundwater. *Environmental Science and Technology* 41(10):3408-3414.

Gilliom, R. J., J. E. Barbash, C. G. Crawford, P. A. Hamilton, J. D. Martin, N. Nakagaki, L. H. Nowell, J. C. Scott, P. E. Stackelberg, G. P. Thelin, and D. M. Wolock. 2006. *The quality of our nation's waters: Pesticides in the nation's streams and ground water, 1992-2001.* Circular 1291. Reston, VA: U.S. Department of Interior and U.S. Geological Survey. http://pubs.usgs.gov/circ/2005/1291 (accessed November 25, 2014).

Gordon, L. M., S. J. Bennett, C. V. Alonso, and R. L. Binger. 2008. Modeling long-term soil losses on agricultural fields due to ephemeral gully erosion. *Journal of Soil and Water Conservation* 63:173-181.

Greene, C. R. 2001. *U.S. organic farming emerges in the 1990s: Adoption of certified systems.* Agriculture Information Bulletin No. 770. Washington, DC: U.S. Department of Agriculture, Economic Research Service, Resource Economics Division.

Grube, A., D. Donaldson, T. Kiely, and L. Wu. 2011. *Pesticide industry sales and usage: 2006 and 2007 market estimates.* Washington, DC: U.S. Environmental Protection Agency. http://www.epa.gov/opp00001/pestsales/07pestsales/market_estimates2007.pdf (accessed November 25, 2014).

Hanks, J., and J. T. Ritchie. 1991. *Modeling plant and soil systems.* Madison, WI: Society of Agronomy, Crop Science Society of America, and Soil Science Society of America.

Hanley, N., S. Banerjee, G. D. Lennox, and P. R. Armsworth. 2012. How should we incentivize private landowners to "produce" more biodiversity? *Oxford Review of Economic Policy* 28(1):93-113.

Hayes, T. B., A. Collins, M. Lee, M. Mendoza, N. Noriega, A. A. Stuart, and A. Vonk. 2002. Hermaphroditic, demasculinized frogs after exposure to the herbicide atrazine at low ecologically relevant doses. *Proceedings of the National Academy of Sciences of the United States of America* 99:5476-5480.

Hayes, T. B., P. Falso, S. Gallipeau, and M. Stice. 2010. The cause of global amphibian declines: A developmental endocrinologist's perspective. *Journal of Experimental Biology* 213:921-933.

Heap, I. 2014. *International Survey of Herbicide Resistant Weeds. Weeds resistant to EPSP synthase inhibitors (G/9).* http://www.weedscience.org/summary/MOA.aspx?MOAID=12 (accessed November 25, 2014).

Heathcote, A. J., C. T. Filstrup, and J. A. Downing. 2013. Watershed sediment losses to lakes accelerating despite agricultural soil conservation efforts. *PLoS ONE* 8(1):e53554.

Helmers, M. J., X. Zhou, H. Asbjornsen, R. Kolka, M. D. Tomer, and R. M. Cruse. 2012. Sediment removal by prairie filter strips in row-cropped ephemeral watersheds. *Journal of Environmental Quality* 41:1531-1539.

Henry, M., M. Beguin, F. Requier, O. Rollin, J.-F. Odoux, P. Aupinel, J. Aptel, S. Tchamitchian, and A. Decourtye. 2012. A common pesticide decreases foraging success and survival in honey bees. *Science* 336:348-350.

Hertel, T. W., W. E. Tyner, and D. K. Birur. 2010. The global impacts of biofuel mandates. *Energy Journal* 31(1):75-100.

Hunt, J. W., B. S. Anderson, B. M. Phillips, P. N. Nicely, R. S. Tjeerdema, H. M. Puckett, M. Stephenson, K. Worcester, and V. de Vlaming. 2003. Ambient toxicity due to chlorpyrifos and diazinon in a central California coastal watershed. *Environmental Monitoring and Assessment* 82(1):83-112.

IPCC (Intergovernmental Panel on Climate Change). 2013. *Fifth assessment report: Climate change 2013*. http://www.ipcc.ch/report/ar5 (accessed November 25, 2014).

Konikow, L. F. 2013. *Groundwater depletion in the United States (1900–2008). Scientific Investigations Report*. Reston, VA: U.S. Department of the Interior, U.S. Geological Survey. http://pubs.usgs.gov/sir/2013/5079/SIR2013-5079.pdf (accessed November 25, 2014).

Larson, S. J., R. J. Gilliom, and P. D. Capel. 1999. *Pesticides in streams of the United States—initial results from the National Water-Quality Assessment Program*. U.S. Geological Survey Water-Resources Investigations Report No. 98-4222. Sacramento, CA: U.S. Geological Survey.

Li, C. S., W. Salas, R. H. Zhang, C. Krauter, A. Rotz, and F. Mitloehner. 2012. Manure-DNDC: A biogeochemical process model for quantifying greenhouse gas and ammonia emissions from livestock manure systems. *Nutrient Cycling in Agroecosystems* 93(2):163-200.

Lindenmayer, D. B., and G. E. Likens. 2011. Direct measurement versus surrogate indicator species for evaluating environmental change and biodiversity loss. *Ecosystems* 14:47-59.

Loewenherz, C., R. A. Fenske, N. J. Simcox, G. Bellamy, and D. Kalman. 1997. Biological monitoring of organophospate pesticide exposure among children of agricultural workers in central Washington State. *Environmental Health Perspectives* 105(12):1344-1353.

Losey, J. E., and M. Vaughan. 2006. The economic value of ecological services provided by insects. *Bioscience* 56:311-323.

Lund, J., E. Hanak, W. Fleenor, W. Bennett, R. Howitt, J. Mount, and P. Moyle. 2008. *Comparing futures for the Sacramento-San Joaquin Delta*. San Francisco: Public Policy Institute of California. http://www.ppic.org/content/pubs/report/R_708EHR.pdf (accessed November 25, 2014).

Ma, S., S. M. Swinton, F. Lupi, and C. B. Jolejole-Foreman. 2012. Farmers' willingness to participate in payment-for-environmental-services programmes. *Journal of Agricultural Economics* 63(3):604-626.

Magdoff, F., and H. van Es. 2009. *Building soils for better crops: Sustainable soil management*, 3rd ed. Waldorf, MD: U.S. Department of Agriculture, Sustainable Agriculture Research and Education Program.

McSwiney, C. P., and G. P. Robertson. 2005. Nonlinear response of N_2O flux to incremental fertilizer addition in a continuous maize (*Zea mays* L.) cropping system. *Global Change Biology* 11(10):1712-1719.

Meade, J. E. 1952. External economies and diseconomies in a competitive situation. *The Economic Journal* 62(245):54-67.

Michalak, A. M., E. J. Anderson, D. Beletsky, S. Boland, N. S. Bosch, T. B. Bridgeman, J. D. Chaffin, K. Cho, R. Confesor, I. Daloğlu, J. V. DePinto, M. A. Evans, G. L. Fahnenstiel, L. He, J. C. Ho, L. Jenkins, T. H. Johengen, K. C. Kuo, E. LaPorte, X. Liu, M. R. McWilliams, M. R. Moore, D. J. Posselt, R. P. Richards, D. Scavia, A. L. Steiner, E. Verhamme, D. M. Wright, and M. A. Zagorski. 2013. Record-setting algal bloom in Lake Erie caused by agricultural and meteorological trends consistent with expected future conditions. *Proceedings of the National Academy of Sciences of the United States of America* 110(16):6448-6452.

Mineau, P. 2002. Bird impacts. In *Encyclopedia of pest management*, edited by D. Pimentel. New York: Marcel Dekker. Pp. 101-103.

Montgomery, D. R. 2007. Soil erosion and agricultural sustainability. *Proceedings of the National Academy of Sciences of the United States of America* 104:13268-13272.

Mortensen, D. A., J. F. Egan, B. D. Maxwell, M. R. Ryan, and R. G. Smith. 2012. Navigating a critical juncture for sustainable weed management. *Bioscience* 62:75-84.

Nazarko, O. M., R. C. van Acker, and M. H. Entz. 2005. Strategies and tactics for herbicide use reduction in field crops in Canada: A review. *Canadian Journal of Plant Science* 85:457-479.

Nickerson, C., R. Ebel, A. Borchers, and F. Corriazo. 2011. *Major uses of land in the United States, 2007*. Economic Information Bulletin No. (EIB-89). Washington, DC: U.S. Department of Agriculture, Economic Research Service. http://www.ers.usda.gov/publications/eib-economic-information-bulletin/eib89.aspx#.UtQZsPa6X2A (accessed November 25, 2014).

Norris, P. E., D. B. Schweikhardt, and E. A. Scorsone. 2008. The instituted nature of market information. In *Alternative institutional structures: Evolution and impact*, edited by S. S. Batie and N. Mercuro. London, UK: Routledge. Pp. 330-348.

NRC (National Research Council). 1996. *Ecologically based pest management: New solutions for a new century*. Washington, DC: National Academy Press.

NRCS (Natural Resources Conservation Service). 2013. *Summary report: 2010 National resources inventory*. Washington, DC: Natural Resources Conservation Service. http://www.nrcs.usda.gov/Internet/FSE_DOCUMENTS/stelprdb1167354.pdf (accessed November 25, 2014).

Parton, W. J., D. S. Schimel, C. V. Cole, and D. S. Ojima. 1987. Analysis of factors controlling soil organic-matter levels in Great Plains grasslands. *Soil Science Society of America Journal* 51(5):1173-1179.

Peoples, M. B., D. F. Herridge, and J. K. Ladha. 1995. Biological nitrogen fixation: An efficient source of nitrogen for sustainable agricultural production? *Plant and Soil* 174:3-28.

Pettis, J. S., D. van Engelsdorp, J. Johnson, and G. Dively. 2012. Pesticide exposure in honey bees results in increased levels of the gut pathogen *Nosema*. *Naturwissenschaften* 99:153-158.

Pimentel, D., P. Hepperly, J. Hanson, D. Douds, and R. Seidel. 2005. Environmental, energetic, and economic comparisons of organic and conventional farming systems. *Bioscience* 55:573-582.

Pinder, R. W., P. J. Adams, and S. N. Pandis. 2007. Ammonia emission controls as a cost-effective strategy for reducing atmospheric particulate matter in the eastern United States. *Environmental Science and Technology* 41:380-386.

Pope, C. A. III, M. Ezzati, and D. W. Dockery. 2009. Fine-particulate air pollution and life expectancy in the United States. *New England Journal of Medicine* 360:376-386.

Potts, S. G., J. C. Biesmeijer, C. Kremen, P. Neumann, O. Schweiger, and W. E. Kunin. 2010. Global pollinator declines: Trends, impacts, and drivers. *Trends in Ecology and Evolution* 25(6):345-353.

Power, A. G. 2010. Ecosystem services and agriculture: Tradeoffs and synergies. *Philosophical Transactions of the Royal Society, Series B* 365:2959-2971.

Ragsdale, D. W., D. A. Landis, J. Brodeur, G. E. Heimpel, and N. Desneux. 2011. Ecology and management of the soybean aphid in North America. *Annual Review of Entomology* 56:375-399.

Rivera-Ferre, M. G., M. Ortega-Cerda, and J. Baugartner. 2013. Rethinking study and management of agricultural systems for policy design. *Sustainability* 5:3858-3875.

Robertson, G. P., and S. M. Swinton. 2005. Reconciling agricultural productivity and environmental integrity: A grand challenge for agriculture. *Frontiers in Ecology and the Environment* 3(1):38-46.

Rohr, J. R., and K. A. McCoy. 2010. A qualitative meta-analysis reveals consistent effects of atrazine on freshwater fish and amphibians. *Environmental Health Perspectives* 118:20-32.

Rotz, C. A., F. Montes, and D. S. Chianese. 2010. The carbon footprint of dairy production systems through a partial lifecycle assessment. *Journal of Dairy Science* 93:1266-1282.

Scanlon, B. R., C. C. Faunt, L. Longuevergne, R. C. Reedy, W. M. Alley, V. L. McGuire, and P. B. McMahon. 2012. Groundwater depletion and sustainability of irrigation in the US High Plains and Central Valley. *Proceedings of the National Academy of Sciences of the United States of America* 109:9320-9325.

Schaible, G. D., and M. P. Aillery. 2012. *Water conservation in irrigated agriculture: Trends and challenges in the face of emerging demands.* Economic Information Bulletin No. (EIB-99). Washington, DC: U.S. Department of Agriculture, Economic Research Service.

Schmid, A. A. 2004. *Conflict and cooperation: Institutional and behavioral economics.* Oxford, UK: Blackwell.

Schneider, U. A., B. A. McCarl, and E. Schmid. 2007. Agricultural sector analysis on greenhouse gas mitigation in U.S. agriculture and forestry. *Agricultural Systems* 94:128-140.

Searchinger, T., R. Heimlich, R. A. Houghton, F. Dong, A. Elobeid, J. Fabiosa, S. Tokgoz, D. Hayes, and T. Yu. 2008. Use of U.S. croplands for biofuels increases greenhouse gases through emissions from land-use change. *Science* 319:1238-1240.

Secchi, S., L. Kurkalova, P. W. Gassman, and C. Hart. 2010. Land use change in a biofuels hotspot: The case of Iowa. *Biomass and Bioenergy* 35:2391-2400.

Segerson, K. 2013. When is reliance on voluntary approaches in agriculture likely to be effective? *Applied Economic Perspectives and Policy* 35(4):565-592.

Shaw, S. L., F. M. Mitloehner, W. Jackson, E. J. DePeters, J. G. Fadel, P. H. Robinson, R. Holzinger, and A. H. Goldstein. 2007. Volatile organic compound emissions from dairy cows and their waste as measured by proton-transfer-reaction mass spectrometry. *Environmental Science and Technology* 41:1310-1316.

Shcherbak, I., N. Millar, and G. P. Robertson. 2014. Global metaanalysis of the nonlinear response of soil nitrous oxide (N_2O) emissions to fertilizer nitrogen. *Proceedings of the National Academy of Sciences of the United States of America* 111(25):9199-9204.

Smith, H. F., and C. A. Sullivan. 2014. Ecosystem services within agricultural landscapes—farmers' perceptions. *Ecological Economics* 98:72-80.

Steward, D. R., P. J. Bruss, X. Y. Yang, S. A. Staggenborg, S. M. Welch, and M. D. Apley. 2013. Tapping unsustainable groundwater stores for agricultural production in the High Plains Aquifer of Kansas, projections to 2110. *Proceedings of the National Academy of Sciences of the United States of America* 110(37): E3477-E3486.

Swinton, S. M., F. Lupi, G. P. Robertson, and S. Hamilton. 2007. Ecosystem services and agriculture: Cultivating agricultural ecosystems for diverse benefits. *Ecological Economics* 64(2):245-252.

USDA (U.S. Department of Agriculture). 2008. *User's reference guide: Revised Universal Soil Loss Equation Version 2 (RUSLE2).* Washington, DC: USDA/Agricultural Research Service.

USDA. 2009. *2007 Census of agriculture farm and ranch irrigation survey (2008)*. Washington, DC: U.S. Department of Agriculture, National Agricultural Statistics Service. http://www.agcensus.usda.gov/Publications/2007/Online_Highlights/Farm_and_Ranch_Irrigation_Survey/fris08.pdf (accessed November 25, 2014).

USDA. 2012. *Water erosion prediction project (WEPP)*. Washington, DC: USDA/Agricultural Research Service. http://www.ars.usda.gov/Research/docs.htm?docid=10621 (accessed November 25, 2014).

USDA. 2014a. *Agricultural Act of 2014: Highlights and implications*. http://www.ers.usda.gov/agricultural-act-of-2014-highlights-and-implications.aspx#.VAsz-BaNaul (accessed November 25, 2014).

USDA. 2014b. *2012 Census of agriculture. United States*. Washington, DC: USDA.

USGS (U.S. Geological Survey). 2014. *Pesticide national synthesis project: Glyphosate*. Reston, VA: U.S. Geological Survey, National Water-Quality Assessment Program. http://water.usgs.gov/nawqa/pnsp/usage/maps/show_map.php?year=2011&map=GLYPHOSATE&hilo=L&disp=Glyphosate (accessed November 25, 2014).

Vandenberg, L. N., T. Colborn, T. B. Hayes, J. J. Heindel, D. R. Jacobs, Jr., D. H. Lee, T. Shioda, A. M. Soto, F. S. vom Saal, W. V. Welshons, R. T. Zoeller, and J. P. Myers. 2012. Hormones and endocrine-disrupting chemicals: Low-dose effects and nonmonotonic dose responses. *Endocrine Reviews* 33:378-455.

Wakatsuki, T., and A. Rasyidin. 1992. Rates of weathering and soil formation. *Geoderma* 52:251-262.

Waldman, K. B., and J. M. Kerr. 2014. Limitations of certification and supply chain standards for environmental protection in commodity crop production. *Annual Review of Resource Economics* 6(1):429-449.

Weersink, A., S. Jeffrey, and D. J. Pannell. 2002. Farm-level modeling for bigger issues. *Review of Agricultural Economics* 24(1):123-140.

Weston, D. P., Y. Ding, M. Zhang, and M. J. Lydy. 2013. Identifying the cause of sediment toxicity in agricultural sediments: The role of pyrethroids and nine seldom-measured hydrophobic pesticides. *Chemosphere* 90:958-964.

Woodward, R. T. 2011. Double-dipping in environmental markets. *Journal of Environmental Economics and Management* 61(2):153-169.

Zhan, Y., and M. Zhang. 2012. PURE: A web-based decision support system to evaluate pesticide environmental risk for sustainable pest management practices in California. *Ecotoxicology and Environmental Safety* 82:104-113.

Zhan, Y., and M. Zhang. 2014. Spatial and temporal patterns of pesticide use on California almonds and associated risks to the surrounding environment. *Science of the Total Environment* 472:517-529.

Zhang, W., T. H. Ricketts, C. Kremen, K. Carney, and S. Swinton. 2007. Ecosystem services and dis-services to agriculture. *Ecological Economics* 64(2):253-260.

5

Social and Economic Effects of the U.S. Food System

As with the environmental and health indicators discussed in earlier chapters, most social and economic outcomes reflect complex causal processes, and they can vary widely based on time period, spatial organization, market conditions, regulatory forces, and adaptive mechanisms of actors in the system. In this section, we outline major classes of social and economic effects that can be linked to characteristics of the U.S. food system and present summary information about the overall performance of the system. We focus on three broad classes of social and economic effects:

- Levels of income, wealth, and distributional equity;
- Broader indicators of quality of life, such as working conditions, job satisfaction, and freedom of choice to pursue taste and lifestyle preferences; and
- Associated impacts on worker health and well-being.

Affected individuals fall into three groups: (1) people involved directly in agricultural food production (e.g., farmers); (2) people involved in the rest of the food system (e.g., processing, manufacturing, food service, and retailing); and (3) consumers. Food production, processing, and availability also can affect community-level measures, such as economic growth and social infrastructure.

Although social and economic dimensions of effects are distinct, they are more closely interrelated than other dimensions. For this reason, we are presenting them in one chapter. This chapter begins with an overview of the social and economic impacts of the food system on key sectors of the food system. To discuss these impacts, select data sources and metrics are described. Tables B-1 through B-4 in Appendix B provide more details on these data sources. The committee has focused in this chapter on market-based economic effects, including measurable changes in the financial well-being of key actors in the food system and broader indicators of market performance by sector (e.g., output, efficiency), but it did not attempt to estimate non-market economic values for social impacts. However, a discussion of non-market valuation methods for environmental effects is included in Chapter 4. In addition, while the chapter identifies the importance of capturing differential impacts on distinct social groups (e.g., women, minorities, immigrants), the committee did not review the moral and ethical or legal aspects of different outcomes. Consideration of whether particular types of social and economic effects are better than others should be guided by the best available information about those effects and by the cultural, political, and ethical views of stakeholders and decision makers.

POTENTIAL SOCIAL AND ECONOMIC EFFECTS ON THE FOOD PRODUCTION SECTOR

Income, Wealth, and Distributional Equity

The food production sector includes farmers, ranchers, fishers, hired workers, their family members, and residents in the communities in which these individuals reside (primarily, but not exclusively, rural or small town). Occupations in this sector involve planting, caring for, and harvesting raw food items, livestock, and seafood (FCWA, 2012). About 40 percent of the U.S. land area is used for farming, with 2.1 million farm operations generating nearly $400 billion in sales (55 percent from crops and 45 percent from livestock) and more than $100 billion in net farm income in 2013 (ERS, 2014i; USDA, 2014b).

Taken as a whole, the U.S. farm sector has experienced remarkable growth in output, rising by 2.5 times over the past 60 years (see Figure 5-1). More impressive is the fact that this growth in output has occurred with relatively little increase in the total combined use of factor inputs (capital, labor, purchased inputs) (Wang and Ball, 2014). The increase in output can be attributed mostly to an increase in the quality of labor, capital, and technology inputs. As a result the "factor productivity" (the amount of output per unit of input) of U.S. farming has grown by an average of 1.49 percent per year since 1948 (ERS, 2014a), although it has slowed noticeably during the past 20 years, declining to significantly less than 1 percent over the most recent decade. Declines in the rate of productivity increase have been linked to reductions in agricultural research investments (particularly by the

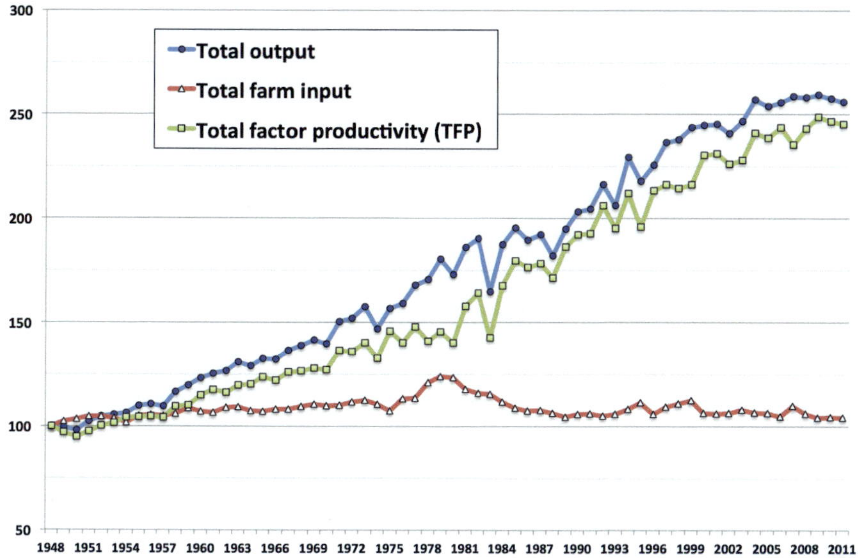

FIGURE 5-1 Indexes of total farm output, input use, and factor productivity in the United States, 1948-2011.
SOURCES: ERS, 2014a; Wang and Ball, 2014.

public sector) and possible biological yield plateaus of major agricultural crops (Alston et al., 2009).

Interestingly, the mix of inputs used to produce growth in food output has changed dramatically since the mid-20th century (see Figure 5-2). Specifically, the use of labor has declined by nearly 80 percent, the use of capital inputs has remained roughly the same (a decrease of 12 percent), and the use of purchased variable inputs has more than doubled. The mix of capital inputs has also shifted, with land inputs slowly declining throughout the past 60 years but the importance of capital equipment growing rapidly through the 1970s, then declining in importance in the latter 20th century. Finally, the use of fertilizer accounts for a significant portion of the increased use of purchased inputs—growing nearly three-fold by the mid-1970s and then remaining at that level (with significant annual fluctuations) through 2011. It appears that the reduced impact in productivity growth from a decline in the use of labor and land inputs has been offset by the positive impact of increased use of other inputs (e.g., technology, computerization, fertilizer, pesticide).

Economic returns and competitiveness in U.S. agriculture are shaped

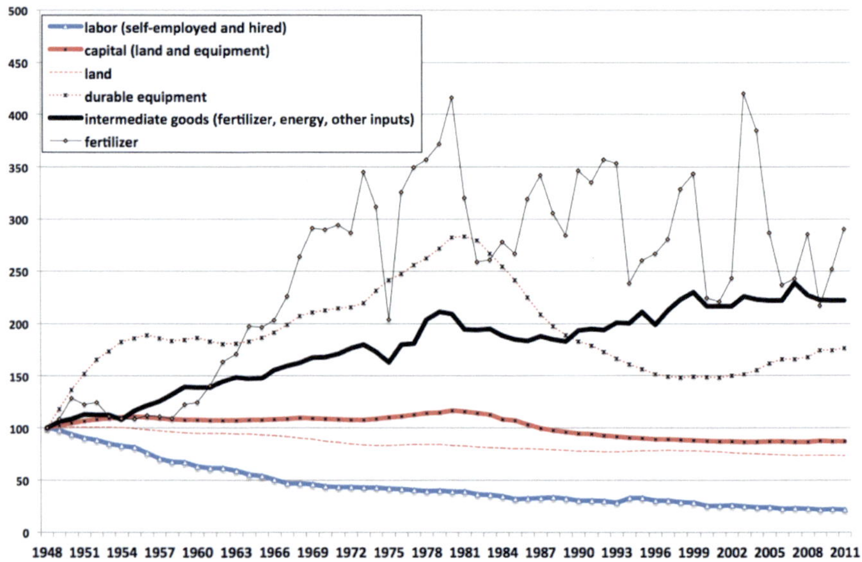

FIGURE 5-2 Index of use of different farm inputs by type in the United States, 1948-2011.
SOURCE: ERS, 2014a.

by heterogeneous public policies that support commodity prices, subsidize crop insurance, promote export markets, and influence labor and environmental practices (see Chapter 2). Public investments in infrastructure for energy, transportation, communication, price information, market coordination, financing opportunities, and tax benefits also shape farm sector performance. Public investments in basic and applied research throughout most of the 20th century have provided high rates of economic return to taxpayers and undergirded a period of rapid technological change and increases in productivity (Fuglie and Heisey, 2007; Kinsey, 2013).

Despite significant increases in total output and factor productivity over this period of time, after adjusting for inflation, aggregate net income in the U.S. farm sector has remained relatively stable over the past 40 years (see Figure 5-3). Because their largest asset is usually land, farm businesses have gained significant wealth over the past 50 years from capital gains associated with rising asset values that increased by 170 percent in real terms between 1960 and 2012.

The distribution of net farm income varies widely by farm type and

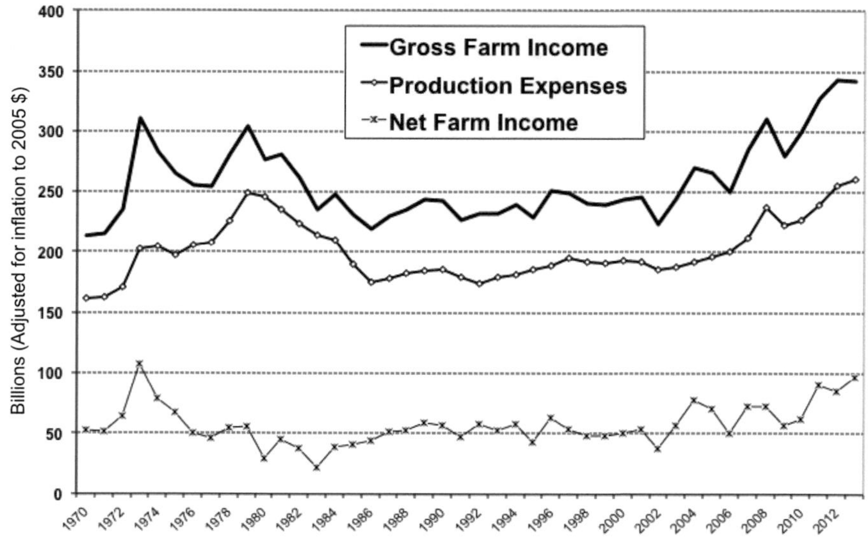

FIGURE 5-3 Inflation-adjusted value of gross farm sales, production expenses, and net farm income, 1970-2013.
SOURCE: ERS, 2014i.

farm size (O'Donoghue et al., 2011). The largest farms in the United States (with gross sales of more than $1 million) represented roughly 4 percent of operations in 2012 but generated about 66 percent of the total market sales of U.S. farm products and accounted for an even larger share of the aggregate total national net farm income in that year (USDA, 2014b).

As a group, farm-operator households have seen their economic well-being rise in recent decades, particularly relative to the average U.S. household (see Figure 5-4) (ERS, 2014b). However, these average statistics for the sector as a whole mask considerable variation among actual farm households and the fact that most farm households rely on off-farm income as the principle basis for household survival (see Figure 5-4). For instance, 57 percent of U.S. farm operations in 2012 had gross farm sales below $10,000, and these operations typically reported net losses from their farming business (USDA, 2014b). Some of these farms are operated as hobbies by urban dwellers who are employed in other occupations and rely on off-farm income (Fernandez-Cornejo, 2007; Hoppe et al., 2010). For farms with less than $250,000 in gross sales, nearly all of the roughly $70,000 gross average household income comes from off-farm employment and

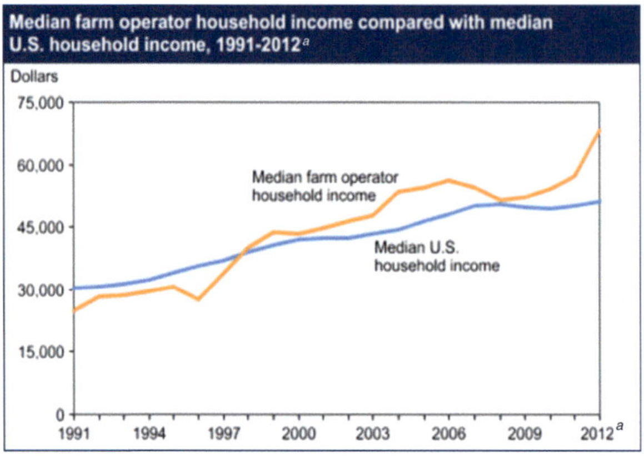

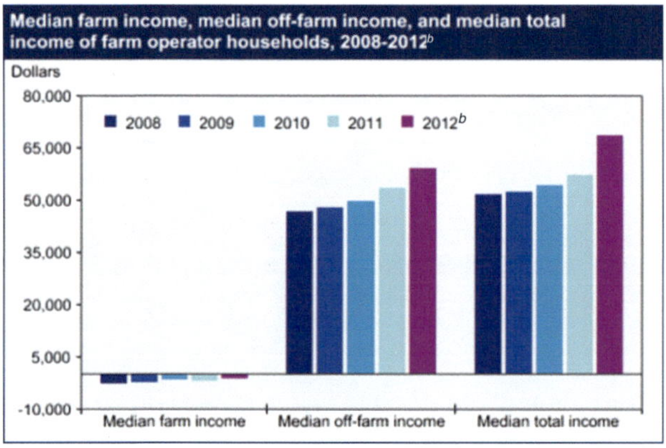

FIGURE 5-4 Farm operator household income and average household income of family farms.
NOTE: Data as of November 26, 2013.

[a] Differences between 2012 estimates and estimates from prior years reflect changes in survey methodology and implementation associated with the 2012 Agricultural Resource Management Survey in addition to changes in the economic situation of farm households. Source: USDA, Economic Research Service and National Agricultural Statistics Service, Agricultural Resource Management Survey and U.S. Census Bureau, Current Population Survey.

[b] Differences between 2012 estimates and estimates from prior years reflect changes in survey methodology and implementation associated with the 2012 Agricultural Resource Management Survey in addition to changes in the economic situation of farm households. Source: USDA, Economic Research Service and National Agricultural Statistics Service, Agricultural Resource Management Survey.
SOURCE: ERS, 2014b.

unearned income (Hoppe et al., 2010). In the latest estimates from the U.S. Department of Agriculture (USDA), roughly 60 percent of off-farm income in farm households comes from wages and salary payments to the operator or other adults in the household. Another 20 percent is derived from transfer payments (e.g., Social Security) or interest and dividends on investments. Most of the remaining portion is from non-farm business income (ERS, 2014b). By contrast, among commercial farms with gross sales greater than $350,000, the average farm household in 2012 made more than $200,000 in total income, with nearly 75 percent of this total accounted for by net farm income (ERS, 2014b).

As the U.S. food system has evolved, the overall efficiency and relative economic power of each subsector in the food supply chain has shifted (Marion, 1986; Reardon and Timmer, 2012; Sexton, 2000, 2013). As discussed in Chapter 2 (see Figure 2-5), the farming sector receives an average of 17 percent of the consumer food dollar as gross farm receipts, down from about 40 percent of consumer food spending in 1950 (Schnepf, 2013). The change primarily reflects the pronounced shift toward food consumed away from home (where a higher share of food expenditures cover the cost of preparation and service), but it also reflects an increased number and technical sophistication of processing and marketing channels between farmers and consumers. Although a smaller fraction of consumer food dollars flow into agriculture, the economic well-being of farm households has not always suffered. Large commercial farmers typically earn incomes higher than the average U.S. household, and many are wealthy. The largest and most technically sophisticated farming operations provide an increasingly large share of the nation's output, and they are better equipped to meet the demands of first line handlers and processors (as transaction costs are lower when larger volumes of consistent quality product can be acquired from fewer producers). However, changes in the structure of first-line handlers and processors can affect returns to some farmers. For example, in the highly consolidated meat and poultry industry, the processors/manufacturers can wield both monopsony and monopoly power. That is, they can set the prices they pay for supplies and the prices they charge for their products (MacDonald, 2008). In this sector, payment for farmers' product has evolved into a "tournament system" whereby poultry producers are paid according to their productivity relative to other farmers. In this system, farmers have much less certainty about the price they will receive at the end of a season (Leonard, 2014). Other concerns with increased concentration of market shares in the hands of few firms are the potential loss in competition and decline in the transparency of markets. In the meat packing sector, a small number of firms control most of the business and independent farmers (without production contracts from packing firms) can find it difficult to access open and competitive markets for their livestock

(Key and McBride, 2007; Marion and Geithman, 1995; McEowen et al., 2002). Recent reviews of the literature suggest that adverse impacts on meat prices or consumer welfare have been relatively small, but the distribution of economic returns among different-sized actors or segments of the food supply chain can be affected (Sexton, 2013; U.S. GAO, 2009).

Because many workers on U.S. farms are unpaid family members of farm operators, it is difficult to determine the exact number of people involved in production agriculture. The 2012 Census of Agriculture estimated 3.2 million self-described "operators" on the nation's 2.1 million farms (USDA, 2014b). Combined with unpaid family laborers and paid employees, a recent study by the University of Minnesota's Food Industry Center estimated a total of nearly 6 million workers in the farm sector, or 5 percent of the nation's work force (TFIC, 2014). By contrast, the Farm Labor Survey of the National Agricultural Statistics Service estimates that roughly 2 million self-employed operators and family members work on the nation's farms, and slightly more than 1 million people are hired non-family farm workers (ERS, 2013b).

Although hired workers are a minority of the overall farm workforce, many farm operators and family members do not work full time on their farms, and hired farm workers are now estimated to contribute nearly 60 percent of total full-time equivalent labor on U.S. farms (Martin and Jackson-Smith, 2013); their contributions are increasingly important (Henderson, 2012; O'Donoghue et al., 2011; Sommers and Franklin, 2012). Between 60 to 80 percent of hired farm workers are employed on crop farms, most are foreign born, and more than half are unauthorized to work in the United States (Martin, 2013; Wainer, 2011).

Hired farm workers in the United States tend to work for relatively low wages and for fewer days a year than most of the U.S. workforce, which has led to chronic levels of underemployment, unemployment, and poverty in many farm worker households. The vast majority of hired crop workers are engaged in the fruit, vegetable, and horticulture industries, where labor-intensive crop management practices are still widespread. In 2010, the average hired crop worker earned less than $10 per hour, and median weekly earnings were about two-thirds of the average U.S. wage or salary worker's (Martin and Jackson-Smith, 2013). As a result, poverty rates for farm workers are estimated at between 30 and 40 percent, among the highest of any occupational category in the United States (Pena, 2010; USDOL, 2005). Poverty rates for noncitizen farm laborers are even higher, nearly triple that of citizen farm workers (Kandel, 2008).

Quality of Life

Farm Owners

Because economic returns to agriculture have generally been volatile and below prevailing market rates of return to capital and labor (Cochrane, 1993), economists and sociologists have long sought to understand the motivation of farm operators to persist in farming (Gardner, 2002; Reinhardt and Barlett, 1989). Motivations to enter and remain in farming include a desire to maintain a family tradition, be one's own boss, work outdoors, and spend time with and teach work ethics to one's children (Barlett, 1993; Gasson and Errington, 1993).

Concern is growing, however, that the high capital costs and uncertain economic returns associated with modern agriculture have made it difficult for young farmers to successfully enter the sector. The average age of U.S. farmers has risen from 50 in 1978 to 58 in 2012, and a diminishing fraction of U.S. principal farm operators are younger than age 35 (see Figure 5-5) (USDA, 2014b). To some extent, this shifting demographic reflects the overall aging of the population, but it also results from a steady decline in the rate of new farm entry and the reduced number of transfers of family farm businesses across generations over the past 40 years.

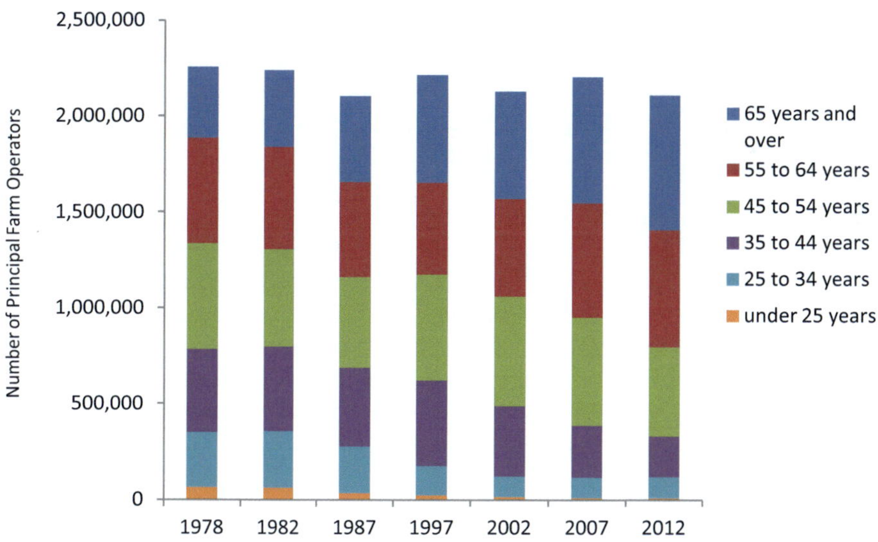

FIGURE 5-5 Age distribution of principal farm operators.
SOURCES: USDA, 2009, 2014b.

Although qualitative research on farm households in the United States consistently underscores the importance of quality of life outcomes to farm sector dynamics, quantitative indicators of positive quality of life effects on farmers and farm households are more difficult to find. One indicator is the degree of decision-making control that farmer operators have over day-to-day work allocation or production practices. A major example is the steady rise of contract production in U.S. agriculture, where production and marketing contracts now cover nearly 40 percent of U.S. production (MacDonald and Korb, 2011). In some livestock sectors—particularly beef cattle, hogs, and poultry—the vast majority of production is marketed under contract. The traditional spot market (non-negotiated) transactions by independent producers (Lawrence, 2010) has shifted to marketing contracts to highly consolidated meat packing industry and, eventually, to vertical integration (see Chapter 2 and below), which has both benefits and costs. Some of the benefits from vertical integration are higher efficiencies and a reliable supply of product (for the integrators) and more price certainty and aid with decisions about inputs and planting/management strategy (for the farmers). Other benefits or costs vary by contract (ERS, 1996). Farmers, however, have lost some entrepreneurial autonomy and decision-making power over assets due to unbalanced relationships in bargaining power with agribusiness firms (Stofferahn, 2006). For example, producers often assume most of the fixed capital investment costs, but they have less control over production practices and depend on the availability of future contracts to survive (MacDonald and Korb, 2008; MacDonald and McBride, 2009). In addition, independent farmers find it increasingly difficult to gain access to competitive cash markets for their products (Key and McBride, 2007; MacDonald and McBride, 2009; Marion and Geithman, 1995; Sexton, 2000; Ward, 2007).

Farm Workers

Hired farm laborers face particularly difficult working conditions and experience a quality of life that is well below that of most others in the U.S. population. Many farm workers live in substandard housing and have relatively little control over their work schedule or labor practices. About 15 percent of U.S. crop workers migrate from farm to farm to find continuous employment (Seattle Global Justice, 2014). This can disrupt family structure and educational experiences for children (Kandel, 2008).

As noted above, more than half of the farm worker population is foreign born, and many do not have legal permission to work in the United States. The insecure citizenship and immigration status of many farm workers often results in a lack of economic and political power and leaves them vulnerable to exploitation (Hall and Greenman, 2014). Estimates from the Bureau of Labor Statistics indicate that unions represent only 1.2 percent of all private-sector employees in agriculture and related industries, and 1.8 percent of employees in food service and beverage establishments (BLS, 2014c). Good estimates of the number of foreign born or illegal farm workers affiliated with unions are lacking, but groups such as the United Farm Workers of America, founded in 1962 by migrant farm laborer Cesar Chavez, are still organizing to improve working conditions and wages for farm workers.

Women and Racial/Ethnic Groups

According to the 2012 Census of Agriculture, almost 83 percent of "primary" farm operators in the United States are white and male (USDA, 2014b). However, women are the principal operators of another 14 percent of all U.S. farms, up from roughly 5 percent in 1982 (Hoppe and Korb, 2013). Moreover, when principal, secondary, and tertiary operators are counted, nearly 1 million women (of all races) were engaged in running U.S. farms in 2012 (30 percent of the total) (USDA, 2014b). The role of women in U.S. agriculture has always been significant, though their presence in official statistics has often underestimated their contributions because until recently the Census only enumerated characteristics of the primary farm operator on each farm (Hoppe and Korb, 2013).

Farmers from racial and ethnic groups that are historically underrepresented in farming have also shifted in recent years. Historically, the number of African American farmers and sharecroppers in the United States declined by 98 percent since 1920 (Banks, 1986), a trend that is linked to political, economic, and cultural discrimination (Wood and Gilbert, 2000). More recently, the number of farms owned by Hispanics, American Indians, African Americans, and Asians all increased over the number owned by each of these subpopulations in 2007 (USDA, 2014b). The number of Hispanic-owned farms, in particular, has increased by 21 percent between 2007 and 2012. Although the share of farms operated by women and these racial and ethnic groups has increased over time, many of these farms had sales below $50,000 (an indication of smaller farms) (USDA, 2014b). Specifically, the percentage of farms that made less than $50,000 was 91 percent for women-owned farms, 85 percent for Hispanic-owned farms, 92 percent for American Indian-owned farms, 94 percent for black-owned farms, and 65 percent for Asian-owned farms.

Rural Communities

The economic performance and quality of life for farm operators and hired farm workers can be an important contributor for community life and well-being, particularly in rural areas where farming is a major driver of local social and economic activity. Researchers know that rural communities that rely most heavily on farming for their local economic base are more likely to experience economic stagnation and population declines (Isserman et al., 2009). Growing farm size and specialization of production may be associated with declining local purchasing patterns and reduced landscape amenities that could attract non-farm development (Foltz et al., 2002; McGranahan and Sullivan, 2005). Traditionally, family farming systems with relatively equitable patterns of asset ownership and reliance on a family labor force have been linked to healthy dynamics in community social arenas and local businesses (Goldschmidt, 1978; Labao and Stofferahn, 2008; Lyson, 2004). Evidence also suggests that more diversified farming systems can generate ecological and aesthetic landscape benefits and increase reported quality of life (Deller et al., 2001; Flora, 1995; Santelmann et al., 2004).

Rural communities that host large farm worker populations often struggle to meet this group's unique social service and educational needs (Findeis et al., 2002). Farm worker towns in the Central Valley of California experience some of the lowest per capita income, poorest public services, and most stressed local fiscal conditions of any rural communities in America (Martin, 2009).

Health

Access to Health Care and Health Care Benefits

Farm operators and households Farm operators and their families, like millions of other Americans, deal with issues related to accessing affordable health care as well as health and safety considerations specific to this occupation. Patterns of health insurance coverage are changing for most individuals and families in the United States with implementation of the Patient Protection and Affordable Care Act (ACA).[1] Presumably, farm households that lacked access to affordable health insurance are now eligible to obtain coverage through the ACA. A comprehensive report by USDA found that before implementation of the ACA, 9.3 percent of all people living in farm-operator households did not have health insurance, a lower share than in the U.S. population as a whole (ERS, 2014j). Households where farming was the primary occupation, such as in the dairy industry, were the most likely to lack health insurance (ERS, 2014j). Farm households without

[1] Patient Protection and Affordable Care Act, Public Law 111-148, 111th Cong., 2nd session (March 23, 2010).

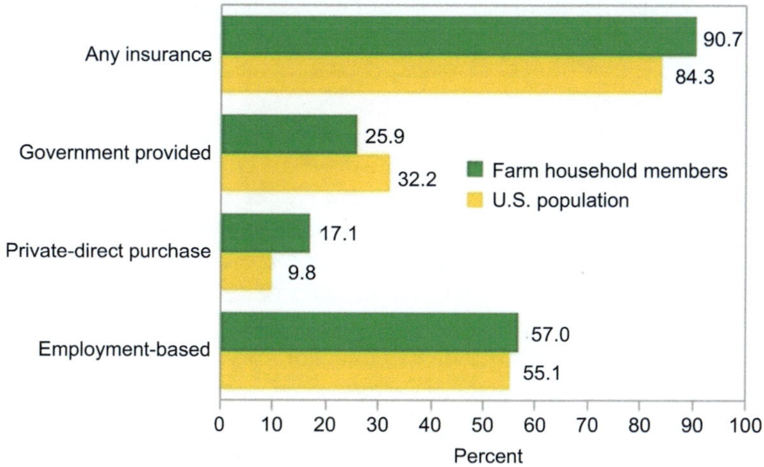

FIGURE 5-6 Source of health insurance coverage for farm and U.S. persons.
NOTE: Individuals may have more than one source of health insurance.
SOURCE: http://www.ers.usda.gov/data-products/chart-gallery/detailaspx?chartId=33728 (accessed November 24, 2014).

access to employer-sponsored health insurance (typically from non-farm work) paid an average of $6,000 annually in insurance premiums.

A large body of literature has documented unequal access to health care by individuals who live in rural areas (Murray et al., 2006; Probst et al., 2007; Syed et al., 2013). Because most farmers reside in rural areas, many of them must travel significant distances to interact with the medical system. Approximately 60 percent of farm-operator households are located in rural areas, which have known physician shortages (Jones et al., 2009b). According to data from the U.S. Department of Health and Human Services' Health Professional Shortage Areas, 17 percent of the farm population resides in shortage areas for primary care access (HRSA, 2014; Jones et al., 2009a). Dental and mental health care is also not easily accessible to farmers compared to the general population (Jones et al., 2009a). However, prior to the ACA, farm households had health insurance coverage at about the same rate as the general U.S. population (see Figure 5-6).

Farm laborers Migrant and seasonal farm workers are distinct worker populations: most migrant workers are foreign born, typically from Mexico and Central America, and live in temporary housing, whereas seasonal workers are primarily U.S. born and are permanent residents of a community (Seattle Global Justice, 2014). Both face challenges in accessing social and health care services. For instance, few migrant workers are provided with health insurance. Lack of transportation, inconvenient hours, cost, language barriers, and frequent relocation are other barriers (Seattle Global Justice, 2014). Delaying care because of concerns related to immigration status results in worsened health conditions (Bail et al., 2012).

In addition to low wages, seasonal farm workers and migrant workers rarely have access to important protections such as workers' compensation (NCFH, 2012). According to data compiled by the advocacy group Farmworker Justice, only 13 states plus the District of Columbia, Puerto Rico, and the Virgin Islands require employers to provide workers' compensation insurance or equivalent benefits to migrant and seasonal workers; this coverage is optional in 16 states (Farmworker Justice, 2009). This lack of coverage is important because when workers are sick or injured, they do not receive compensation; workers who miss work also are likely to lose their job. Most food system workers, including farm laborers, do not have paid sick days or do not know if they do and have worked when sick (FCWA, 2012). Non-American citizens cannot obtain insurance under the ACA, and because the food system employs so many undocumented immigrants, they will remain part of the uninsured population (NILC, 2014). Immigrants who are lawfully present in the United States may receive only limited federal coverage for health care (NILC, 2014).

Health and Safety Effects

Agricultural production has recognized health and safety risks. Modern agriculture involves the use of large machinery and potentially dangerous agrichemical inputs. Farming is one of the most hazardous occupations in the United States[2] (McCurdy and Carroll, 2000; NIOSH, 2010). From 2006-2009, the occupational fatality rate for workers in agriculture, forestry, and fishing was significantly higher than for all other industries (see Figure 5-7). Recognizing the hazards in this industry, Congress in 1990 directed the National Institute for Occupational Safety and Health (NIOSH) to develop specific strategies to address the high risks of injuries and illness to agricultural workers and their families. Under the NIOSH portfolio, the Agriculture, Forestry, and Fishing sector has a number of strategic goals to guide research and partnership efforts targeting priority areas, including traumatic injury and hearing loss (CDC, 2014b). Commercial fishing also receives specific attention from NIOSH, as the fatality rate

[2] In 2004, an estimated 9.2 injuries occurred every hour on U.S. farms, with a fatality rate of nearly 26 per 100,000.

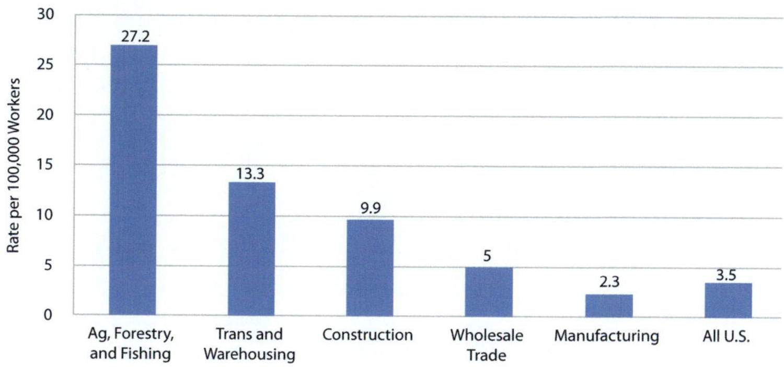

FIGURE 5-7 Occupational fatality rate, 2006-2009.
SOURCE: http://www.cdc.gov/niosh/programs/agff (accessed November 24, 2014).

of 124 per 100,000 workers is well above the overall fatality rate among all U.S. workers of 4 per 100,000 workers (NIOSH, 2014).

Chemical-related exposures also are important, and efforts are underway to conduct better surveillance of these exposures, as episodes of pesticide-related intoxications are not well captured in any national surveillance system (Geiser and Rosenberg, 2006; NIOSH, 2011). According to Calvert and colleagues (2008), the overall incidence of poisoning events was 53.6/100,000 farm workers compared to 1.38/100,000 for non-farm workers. About one-third of the affected workers were pesticide handlers and the rest were farm workers exposed to off-target drift of pesticide applications or exposed to treated plant or animal material. A wide array of signs and symptoms were reported (most of them low severity), with the most frequent being nervous or sensory symptoms, gastrointestinal irritation, eye problems, and skin and respiratory irritation. Acute poisoning is most frequent in processing and packing plant workers compared to other workers in agriculture. The scale of the problem is not easy to track. California, where large numbers of farm workers are employed, is the only state that requires mandatory reporting of pesticide-related intoxications (Geiser and Rosenberg, 2006; NIH/EPA/NIOSH, 2014).

Although farmers have a lower incidence of smoking, cancer, and cardiovascular disease compared to non-farm workers (Jones et al., 2009a), some evidence exists that they also experience high levels of anxiety, stress, depression, and suicide (Fraser et al., 2005; Freire and Koifman, 2013; Roberts et al., 2013). Respiratory disorders, dermatitis, and chronic pain associated with muscle and skeletal damage are also common. Agriculture also is unique among most industries in the significant levels of involvement of children and other family members who work and live on farms, which can lead to additional health and safety risks. Agricultural work may increase their risk of injury, illness, and exposure to toxic chemicals.

POTENTIAL SOCIAL AND ECONOMIC EFFECTS ON THE FOOD INDUSTRY

As noted in Chapter 2, the heterogeneous U.S. food and fiber system accounts for roughly 5 percent of the gross domestic product (GDP) (ERS, 2014e) and nearly one in five jobs in the United States (King et al., 2012). The non-farm sectors of the food industry have become the most significant sources of employment. In 2012, they contributed to approximately 90 percent of the economic value added to the food products purchased by U.S. consumers (see Figure 2-6 in Chapter 2). The primary functions of the non-farm sectors are to transport and transform raw agricultural products into edible foodstuffs. These subsectors (see Figure 2-1 in Chapter 2) are the technology and input suppliers, first line handlers and food manufacturers, wholesale/logistic suppliers, retail food stores, and food service establishments. In addition, a secondary market exists for food recovery in the form of food banks and food shelves plus the food disposal and waste sector.

Income, Wealth, and Social Well-Being of Workers and Communities

In this section, we highlight some of the differences in social and economic outcomes for participants in each of the major post-farming subsectors of the U.S. food supply chain. These sectors are highly interdependent, and changes in any one sector influence the performance of other sectors as well as the price and availability of food. Competitive pressures within each sector (and across sectors) have been major drivers of changes in technology and organizational structure (e.g., consolidation, vertical integration, market expansion, and market differentiation). These, in turn, drive economic efficiencies, opportunities and rewards to labor, and food options to consumers.

A recent study by Robert King et al. (2012) provides an overview of the total and heterogeneous employment opportunities and wages/benefits in each major subsector of the U.S. food industry. They find that about 23 million workers are involved in food system jobs, with average annual earnings of slightly more than $19,000 per year (less than half the average annual income of all workers in the United States in 2007) (see Figure 5-8). By far the largest number of workers is found in the retailing and food service sectors, where annual average earnings tend to be low. Two subsectors—distribution/wholesale and waste recovery—have mean payrolls slightly above the national average income of $41,525; food processing

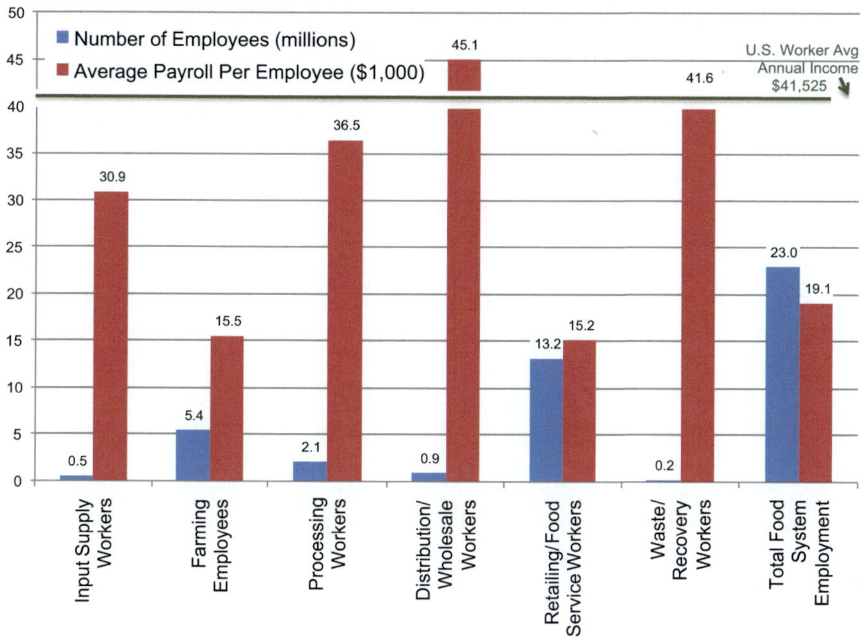

FIGURE 5-8 Number of U.S. food industry employees.
SOURCES: King et al., 2012; data from 2007. http://foodindustrycenter.umn.edu/prod/groups/cfans/@pub/@cfans/@tfic/documents/article/cfans_article_404726.pdf (accessed November 24, 2014).

and manufacturing workers and input supply workers have mean payrolls slightly below.

Technology and Agricultural Input Sector

Farmers in the primary production sector, discussed above, obtain a wide range of materials and services from the agricultural input sector. These inputs include seeds, chemicals, equipment, animal health services, animal breeding/genetics, financing, and information needed for modern commercial farming. As discussed in Chapter 2, over the past few decades, the agricultural input sector has consolidated as a result of numerous mergers and acquisitions. Many agricultural input firms are now global in scope, with diverse types of inputs integrated under relatively few corporate umbrellas.

Structure and profitability of the sector Historically, many first line–handling firms as well as input suppliers were organized as agricultural cooperatives that provided fuel, chemicals, seed, and other inputs to their members. Members of a cooperative are paid a dividend annually that depends on company profits. Cooperative organizations enabled many small producers to band together to gain bulk discounts on farm input purchases and to find markets for their products. The total number of marketing, supply, and service cooperatives declined from 4,663 in 1990 to 2,549 in 2007 as cooperatives merged and farmers shifted to selling through other channels (USDA, 2014a). Concomitantly, the number of members declined from 4.1 million to 2.5 million as net sales rose from $77.3 billion to $127.8 billion. The average returns to the members in 2007 were more than three times as much as they were in 1990 (USDA, 2014a).

Globalization, technological innovation, and organizational restructuring have created competitive advantages for large agribusiness firms with superior products that thrive with economies of scale. In addition to providing inputs, many major agricultural input suppliers contract with farmers to purchase their output. Closer coordination of production, processing, and distribution in vertically integrated operations can lead to gains (e.g., increased efficiency, more uniform food products, and reduced prices for consumers). Consolidation, however, can lead to costs to the workforce (e.g., less employment opportunities in the sector) and to smaller operations that might not have the resources to compete.

Concentration of food and agricultural input firms can lead to shifts in market power and affect the distribution of economic returns among food chain sectors (Myers et al., 2010; Sexton, 2013). Because larger firms generally incur more research and development costs than do most small firms, they must recover these costs as well as capital, regulatory, labor, and other costs. Because these larger firms also experience economies of scale, their ability to raise prices does not always mean that they do raise prices. Moreover, when fewer firms operate in an industry sector, they compete fiercely with each other, which can hold down prices to their customers (Chung and Tostao, 2012; Sexton, 2013). However, in the case of agricultural input suppliers, farmers are willing to pay higher prices if doing so results in greater yields on crops and livestock or results in higher prices for better quality output. As shown in Figure 5-9, the prices of most farm inputs rose more rapidly than the commodity prices received by farmers between 1990 and 2012 (Fuglie et al., 2012).

Workers As shown in Figure 5-8, this sector has relatively few workers compared to other subsectors of the U.S. food supply chain. The average incomes of half a million workers in the farm input sector are the third highest in the overall food industry at about $30,000 per year.

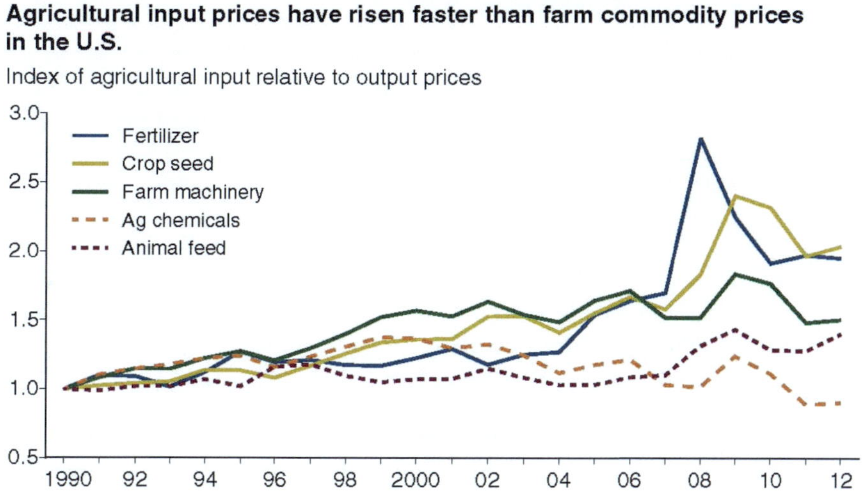

FIGURE 5-9 Agricultural input prices.
NOTE: Prices paid by U.S. farmers for farm inputs divided by prices received from farm commodities (indexes, 1990 = 1.00).
SOURCE: Fuglie et al., 2012.

Given the global nature of many farm input companies, as well as the skills in chemistry and biological systems needed, it seems likely that demand for workers with higher education levels to fill these jobs will grow.

Communities Agricultural input industries have historically contributed to the economic health and employment of rural communities, particularly when they are locally owned and managed or at least maintain production and sales operations in local trade centers. The restructuring of the input industries has led to some consolidation of retail outlets (e.g., for farm machinery and farm chemical inputs), and larger farming operations are known to source their inputs in bulk (at a discount) at greater distances from nonlocal businesses (Foltz et al., 2002; Sfiligoj, 2012). The net result of changes in the structure of both farming and farm input businesses has been to diminish economic opportunities for locally owned agricultural input and supply businesses in many rural communities, particularly those located further from industrial and transportation centers (Drabenstott, 2000; Foltz and Zeuli, 2005; Kilkenny, 2010; Lambert et al., 2009).

Food Processing and Manufacturing

This sector is composed of first line handlers who receive, package, and store raw agricultural products in preparation for shipment to the next party down the food supply chain and of food processors and manufacturers who turn ingredients into edible, packaged, storable, and safe food for final preparation and consumption by consumers or food service establishments (see Chapter 2).

Many companies that buy farmers' goods do so through contracts that guarantee the purchase of a certain amount of product for a predetermined price, assuming that the raw goods meet the quality specifications of the buyer. The benefit of this arrangement is that it alleviates the farmer's risk of not finding a market and of not knowing what the price will be at harvest time. It also can provide an opportunity to hedge against price declines in case of unforeseen market circumstances. The companies' contracts also provide technical advice and set standards of quality and safety that help to ensure a uniform supply of product that will be accepted by the downstream market. The demand from processors and retailers for uniform size and quality of product plays a large role in the benefits from contract farming.

Structure of the sector Changes in the structure of first line handlers can affect competitive pressures and returns to farmers. One example is the livestock supply chain, where vertical coordination has led to changes in the business relationships. In the poultry industry, producers are paid according to their productivity relative to other farmers and have much less certainty about the price they will receive at the end of a season (Leonard, 2014). Concentration of market shares in the hands of few firms can also lead to potential loss in competition and decline in the transparency of markets.

Food processors and manufacturers tend to be large corporations, and many are multinational in scope. They are focused on learning consumer preferences and designing foods to increase their market share. Food and beverage plants in the United States are widely distributed throughout the country, but some areas have seen a decrease in numbers since the 1980s (Edmonson, 2004; ERS, 2014c).

The food processing and manufacturing sector ships about 14 percent of the value shipped by all U.S. manufacturing plants (ERS, 2014c). Food processors and manufacturers are constantly adapting to feedback from retailers' sales and orders. As shown in Figure 2-6 in Chapter 2, food manufacturing adds about 16 percent of all value added in the food supply chain, the second highest amount after the food service sector. In 2011, processing and manufacturing of meat products composed the largest part of that value added by food manufacturers (17 percent), followed by beverages (16 percent), bakery and tortilla products (11 percent), fruits and vegetables (10 percent), and dairy products (10 percent) (ERS, 2014c). The U.S. Census reports 14,487 food processing and manufacturing companies, including 1,510 meat and 421 poultry companies, 3,097 beverage companies, 2,813 bakeries, 1,798 fruit and vegetable preserving companies, 1,007 dairy firms, and 4,050 soft drink manufacturers in 2011 (U.S. Census Bureau, 2014).

Workers Overall, the food processing and manufacturing subsector employs 1.5 million workers. This represents 14 percent of the total manufacturing sector workforce and about 1 percent of the non-farm labor in the United States. Thirty-two percent of these workers are in the meat processing sector, 9 percent are in dairy product manufacturing, 17 percent are in bakery, and 11 percent are in fruits and vegetables (ERS, 2014f). The payroll per employee in the meat and poultry sectors was $41,000 and $29,000, respectively, in 2011 (U.S. Census Bureau, 2014). The payroll per employee in grains and oilseed milling is higher than the national average at $73,000 per year. The payroll per employee in the fruit and vegetable processing sector was $57,000 in 2011 (U.S. Census Bureau, 2014).

Census statistics report that U.S. food manufacturing establishments had an average of 2,661 employees per establishment (plant), with a payroll per employee of $53,090 in 2011. Thirteen percent of the sales receipts were dedicated to payroll in the food manufacturing sector (U.S. Census Bureau, 2014). U.S. manufacturers overall had an average of 2,102 employees per establishment, with an average payroll per employee of $70,000 (U.S. Census Bureau, 2014).

A typical hourly wage worker in a food manufacturing plant earned approximately $12.50 to $14.00 per hour in 2013 (BLS, 2013). At $13.00 per hour, a full-time worker would make an income of $27,040 per year. Plants use a mix of skilled and unskilled labor, though even unskilled workers must be familiar with handling animals, foods, heavy equipment, and/or computerized equipment. Skilled labor requires some formal education in food science, chemistry, management, and marketing.

A recent survey of 2,456 food scientists and technologists, 66 percent of whom were employed in the food industry, shows a median salary of $90,000 in 2013. These employees have degrees in higher education, such as a bachelor's or a graduate degree. About 90 percent reported receiving health insurance and a retirement investment plan (Kuhn, 2014). This illustrates some of the more attractive employment opportunities in this industry. In contrast, this industry also has many part-time workers making minimum wages.

Worker health and safety Food processing workers tend to work in manufacturing facilities and operate equipment that mixes, cooks, or processes ingredients used to manufacture food (BLS, 2014b). The meat and poultry slaughtering and processing industries have long been associated with a high rate of injuries, fatalities, and illnesses (OSHA, 2014). Processing workers are typically exposed to noise as well as extreme heat—for workers interfacing with cooking machinery—or extreme cold—for employees involved with frozen or refrigerated goods. Workers are usually standing for most of these shifts and needing to stretch and reach to clean or operate large equipment. Musculoskeletal injuries, especially low back pain, are therefore a major problem. Injuries related to repetitive motion also are significant, especially in processing plants where employees are working the line and have to conduct the same motion repeatedly during a single shift. Other risks include hazards on the plant floors that increase the risk of slips, trips, and falls.

Communities Because community social and economic well-being is influenced by a wide range of factors, it is often difficult to link community outcomes with the presence or absence of any single business or firm. Because they have relatively small and less diversified economies, rural communities are more affected by changes in local business or employment opportunities. One recent example of this type of change is the dramatic shift in the location of meat processing plants from major urban areas to rural towns during the 1980s and 1990s, which has been linked to a wide range of social and economic impacts (Artz, 2012; Stull et al., 1995).

Wholesale and Logistic Suppliers (Distribution Subsector)

This sector of the food system provides the transportation and warehousing of food and agricultural products between the other sectors. It involves warehousing, trucking and other transportation, and procurement services. This sector is critical to the availability of food in remote areas and in cities far from production location. It also is vital to global trade.

Structure of the sector The total number of companies in the wholesale business related to food, beverage, and agricultural products was 3,810 in 2011 (U.S. Census Bureau, 2014).

On the food service side, traditional wholesalers still dominate because they serve many small retail enterprises with specialized orders. The agricultural input sector also has wholesalers. Nine percent of the wholesale companies listed in the Census data deliver farm supplies and another 9 percent deal in raw farm products destined for processors (U.S. Census Bureau, 2014).

Not traditionally counted among the wholesale sector are the numerous food banks that act as wholesalers to food shelves around the country.

The largest nonprofit wholesaler in this business is Feeding America and its members, such as Second Harvest Heartland. Feeding America has 200 member food banks that collect food and redistribute it to food shelves, soup kitchens, and other charitable feeding establishments in every county in the United States. In 2013, they distributed more than 3,878 million pounds of food (Feeding America, 2014a). This amount is only 0.06 percent of the total edible food listed in Figure 2-2, but it provides more than 3 billion meals per year. In addition to the additional meals provided, food companies and individuals who donate food or cash receive a charitable tax deduction and companies save waste disposal costs.

Workers Wholesale companies related to food and agricultural products employ at least 357,790 people, an average of 78 per establishment (U.S. Census Bureau, 2014). They are among the higher paid workers in the food industry, with an average payroll per employee of $57,000. Six percent of sales receipts is dedicated to payroll in the wholesale sector.

The skills required in the wholesale sector are heterogeneous, from laborers to truck drivers, forklift operators, warehouse managers, computer programmers who optimize the efficiency of loading trucks and truck routes, sales and procurement experts, and food safety experts (e.g., cold chain managers). The distribution of wages across all of these types of workers varies according to their skills, the alternative market for their skills, and where they are located in the country. In addition, Feeding America reports using 8.6 million hours of volunteer labor in 2013 (Feeding America, 2013).

Worker health and safety A significant component of distribution involves transportation, in addition to warehousing (FCWA, 2012). The health and safety risks faced by these workers, especially those involved in warehousing, are repetitive motion and lifting. Warehouse workers have the highest rates of chronic debilitating injuries due to repetitive motion, bending and squatting, and improper lifting techniques (Free Library, 2014). Safety reports indicate a lack of personal protective equipment among these workers, which places them at risk of injury by allowing exposure to injury-producing hazards. Workers load most warehouses and trucks with forklifts that alleviate heavy lifting, but the speed of operation in closed spaces is a potential hazard. Because distribution involves the transport of goods, motor vehicle crashes are a significant cause of death and injury. Motor vehicle-related crashes are the leading cause of work-related fatalities in the United States (CDC/NIOSH, 2014). Truckers who haul food products are exposed to all of the hazards of trucking, including stress and fatigue due to routes and schedules, illness, night driving, and risk of back injuries from heavy lifting.

Retail Food Stores

This subsector includes traditional grocery stores and, increasingly, the large box retailers who sell food as part of a vast mix of general merchandise. Retail stores also include convenience stores and a host of newer venues, such as drug stores, gas stations with convenience stores, specialty foods, and online food companies. Retail food stores had a total of $742.3 billion in sales in 2013. Food sales in retail stores represent 53 percent of all food sales of $1.4 trillion, with the rest of food sales taking place in some form of food service establishment (ERS, 2014d).

Structure of the sector Due in large part to price competition from "big box" stores, stores in this sector have been consolidating to adapt to information and transportation technologies that allow them to minimize in-store inventories. New strategies to attract and hold customers began in the mid-1990s. They involved using information technologies to track customer purchases, instituting loyalty programs, and lowering prices and/or finding market niches that larger stores do not fill. Competition was fierce and the structure of the retail industry began to bifurcate into big companies with generally lower priced goods and companies specializing in smaller stores with specialty products and services at higher prices. In the big box stores, lower food prices can be sustained because they are balanced by more profitable sales of general merchandise. The volume and velocity of turnover of foods that move through retail food stores calls for efficient logistics, efficient aggregation and analysis of data, and energy savings in transportation. It facilitates great buying power, including the power to dictate product quality and safety specifications, quantities, timing, and price. Suppliers are obligated to adapt to the demands of large retailers. For example, roughly one-third of all products sold by major manufacturers are sold through the largest retail company in the United States, which is also the second largest publicly traded company in the world. Retailers are increasingly buying products with their own brand label, further diminishing the market power of food manufacturers with national and international brand names.

Large food retailers (those with more than 100 stores) have developed their own distribution warehouses, cutting out the wholesaler for most products. This enables them to cut costs and compete on price. Nationally, prices at discount stores are 7.5 percent lower than at traditional grocery stores, which puts price pressure on all retail food sellers (ERS, 2014h).

Workers Overall, 56,786 retail food and beverage companies employ more than 2.4 million people, for an average of 43 people per establishment (U.S. Census Bureau, 2014). These employees include stockers, checkers, and managers. This sector also includes workers who cook and prepare food for bakeries and delis within the retail outlets, as well as those who clean the facilities (FCWA, 2012). The payroll per employee is $25,600, or 19 percent of sales receipts. Payroll per employee is lower than in retail businesses in general, where payroll per employee is $28,000, or 11 percent of sales receipts (U.S. Census Bureau, 2014).

The labor in this sector is not generally highly skilled except for management. Although the ubiquitous nature of retail food stores provides employment opportunities in most communities, wages tend to be near minimum wage for many workers. The average earnings of $25,600 is 114 percent of the U.S. poverty level for a single person in 2014 and almost equal to the poverty level of $23,850 for a household of four people (HHS, 2014).

Worker health and safety Jobs in retailing involve heavy lifting and the use of potentially hazardous equipment, which places workers at risk of back injuries and lacerations or amputations. In addition, psychosocial factors, such as work-related stress and shift work, are important considerations for these employees.

Food Service Establishments

This sector includes individually owned restaurants, mid-priced chains, quick service (fast food) establishments, hotels, and beverage establishments. They cater to the tastes of their particular customers and are often leaders of food innovation. Also in this sector are institutional food service establishments such as schools, hospitals, prisons, food (soup) kitchens, and Meals on Wheels.

Structure of the sector The food service sector has at least 125,951 companies and approximately 4 million employees. It employs an average of 32 people per establishment; payroll is more than 27 percent of their sales revenue (U.S. Census Bureau, 2014). It is a labor-intensive business, mostly because it is largely a service business with few opportunities to substitute capital for labor. The cost of the food in most food service places is no more than one-third of their total costs.

In 2013, 47 percent of all food sales were in this sector, consistent with the division of sales over the past several decades (ERS, 2014g). As data from USDA's Economic Research Service show, however, sales at fast food establishments increased the most in the mid-1980s, while institutional food sales were down (see Figure 5-10).

Workers The average income of food service workers, $24,857, is about the same as the poverty level for a household of four persons, $23,850 in

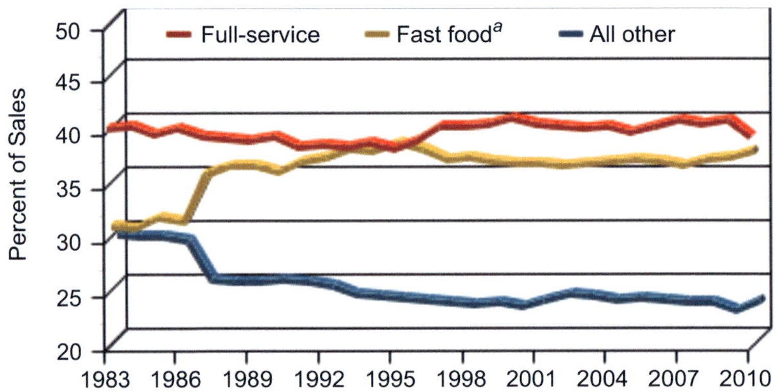

FIGURE 5-10 Sales of food.
[a] Fast food excludes contract feeding and concessions.
SOURCE: ERS, 2014g.

2014 (HHS, 2014; U.S. Census Bureau, 2014). The skill level in this sector is relatively low except for management and a few very skilled chefs. This sector provides employment in nearly every community.

Not surprisingly, turnover also is a problem among retail workers, especially among those who experience wage theft (e.g., not receiving overtime payments, tip misappropriations) (FCWA, 2012). For the most part, these wage inequities are present at the largest companies (Kelly et al., 2012). It is important to note, however, that while many wage violations occur, this sector also demonstrates promising examples of best practices for worker wages, career mobility, and good supply chain policies and programs (Kelly et al., 2012; Liu, 2012).

Worker health and safety Food service workers perform a variety of customer service, food preparation, and cleaning duties. Shift work is very common, and in 2012, about half of these workers were employed part time (BLS, 2014b). Food and beverage serving and related workers are on their feet most of the time and they have to lift heavy objects, such as trays of food. During busy dining periods throughout the day, workers are called to serve customers quickly and efficiently. Injuries among these workers tend to be nonfatal and are mainly due to slips/trips/falls, burns, and lacerations that may lead to time away from work.

Teen workers are overrepresented in this sector, primarily because the option to work various shifts allows for flexible schedules. Young workers have high occupational injury rates, which are partially attributed to the number of injury hazards in food service establishments (e.g., slippery floors and use of knives and cooking equipment) (CDC, 2014c). The rate for occupational injuries of young workers treated in emergency departments from 1998 to 2006 was approximately two times higher than among workers age 25 and older (CDC, 2014c). In addition to these hazards, inexperience and lack of safety training also may increase workplace injury risks for young workers (CDC, 2014c).

Many food service workers also report having no access to paid sick days. One survey of more than 600 food system workers in the United States found that only 21 percent confirmed they had paid sick days (the rest either did not have them or were unaware if they had them) (FCWA, 2012). Reports also have documented working long hours and the inability to take breaks because of a need to maintain the output demands (CDC, 2014a). Employees who work with food when infected by norovirus or other contagious illnesses can spread disease to others by easily contaminating food and drinks that are touched. Because of the lack of sick leave, food service workers have an economic incentive to return to work as soon as possible. Food establishments are generally very busy, and not showing up during a busy time (e.g., holidays and weekends) can potentially lead to losing a job.

Overall Worker Well-Being in U.S. Food System

Poverty and injustice in the food system has been described in the literature for centuries (VanDeCruze and Wiggins, 2008). Evidence shows that 40 percent of food industry jobs provide a wage at the federal poverty level; only 13.5 percent of the jobs provide wages that yield an annual income at 150 percent of the poverty level (FCWA, 2012). As the previous sections of this chapter have described, some food system workers receive a livable wage, but many do not, and they have little or no career mobility in these jobs. Estimates from 2010 indicate that median hourly wages for employees in U.S. food industry sectors vary slightly by segment (median hourly wages of approximately \$9.00 to \$13.00 for workers in production, processing, distribution, and services), but incomes for positions within the sectors vary greatly (Kelly et al., 2012). For example, of the top 100 chief executive officers in the United States, 8 are from the food system and their total salaries in 2012 equaled that of more than 10,300 food service workers (FCWA, 2012).

Among the top five companies taking the lead globally with promising policies and programs, four are European companies. This suggests that U.S. companies can learn important lessons about promoting fair wages, mobility, and other social and economic advancements for food system workers (Kelly et al., 2012). *Fortune* magazine publishes an annual list of the 100 best companies to work for in the United States. In 2014, three grocery companies, two restaurant chains, and two food manufacturing companies were on the list. Among these seven companies, average salaries ranged from $45,684 to $115,007, while the average hourly workers' annual wage income ranged from $26,240 to $52,318. Of note, none of these companies offered wage benefits or paid for health insurance, but amenities that employees praised were flexible work hours, training and upward mobility in the company, on-site child care and fitness centers, or paid health club benefits (*Fortune* magazine, 2014).

Food Company Performance and Contribution to the Economy

Two measures of the performance of companies are size and profitability. The Fortune 500 is an annual list of the top 500 publicly traded companies registered in the United States with U.S. operations. This list does not include privately held companies in any industry, but it serves to compare food firms to firms in other U.S. industries. Firms are ranked by total revenue, and profitability also is reported (*Fortune* magazine, 2014). The profitability of each of these companies indicates their contribution to the economy in general and to the wealth of their stockholders as well as the stability of employment for their employees. For 2013, 39 of the top 500 companies were in the food industry. Annual revenue of these 39 food companies ranged from $6.5 to $469.3 billion. Table 5-1 shows the distribution of Fortune 500 food system companies across the food supply chain. The most numerous firms represent the food manufacturing and retail food sectors.

In general, the largest profits are found in the food manufacturing sector, primarily among large multinational companies and in the food service sector. Economic returns to manufacturing companies and their investors are larger than in most other sectors partly because this sector has relatively high concentration through merger and acquisition and global markets. In the food service sector, consumers pay for experiences and convenience as well as food; several of the chain operations operate on a global scale.

Trends that mitigate the profits in this sector are fluctuating raw commodity prices and the trend toward private retail store labels instead of (inter-) national brands. Rising commodity prices are often hedged forward to reduce uncertainty and smooth out manufacturing costs and wholesale prices of product. Food manufacturers that are producing the products are skilled in selling them under various private labels to mitigate competition from other private store labels. Wholesalers are perhaps the most vulnerable sector and struggle for profitability as retailers contract directly with processors to deliver product to stores and/or set up their own distribution

TABLE 5-1 Number of Food and Agriculture Firms in the Fortune 500 List, Ranking by Total Revenue and Profitability

	# of Firms in Fortune 500	Ranking Range in Fortune 500		Profits as % of Revenue		
		High	Low	Average	Low	High
Agricultural input firms	2	27	69	2.0		
Food manufacturing	18	43	452	6.7	–2.0	19.0
Food wholesale and distribution	4	65	500	2.0	–2.0	5.0
Retail food companies	10	1	378	2.6	–3.0	6.0
Food service	5	111	328	10.0	1.0	20.0
All food system companies	39	27	600			

SOURCE: *Fortune* magazine, 2014.

centers and logistics operations. The exception to this is in the wholesale business for the food service sector.

Retail food stores traditionally struggle for profitability mostly because of fierce horizontal competition. Many stores go out of business as consumers seek the lowest prices for homogeneous products or unique shopping experiences and products in upscale stores. The bifurcation of retailers has been occurring since the 1990s, with the big box stores on one side and unique food offerings like organic and total private labels on the other. Retailers that try to supply middle-of-the-road grocery stores are disappearing. Profits on grocery store sales are traditionally stated as 2 percent, meaning they operate at very small margins (FMI, 2013).

POTENTIAL SOCIAL AND ECONOMIC EFFECTS ON U.S. CONSUMERS

Perhaps the primary indicator of social and economic success in any food system is the ability to provide a population with an abundant supply of affordable, safe, high-quality, and nutritious food. This review suggests that the U.S. food system meets these goals most of the time for most people, but significant diet-related disease (see Chapter 3) and food insecurity point to areas needing improvement. Researchers have understood for decades that all of the decisions made regarding food, purchasing, and consumption depend on multiple variables. These include the communities in which people live; the food available in those communities; the influences to which they are exposed, such as advertising and marketing; and their beliefs about the environment, farming, globalization, and many other factors. The food system is dynamic and the changing eating habits and cultural and environmental dispositions among U.S. consumers over the past several decades signal a shift in preferences. This shift will be necessary to assess in future decades.

Food Costs and Expenditures

Compared to other social and economic variables, income arguably has the strongest marginal impact on dietary behavior: higher-income households spend more for food and eat higher-quality diets; lower-income households buy more generic brands and discounted foods (Contento, 2010) and prepare more of their food at home. In 2009, the lowest quintile households spent $3,500 on food, while households in the highest quintile spent more than three times that at $10,800 (BLS, 2010). However, those in the lowest quintile of income spend a much higher share of their total income on food (nearly 35 percent in 2012) than do those in the highest quintile (7 percent) (BLS, 2014a) (see Figure 5-11), despite the fact that over the past 50 years, the average share of income spent on food has fallen from approximately 18 percent to approximately 10 percent (ERS, 2013a).

The foods purchased and consumed by lower- and higher-income households are different, as is the percentage of food dollars spent on food at home (FAH) compared to food away from home (FAFH). Actual expenditures on all food product categories, including fruits and vegetables (Ludwig and Pollack, 2009), increase at every income level and are 2.5 times higher for the highest income levels (BLS, 2012).

One measure of how the U.S. food system serves the needs of consumers is the rate of change in food prices and the percentage of income required to purchase food. Historically, the Consumer Price Index[3] (CPI) for food at retail stores was below or the same as overall inflation, running at about 2 to 3 percent between 1990 and 2005 (Volpe, 2013). Since 2005, the CPI for food has been more volatile due in part to international market shortages, weather, and other factors. Between 2006 and 2012, the CPI for food rose 20 percent compared to 14 percent overall. This led to the percentage of disposable income spent on food rising from an average of 9.5 to over 10 percent (Volpe, 2013).

The costs of producing, processing, and transporting food to consumers

[3] The Consumer Price Index is the measure of the average change over time in the prices paid by urban consumers for a market basket of consumer goods and services.

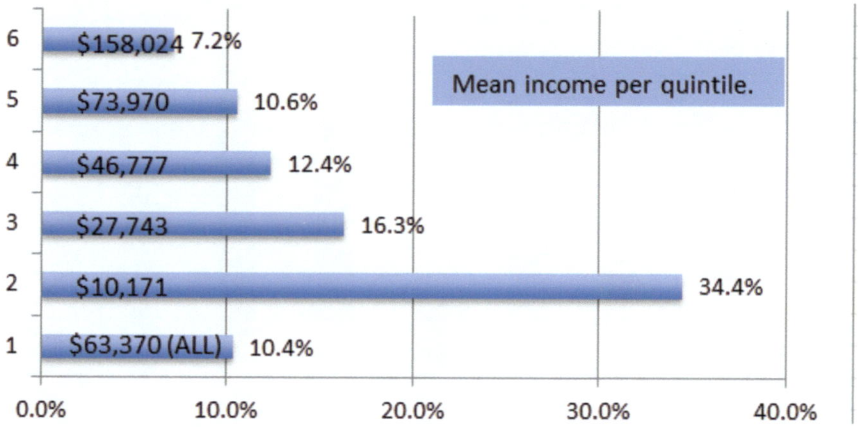

FIGURE 5-11 Food expenditure by income.
NOTE: 1 = Total population; 2 = Lowest income quintile; 3 = 2nd income quintile; 4 = 3rd income quintile; 5 = 4th income quintile; 6 = Highest income quintile.
SOURCE: BLS, 2014a.

all influence the food price and the CPI for food. Reducing these costs can lower food prices and food price inflation. Figure 5-12 displays the CPI for food relative to the overall CPI from 2006 to 2012.

Food Security and Food Access

Most U.S. households are food secure—that is, they have access to a dependable food supply. Since 2000, USDA has monitored the extent and severity of food insecurity through an annual national representative survey (Gundersen et al., 2011). In a 2012 survey documenting food security in the United States (Coleman-Jensen et al., 2013), about 8.8 percent of households (10.6 million) were described as having low food security (reports of "reduced quality, variety, or desirability of diet, with little or no indication of reduced food intake") (USDA, 2014c). Another 5.7 percent of households (7 million) were described as having very low food security in which the food intake of some household members "was reduced and normal eating patterns were disrupted at times during the year due to limited resources" (Coleman-Jensen et al., 2013, p. v). About 10 percent of U.S. households that had children were classified as food insecure. The prevalence of food insecurity was lower in the year 2000 than it is now. It substantially increased in 2007-2008 as the recession started and has been essentially unchanged since then. In 2012, 1.2 percent of households

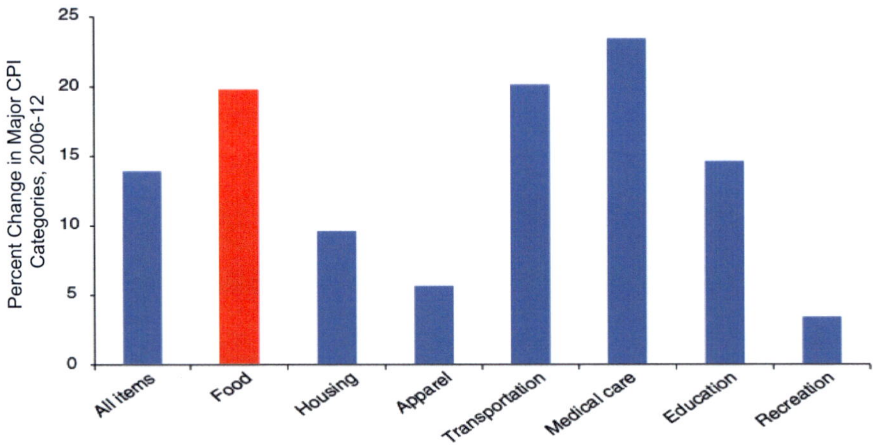

FIGURE 5-12 Consumer Price Index for food.
NOTES: Between 2006 and 2012, food price inflation was greater than overall price inflation. CPI = Consumer Price Index.
SOURCE: Volpe, 2013.

with children experienced very low food security sometime during the year (Coleman-Jensen et al., 2013).

Food insecurity is determined by multiple variables. One of the most important is income; 40 percent of households with incomes lower than the federal poverty level are food insecure, while only 7 percent of households with income above 185 percent of the poverty level are food insecure (Coleman-Jensen et al., 2013). However, income is not the only factor in predicting food insecurity: households without liquid assets are much more likely to be food insecure, and income volatility is associated with food insecurity (Gundersen et al., 2011). Not surprisingly, housing instability is also a factor (Ma et al., 2008). Other characteristics that correlate with food insecure households are those headed by an African American, a Hispanic, a younger person, or a less educated person (Gundersen et al., 2011). Further analysis of data on food insecurity by the Economic Research Service found that three national-level economic measures—changes in unemployment, inflation, and the price of food—accounted for 92 percent of the year-to-year variation in the national prevalence of food insecurity from 2001 to 2012 (Nord et al., 2014).

Numerous studies have shown that food insecurity increases the risk of a range of health and psychosocial problems among children, adolescents, and adults (Gundersen and Kreider, 2009; Huang et al., 2010; Kirkpatrick et al., 2010; Nord, 2009; Seligman et al., 2007, 2010; Whitaker et al.,

2006). Children who are food insecure have increased risk of asthma, cognitive impairment, and behavioral problems; have lower math scores; and are twice as likely to repeat a grade and three times as likely to be suspended from school as children who are food secure (Alaimo et al., 2001). Teens who reported being food insecure were found to be twice as likely to suffer from depression and five times as likely to commit suicide as were food secure teens (Alaimo et al., 2002; Ashiabi, 2005). Food insecure adults have an increased risk of heart disease and depression or anxiety (Seligman et al., 2010; Whitaker et al., 2006) and, under the most severe levels of food insecurity, adults have more than twice the risk of diabetes compared to those who do not experience food insecurity (Seligman et al., 2007). Furthermore, diabetic individuals have more difficulties following a diabetic diet and need more medical attention if they are also food insecure (Nelson et al., 2001; Seligman et al., 2012). Due to these individual-level consequences, low food security also raises societal costs of providing education (e.g., due to higher educational investments needed when children are unable to learn because of food insecurity) and health care (Brown et al., 2007).

It is argued that food insecurity is a market failure that occurs when private markets do not provide enough food even when the benefits of providing it outweigh the social costs (Rocha, 2007). Food itself is a private good, but food security is a public good, so the government has stepped in to help alleviate some of the problem. Approximately 60 percent of food insecure households participate in one or more government nutrition or food programs (Feeding America, 2014b). These programs, such as the Supplemental Nutrition Assistance Program (SNAP), School Lunch Program (SLP), and the Special Supplemental Nutrition Program for Women, Infants, and Children (WIC), contribute to better food security for low-income households, increase revenue to producers and processors, and reduce expenditures on other public services (Kinsey, 2013). In 2013, more than 47 million individuals received SNAP benefits. About 70 percent of participants are families with children and more than 25 percent are households with seniors or people with disabilities (CBPP, 2014). In the same year, for the first time, working-age people made up the majority of households receiving benefits (Yen, 2014). It should be noted that the multiplier effect of SNAP is quite substantial. Taking into account direct and indirect effects, $1 billion of retail food expenditures by recipients generates $267 million in agricultural production, $87 million in value-added processing, and nearly 3,000 food and agricultural jobs (Hanson, 2010).

Even with their SNAP benefits, the typical food insecure households purchased significantly less food than did typical food secure households of the same size and composition in 2012 (Coleman-Jensen et al., 2013). Some of the difference can be explained by three critical barriers that constrain the ability of SNAP payments to guarantee good nutrition among low-income households: (1) a lack of time to prepare foods requires the purchase of value-added or prepared foods in many situations, (2) limited access to outlets (e.g., supermarkets and big box stores) in many areas hampers the ability to purchase nutritious foods at a reasonable cost, and (3) substantial variability in food prices by geographic region means that people living in high-cost areas benefit less from SNAP payments than do those in low-cost areas (IOM, 2013). In addition, the assumptions used to calculate food stamp benefits do not account for changes in other expenditures, such as those for housing, that have increased considerably over past decades, resulting in less money available to purchase adequate diets.

A corollary to food insecurity is limited food access, which has been defined as the inability to purchase nutritious, affordable foods within a prescribed distance from home. There are several different food access issues: a lack of supermarkets in low-income areas; a lack of transportation to supermarkets or superstores; and an abundance of smaller stores, which charge higher prices and carry few healthy foods (Ver Ploeg et al., 2009). This spatially complex phenomenon was first described in Great Britain as a "food desert" and defined variously as a situation where people live more than a certain distance from a supermarket and do not have access to a vehicle (Cummins and Macintyre, 1999). The findings from a study of the problem by a large team of researchers and policy analysts from several USDA agencies suggest that the term food desert is not accurate or useful in many cases (Ver Ploeg et al., 2009). In fact, USDA analysis found that access to a supermarket or a large grocery store is a problem for only a small percentage of low-income households in low-income areas (about 4 percent of the total U.S. population, many of them in rural areas). Also, low-income households shop where food prices are lower when they can. Eighty-two percent of SNAP benefits were redeemed at supermarkets or large grocery stores in 2012 (CBPP, 2014). More recent research has found that in many places around the United States, low-income urban neighborhoods have more grocery stores, supermarkets, and full-service restaurants, along with more fast food restaurants and convenience stores, than do affluent areas (Lee, 2012). However, these findings do not mean that the quality of food in stores in low-income areas is as high as in more affluent areas, and low-income households, especially very low-income families, do not face many barriers in procuring and preparing nutritious meals (Ver Ploeg et al., 2009).

Factors Influencing Food Purchase Decisions

Consumers are the end of the food chain, and their health and wellness is the primary reason food production is absolutely necessary in every society, from a subsistence-livelihood household to the global community. A scan of the literature on contemporary food systems offers many elements that consumers desire from the food system, including a low risk of illness from the consumption of unsafe food, a wide availability of a variety of food choices, low price, foods that meet taste preferences, foods that offer various types of convenience, the ability to act on desires for foods produced in environmentally sound ways that have not unduly harmed natural resources, accessibility to culturally desired food products and ingredients, and access to innovative culinary trends. These indicators are reflected in both the research findings over many decades of the major determinants of food choices (Contento, 2010) and the responses made year after year to the IFIC Foundation's nationally representative Food and Health Survey (IFIC, 2014a). In the most recent survey, in response to a question about what factors have a significant or great impact on a decision to buy foods and beverages, the first choice is taste (90 percent choosing this). The second is price (73 percent), then healthfulness (71 percent), convenience (51 percent), and sustainability (38 percent) (IFIC, 2014a). These factors are described below.

Taste

Humans are born with a predisposition to like sweet and to reject sour or bitter flavors, and over time, they develop preferences for salt and fat (Contento, 2010). However, these biologically inherent tastes are not determinative. People's likings for specific foods are largely learned. With repeated consumption a preference for a novel food tends to increase. Therefore if children (or adults) are frequently exposed to foods that are high in sugar, fat, and salt, they will become familiar and preferred over foods that are relatively unfamiliar (Contento, 2010). These research findings explain in part the heightened concern about television advertising to children of foods of low nutritional quality that are high in fat, added sugars, and sodium. In 2009, food advertisers spent $1.8 billion on marketing to youth ages 2 to 17 (Powell et al., 2013). People tend to like calorie-dense foods, which would have been adaptive when such food was scarce but is maladaptive where food is readily available (Contento, 2010). Retraining the U.S. palate to expect and accept foods and beverages with less salt and sugar is under way by many food companies, but it progresses slowly (Kinsey, 2013). Nutrition educators have been engaged in related efforts for many decades, but with quite limited resources compared to those of the food industry (Contento, 2010).

Price

Food prices change frequently for a number of reasons. Between 1980 and 2010, CPIs were much lower compared to the CPI over time for carbonated drinks, nonalcoholic beverages, and whole milk, and they were quite a bit higher for all fruits and vegetables and even higher for fresh fruits and vegetables (Wendt and Todd, 2011). A study by researchers at USDA, however, shows that the prices of many staple fruits and vegetables have not had disproportionate price increases (Kuchler and Stewart, 2008). Furthermore, when measured on either a weight or a serving basis, healthy foods can cost less than less healthy foods—defined as being high in saturated fat, added sugars, and sodium, or contributing little to meeting dietary recommendations (Carlson and Frazão, 2012).

Complementing the data on price indexes is a review of multiple estimates of price elasticities calculated between 1938 and 2007 (Andreyeva et al., 2010). Price elasticity is defined as the percentage change in quantity purchased as a result of a 1 percent change in the price of a product. Over time, the highest price elasticities are for food away from home, soft drinks, juices, beef, and pork. The lowest price elasticities are for fats and oils, cheese, sweets and sugars, and eggs, suggesting that purchase of the latter foods are more resistant to price changes.

Older, higher-income consumers and men are less likely to be influenced by price than are younger, low-income consumers and women (IFIC, 2013). Just and Payne (2009) argue that most consumers are not very responsive overall to changes in price and income, but that they tend to be more responsive to changes (especially a lowering) in the price of foods high in fat, salt, and sugar. Lowenstein (2013) reports that between 1980 and 2000 the relative price of food fell nearly 15 percent, and processed food prices declined the most. He states that several economic reports assign most of the increase in obesity over that time to the increase in calorie intake that resulted from the change in prices (Lowenstein, 2013).

Healthfulness

Healthfulness includes nutritional value as well as food safety from microbial contamination or elements such as pesticide residues and other toxicants. In the most recent IFIC survey (IFIC, 2014a), the importance of healthfulness as a factor affecting food and beverage purchases increased significantly over the prior 2 years. Higher-income shoppers, on average, purchase slightly more healthful foods than do lower-income shoppers, but all subgroups fall far short of purchasing a food basket that meets USDA dietary guidelines (Volpe and Okrent, 2012). Women and older consumers are more likely to use healthfulness as a key factor in food purchasing.

However, few consumers understand health issues at more than a superficial level (Just, 2013), and they may choose many products that are not health enhancing. Manufacturers and marketers study and analyze models of consumer behavior, including deliberate and slow purchases versus those that are emotional and heuristic (Shiv and Fedorikhin, 1999). Manufacturers understand that consumers respond to a variety of factors, such as the price, the price of substitutes and complements, the number of calories, the size of a portion, the shape and color of containers, product placement, and others, and can make changes in their marketing approaches if they wish to do so (Just, 2013).

Convenience

Beginning in the 1950s, the growing presence of women in the workforce and other social and cultural changes created a demand for foods that would be easy to acquire and convenient and quick to prepare. Since then, convenience foods have become a staple feature of the food landscape. Convenience foods—defined as those processed foods that need little preparation, are preprepared, and are preserved for long-term storage—are popular among consumers because meal preparation requires little time and effort, and some are less expensive than their home-prepared counterparts (Kinsey, 2013). Consumers recognize that these foods are shelf stable and amenable to long-distance transportation and long-term storage in the home and other institutions (Kinsey, 2013). In the latest IFIC survey, three-quarters of respondents believe that processing can help food stay fresh longer; 63 percent believe they benefit from modern food production and processing, with the top two benefits being improved food safety and prolonged freshness (IFIC, 2014a).

Convenience foods also are popular among food manufacturers because these products are very high earners. For example, of the 10 most profitable food production categories in the United States, 6 are convenience/snack foods: snack foods; cookies, crackers, and pasta; chocolate; sugar processing; ice cream; and candy (Cohen, 2013). The majority of these foods are high in sugar, salt, saturated fat, or total fat, or they are of low nutrient density. Food companies are continually expanding their offerings of convenience foods through line extensions, new packaging, and some genuinely new products. The average number of new food and beverage products introduced to the market between 2006 and 2010 was 21,368 per year (ERS, 2013c). This proliferation of processed and convenience foods means that food corporations have increasingly shaped what and how consumers eat (Belasco and Scranton, 2002). Because the number of items in stores is so high, consumers must spend much more time in the store making decisions (Kinsey, 2013). Furthermore, consumers make more than 200 food-related decisions every day, and often fall back on habits and perceptions or misperceptions that lead them to make poor choices (Wansink and Sobal, 2007).

Meeting the desire for convenience has also led to the rise of fast food outlets and the ubiquitous presence of food for sale in all types of stores and public places. In addition, busy lives mean that consumers are increasingly combining eating with other activities, such as working, driving, watching TV, and interacting with the Internet, e-mail, or phones (Kinsey, 2013), thus increasing the desire for foods that are convenient and easy to eat. These behaviors appear to have contributed to the obesity problem in the United States (Harvard School of Public Health, 2012).

One way to consider the growing importance of convenience in food choices is to examine the relative expenditures on food at home and food away from home. In 2012, the average share of total food expenditures spent on FAFH by U.S. households was 49.5 percent (see Chapter 2, Figure 2-3). Of the total dollars spent on food in the lowest-income households, 30 percent was spent on FAFH and 70 percent on FAH, while in the highest income quintile the expenditures were closer to 50 percent in each category (BLS, 2014a).

Between 1977-1978 and 2005-2008, the share of calorie intake from FAFH increased from 18 to 32 percent (Lin and Guthrie, 2012). In addition, the percentage of fat calories of FAH declined substantially compared to fat from FAFH during that time. The highest percentage of calories from saturated fat occurred in fast foods compared to the percentage in restaurant foods, school food, and FAH (Lin and Guthrie, 2012).

Concurrent with the increase in eating at restaurants and fast food establishments, the percentage of time spent on food preparation, along with the daily number of calories consumed from food eaten at home, decreased in all socioeconomic groups from 1965 to 2008 (Smith et al., 2013). The largest decline occurred between 1965 and 1992 and has leveled off since, but many Americans do not know how to cook anymore. Other research indicates that changes in time spent on preparing food may differ by income, for one study found that more than 60 percent of low-income consumers prepare main meals from scratch an average of four times per week (more often than do moderate-income families), and they use some forms of preprepared foods twice per week (Share Our Strength, 2012).

Sustainability

A loss of confidence in the safety and healthfulness of food (short term and long term), as well as the government's apparent inability to ensure it, has led consumers to look for foods that espouse certain priorities, including organic production practices, humane treatment of animals and fish, and many different sustainability practices (Kinsey, 2013). The percentage of consumers who claim to know something about sustainability has continued to rise and many say that sustainability is somewhat or very important to them (IFIC, 2014a). The aspects of sustainability reported as most important are conserving the natural habitat, ensuring an affordable and sufficient global food supply, and reducing the amount of pesticides (IFIC, 2014a). Another national survey (Cone Communications, 2014) has found that 77 percent of the U.S. population says that sustainability does factor into their food purchasing decisions. Thirty-five percent of consumers report that they purchase foods and beverages advertised as local, 32 percent buy foods and beverages labeled as organic, and 20 percent purchase foods and beverages in recycled or recyclable packaging, despite the price premium that is often attached to these products (IFIC, 2014b).

In 2011, 78 percent of U.S. adults were buying organic foods at least occasionally and 40 percent were buying more organic food than they had in the past year (OTA, 2011). Fruits and vegetables are approximately 35 percent of all organic food sales, and the preponderance is fresh produce (OTA, 2014). Organic food sales were $32 billion in 2013, equal to 4 percent of all sales of food at home (OTA, 2014). Studies have found that consumers who have higher levels of education are more likely to buy organic products than are less educated consumers, but other factors (e.g., race) do not have a consistent effect on purchasing organic products (Dimitri and Oberholtzer, 2009). For example, African Americans are somewhat less likely to purchase organic foods, but when they do they purchase much greater quantities than do white consumers (Stevens-Garmon et al., 2007).

Questions about the ability of organic agriculture to produce comparable food yields have persisted for many years. However, a large analysis, including almost 300 research comparisons between organic and nonorganic production around the world, shows that the yield indexes were similar between the two different production methods (Badgley et al., 2007). However, a recent comprehensive meta-analysis shows that, overall, organic yields are typically lower than conventional yields, with the differences depending on the site and systems characteristics (Seufert et al., 2012). The debate about this will continue as other analyses are completed on organic as well as other alternative/sustainable food production systems. The debate is important because using organic methods versus nonorganic practices involves trade-offs in other domains that should be explored. For example, choosing organic methods might result in lower productivity, but also in better outcomes in the health and environmental domains; these trade-offs are important but challenging to measure (e.g., see Chapter 7, Annex 4, "Nitrogen in Agroecosystems"). A comparison of multiple environmental effects measured in Europe demonstrated significant differences between organic and conventional systems: organic systems were higher in soil organic matter and lower in energy use. Conventional systems were lower in nitrogen leaching, nitrous oxide emissions, and land use. The authors also report that most studies that compared biodiversity demonstrated lower impacts from organic farming (Tuomisto et al., 2012). The use of synthetic pesticides in nonorganic systems—to control or kill potential disease-causing organisms—pose a number of concerns for environmental health, including water quality impairment by pesticides in 90 percent of water bodies in the United States, in 80 percent of the fish that have been studied, and in 33 percent of major aquifers (U.S. Fish and Wildlife Service, 2014). Pesticides also are producing negative effects on endangered and threatened species and on pollinators (EPA, 2014).

Some consumers express concerns about the perceived loss of direct social and economic ties to local producers and business owners, an increasingly homogenized food retail environment, and lack of transparency in how food is produced and distributed. Local food, which has no generally accepted definition, is a small but growing sector in the United States. In 2008, local sales were $4.8 billion, or about 1.9 percent of total gross farm sales (Low and Vogel, 2011). Most sales are made in metropolitan areas, and in the Northeast and on the West Coast (Tropp, 2014). The majority of local food sales are made through intermediated commercial markets—less than 25 percent come from direct marketing, such as in farmers' markets (Low and Vogel, 2011). About 75 percent of consumers consume locally produced food at least once per month, and almost 90 percent think local foods are very or somewhat important (Tropp, 2014). The motivations for local purchasing, according to a number of surveys, are freshness/superior quality, support for the local economy and local farms, and knowing the source of a product (Martinez et al., 2010).

Consumer concerns about sustainability have contributed to greater calls for corporate social responsibility among mainstream food supply chain firms. Corporate social responsibility (sustainability) programs aimed to improve social and environmental performance have led to significant (and largely unanticipated) changes in the practices of many food processors and retailers. Decisions by retail firms to demand certification of the use of sustainable production and business practices from their suppliers has become one of the most significant drivers of change in the modern U.S. food system.

COMPLEXITIES OF THE SOCIAL AND ECONOMIC EFFECTS

As this chapter shows, any food system configuration will generate positive and negative social and economic effects, and the selection of any of them will invariably result in various trade-offs that need to be compared. Comparing alternative configurations of the U.S. food system is complicated by the fact that, for any one configuration, the various populations and industry sectors might be affected in different ways, both positively and negatively. For example, the efficiencies in the system that have reduced costs for the industry and food prices for consumers have had trade-offs, such as lost jobs and low food-worker wages. These complexities, then, have implications for the methodological approaches used to estimate effects, as it is challenging to tease apart multiple influences and determine the effects of combined exposures. In this section, we highlight some representative examples of the distributions of costs and benefits that occur within the social and economic dimensions as well as interactions that occur between this and the health and environmental dimensions.

Diversity of Impacts

Differences Across Social Groups

The social and economic effects explored in this chapter differentially affect individuals across sociodemographic groups. These disparities have been extensively documented, particularly regarding their effects on health (NIH/HHS, 2014). To appreciate the influence of sociodemographic factors—such as income, race, ethnicity, gender, and citizenship status—when exploring the social and economic effects of the food system, one must acknowledge the statistical correlation of race and ethnicity with socioeconomic status (SES, a construct measuring education, income, and occupation) (LaVeist, 2005). For example, SES tends to be lower among African Americans and Hispanic Americans than white Americans (LaVeist, 2005). In addition, racial residential segregation among the U.S. population has been linked to health and economic disparities (White et al., 2012; Williams and Collins, 2001). The social and economic effects and differences that result from education, occupational working conditions, income, or other factors are closely tied to where people live (LaVeist et al., 2011). Thus, along with the confounding effects of social factors, the geographic and community- or neighborhood-level effects are important to consider when understanding and determining the social and economic effects of the food system. As these effects are measured when applying the framework that the committee developed (see Chapter 4), it is important to at least acknowledge that these social and economic complexities exist and, when feasible, adequately account for them using appropriate statistical methods.

Regional and Global Differences in Impacts on Food Availability and Access

In 2012, the food system produced, on average, 3,688 calories per person per day in the United States (Economist Intelligence Unit, 2013) and approximately 2,700 calories per person per day, globally. As discussed above, this average availability is not distributed equally (Coleman-Jensen et al., 2013; Economist Intelligence Unit, 2013). The accessibility to and affordability of foods globally also is highly diverse. Approximately 842 million people are food insecure worldwide, but the level of insecurity varies substantially depending on the area of the world, with the majority of them living in developing areas (FAO, 2013). In addition, countries differ in the progress made over the years (FAO, 2013). The poverty level is well correlated with the prevalence of undernourishment (FAO, 2013), a factor that can create detrimental feedbacks. The Global Food Security Index (GFSI), created by the Economist Intelligence Unit in 2012, is a measure of food security across the three dimensions of affordability, availability, and use (quality and safety) that integrates 27 indicators.[4] Measured by the GFSI, Asia/the Pacific and sub-Saharan Africa are the areas with the most food insecure people, by numbers and concentration, respectively (Economist Intelligence Unit, 2014).

On the other side of the spectrum are developed countries, namely, the United States and most northern European countries. In each country, the mechanisms for differences in the indicators are rooted in many circumstances related to social, political, and economic drivers that lead to poverty and food insecurity. However, against this background, food-related interventions in developed countries also can have important reverberations in other parts of the world, affecting the poor severely. For example, the global food crisis of 2008 stemmed in part from U.S. biofuels policies. The increase in food prices disproportionally affected some countries like Cambodia, a net importer of rice, where most citizens are net buyers who are already close to the poverty line. The increase in rice prices in 2007-2008 led many Cambodians to levels below the poverty line (Maltsoglou et al., 2010). In addition, the FAO reports that food producers, and especially small holders, are more vulnerable to price increases than are consumers.

Another indicator of global food security is the safety and quality of food. Compared to poorer countries, improvements in diversity and safety of the food supply in the developed world have resulted in much improvement in the adequacy of diets. In developing countries, however,

---

[4] As an example, food affordability is measured by food consumption as a percentage of total household expenditure, proportion of the population living under the poverty line, GDP per capita, agricultural import tariffs, presence of food safety net programs, and access to financing for farmers.

micronutrient availability, protein quality, and diet diversification are more problematic (Economist Intelligence Unit, 2013). A recent paper warned about the increased similarity in diets worldwide being a threat to health and food security, as many countries, especially those less developed, are forsaking traditional crops in favor of a more narrow diversity of crop species (Khoury et al., 2014).

Regional Differences in Social and Economic Impacts of Structural Change

The impacts of structural changes in size and organization of firms in the food supply chain are not experienced equally in all places. In general, rural areas are disadvantaged and have a relatively difficult time adjusting to economic changes associated with industry integration, consolidation, and globalization. This is because their economies are less diversified, lack the agglomeration benefits of urban areas, and offer fewer options to individual employees or firm owners who are displaced by competitive forces. Rural areas are more expensive to service, and it is rare for more than one major retail grocery chain to be able to survive in one area, leading to lower levels of competition, less diverse offerings, and higher prices for many food products.

Different regions also have fared better or worse during recent periods of change. Areas with good soils, favorable climatic conditions, and well-developed agribusiness infrastructure have seen more rapid consolidation in farming and concentration of high-value production systems. Those with better proximity to urban markets have been better able to capitalize on the growth of local and regional food marketing opportunities. Trends that benefit particular commodities will provide benefits for regions that specialize or have competitive advantages in the production of those commodities. For example, the rapid rise of the corn ethanol market in the 2000s could result in significant gains for corn-producing areas but also drive up costs of production and reduced profitability in livestock production regions that had used corn as a major feed source.

Interactions Among Social, Economic, and Environmental Effects

There are many trade-offs between environmental outcomes and the level of profitability or efficiency across the food supply chain. In providing an abundant supply of inexpensive food, the U.S. food system also generates significant impacts on the environment. Conversely, efforts to address environmental problems associated with agricultural production are likely to increase costs to consumers and reduce production efficiencies. Not all gains in environmental performance come at the expense of efficiency, however. For example, using nutrient inputs more efficiently (e.g., matching nutrient applications to crop needs more precisely) may reduce the risk of nutrient losses to the environment. The use of "precision agriculture" techniques can save producers some variable input costs and potentially reduce environmental damage, though rates of adoption have been slower than anticipated (Schimmelpfennig and Ebel, 2011).

Because agriculture is the dominant land use in most regions of the United States, the quality of life by rural residents can be affected by changes in production practices and cropping patterns. Traits of high-output, high-efficiency production systems (e.g., confinement agricultural operations or large-scale monoculture of field crops) can diminish landscape amenity qualities that make rural places desirable to nonagricultural residents. One environmental issue that is affecting producers and consumers alike is the diminished quantity and quality of water. Changes in water associated with farm production and food manufacturing have direct impacts on the cost and quality of water available to small town and urban residents (see also Chapter 3 on the interactions among social, economic, and health effects, and Chapter 7, Annex 4 for a detailed description of the trade-offs among crop productivity and environmental and health effects with different nitrogen management approaches).

Interactions Among Social, Economic, and Health Effects

Health, income, and SES are interrelated in multiple ways. On average, higher-income individuals live longer and are healthier than are lower-income individuals (Deaton and Paxson, 2001). This is in part because they spend more on safety (e.g., drive newer, bigger, safer cars; live in less polluted, safer neighborhoods) and may have better access to health care and insurance. Healthier individuals also may earn more because they lose fewer workdays to disability and illness and may have lower medical expenses, but this effect cannot explain the strength of the income–health relationship (Smith, 1999), nor can it explain the better health of children born to higher-income parents (Case et al., 2002). SES is related to health even after controlling for income (Marmot, 2002). One reason may be the adverse health effects of stress related to lack of control over one's daily activities (e.g., a lower-status employee has less flexibility at work). Some of the associations between health and income and SES may also be related to education, as research shows that better educated individuals have better paying and safer jobs, a lower risk of chronic disease, positive health behaviors, and longer lives than do those with less education (RWJF, 2013).

METHODOLOGIES TO LINK THE FOOD SYSTEM WITH SOCIAL AND ECONOMIC EFFECTS

Determining the social and economic effects of the food system should involve the use of valid and reliable data measured at the necessary scale (e.g., national, regional, or local). However, several current data needs and gaps challenge the ability to accurately measure these effects. A more thorough discussion of the methods needed to comprehensively explore the effects of the food system is presented in Chapter 7. Here, we describe some of the key methodological issues that should be considered when measuring the social and economic effects of the food system.

Data Needs, Metrics, and Analytical Methodologies

To conduct an assessment of the social and economic effects of alternative configurations of the food system and propose interventions (see examples of interventions in Box 5-1), it is necessary to identify key metrics or indicators of social and economic effects. The broad categories outlined in Box 5-2 are well-documented examples of those metrics.

A wide range of food and agricultural data—including prices, costs, inputs, production levels, incomes, food availability, and environmental effects—are compiled by USDA and made available to the public by the National Agricultural Statistics Service and the Economic Research Service. Consumer food expenditures are available from annual surveys by the Bureau of Labor Statistics (BLS). A food prices database is available from USDA's Center for Nutrition Policy and Promotion. Information on food producers is available from USDA surveys and Agricultural Census Data. The Agricultural Resource Management Survey tracks agricultural practices, including chemical and mechanical input use that affect agricultural productivity and environmental outcomes. Other federal agencies, including the BLS and the Centers for Disease Control and Prevention, collect data on occupational safety and health for workers across the food sector, although data are often at the industry level and not always by occupations. Appendix B includes information on where to find some of these key databases, as well as metrics to measure these effects.

However, many data gaps exist. Many of the current national datasets allow for aggregate estimates of economic and social outcomes, such as total number of workers, sector output, productivity, and profitability, especially for large-scale farms. Similar estimates are not easily generated for small-scale farms and by geography, over time, and for certain sectors due to lack of data. In addition, although some of the existing national datasets present data by key sociodemographic factors, such as race, ethnicity, gender, and immigration status, these measures are often lacking at the regional

BOX 5-1
Examples of Interventions with Social or Economic Effects

Policies

- Employment and Training program of the Farm Bill (Agricultural Act of 2014), which reallocates farm bill spending to emphasize rural community development over subsidies to farm operations.
- State minimum wage laws.
- Fair Labor Standards Act, which contains restrictions for minimum age for employment, the times of day youth may work, and the jobs they may perform.
- Government food assistance programs (e.g., SNAP [Supplemental Nutrition Assistance Program], WIC [Special Supplemental Nutrition Program for Women, Infants, and Children]).
- Nutrition Labeling and Education Act, which provides for the Nutrition Facts label to inform consumers about the nutrient content of packaged food products.
- Establishment of OSHA (Occupational Safety and Health Administration) in 1970 to ensure safe and healthful conditions for working men and women for some sectors.
- Immigration laws that might change the availability and cost of foreign-born workers for farm and food system employment.
- Labor laws that would increase protection of the health and safety of farm and food system workers.
- Antitrust regulation that ensure competitive marketing opportunities for independent livestock operators.
- Access to affordable health insurance through the ACA (Patient Protection and Affordable Care Act). (Does not apply to non-American citizens.)
- National Institute for Occupational Safety and Health (NIOSH) strategies to address the high risks of injuries and illness to agricultural workers, commercial fishers, and their families (e.g., efforts to conduct better surveillance of chemical-related exposures).
- NIOSH NORA (National Occupational Research Agenda) program that sets priorities for sector-specific workplace health and safety research to guide policy and practice.

Voluntary Programs

- Increased public investments in infrastructure and institutional support for emerging local food processing and marketing.

Education Efforts

- Nutritional information on the front of the product package to inform consumers about salient benefits of the products.
- NIOSH Education Research Centers and Agricultural and Safety Health Centers.

BOX 5-2
Selected Broad Categories of Metrics of Social and Economic Effects

Income, Wealth, and Equity

- Gross output (gross domestic product)
- Factor productivity
- Sector profitability
- Average net farm income
- Average and median household income
- Industry concentration
- Worker compensation
- Poverty rate
- Unemployment rate

Quality of Life

- Working conditions (hours, benefits, turnover, safety)
- Community well-being
- Entrepreneurship/managerial control (contracting, debt, vertical integration)
- Gender and racial equality
- Economic power (citizenship status, unionization)
- Occupational injury rates (nonfatal and fatal)

Food Availability

- Food costs and expenditures
- Food security
- Food access
- Food quality (taste, healthfulness, convenience, sustainability traits)

and local levels. Thus, the ability to produce stratified estimates by scale along with key sociodemographic factors for social and economic effects is also limited. As a result, when these measures are of interest, analyses often have to extrapolate findings from one scale to another to generate estimates of the effects. Furthermore, sometimes data are not even available to allow for extrapolation. For example, valid and reliable measures of variables that address some important social effects, such as a sense of well-being and career mobility opportunities, are lacking. These metrics are even more difficult to identify for immigrant populations, who are heavily represented among the farm worker population. Levels of income, wealth, and distributional equity also are challenging to measure. These measures are almost always self-reported, and several datasets display a high degree of missing data for these variables because respondents consider the data too private or sensitive or they may not know their income (Davern et al., 2005). When data are missing, it is important to determine whether the data are missing at random and whether imputation techniques could be validly applied.

These gaps in existing data support a need to collect primary data using both quantitative methods (e.g., survey) and qualitative methods (e.g., focus groups and key informant interviews). Although primary data collection may be labor and resource intensive, collecting them is extremely valuable to fill data gaps as well as to add context to existing discrete secondary data. For example, in 2013, USDA published findings from in-depth interviews with SNAP households exploring their use of SNAP and overall food security (USDA, 2013). Many resources describe qualitative data collection and analysis, and investigators should review them before employing this methodology (Creswell, 2007; Miles and Huberman, 1994; Richards and Morse, 2012).

When it comes to consumers, information on freedom of choice to pursue taste and lifestyle preferences also are lacking from some datasets. However, methods that can be used to measure important economic principles have been published in numerous economics journals (Capps and Schmitz, 1991; Huang and Haidacher, 1983; Nelson, 1994; Phillips and Price, 1982; Reed and Levedahl, 2010; Reed et al., 2005; Richards and Padilla, 2009; Talukdar and Lindsey, 2013; Unnevehr et al., 2010). The economic theory of consumer behavior says that the quantity of a good (e.g., a food) will vary inversely with its price and directly with the consumer's income. Price and income are the key variables in a consumer demand model typically analyzed using linear and nonlinear regression techniques—standard statistical tools. The quantity demanded is modeled as a function of price and income, along with other sociodemographic (e.g., gender, individual or household income) or environmental variables. Including these measures can help answer an important question when measuring economic effects: What is the percentage change in quantity that accompanies a 1 percent change in price or income? Demand analysis, a concept of market demand rather than individual behavior, is most useful in examining market trends and behavior. Time series datasets are typically used for this analysis. Appendix B provides a more detailed list of potential data, metrics, and methodologies.

Although price and income are useful variables, they do not entirely explain consumer food choices. Thus, analysts have used regression techniques to look at food consumption patterns and food choices/purchases/sales with numerous variables that may or may not include price and income. These techniques provide insight into the degree of correlation that exists among variables, such as specific nutrient consumption and age, gender, or location. Because these models are not grounded in economic theory, they are not technically demand analysis, but they have been widely used to help understand how consumers choose food and how those choices affect their health and well-being. Data used for these models are typically cross-sectional measures on individual consumers or households and are usually collected by surveys. These types of data have several caveats, including recall bias that results in understatements of the amount of food eaten.

In addition to the traditional consumer demand and consumption studies, some investigators have conducted studies that use the theory of household economics, which incorporates "value of time" into the analysis (Andorka, 1987; Becker, 1965; Deaton and Paxson, 1998; Juster and Smith, 1997; Kinsey, 1983; Whitaker, 2009). This line of analysis, pioneered by Gary Becker, also has been used to study food consumption, as the amount of time required to obtain food is relevant to household food choices. The data used to analyze these models are almost always survey data on individual or household choice and behavior.

More recently, the theories of behavioral economics (Just and Wansink, 2009; Kahneman and Tversky, 1979; List, 2004; Riedl, 2010; Smith, 1985; Umberger and Feuz, 2004; Wansink, 2006) have informed the understanding of consumer choices of food. This is a combination of economics and psychology that improves the explanatory power of demand/consumption analysis by shedding light on why consumers make choices that appear irrational (e.g., they make choices that differ from what they say they want or for short-run gratification in the face of long-term harm). Prospect theory, which includes studies of how people manage risk and uncertainty, helps to inform this behavior.

One of the issues in analyzing food demand and food choices is a lack of data needed to answer many current questions. For example, to determine the correlates of obesity, detailed data about individual food consumption, food prices, and household characteristics as well as health habits and diseases is desirable. Rarely do all of these data on individuals occur in one dataset. A lack of secondary data is partly responsible for the growth of experimental economics, where researchers collect primary data through techniques such as auction games.[5]

Data for capturing effects of alternative food systems also are lacking. As research in this area has been limited, metrics related to the social and economic effects as they pertain to consumption patterns, workers, and production also are lacking. These data gaps may hamper the ability to

[5] Auction games are situations in which actors independently bid on a commodity that is sold to the highest bidder.

measure the social and economic effects when proposals for alternative food systems are discussed.

The development and improvement of models to understand dynamics of farm and food markets and the behavior of key actors in the food supply chain are important in supporting efforts to assess the social and economic effects of changes in the food system. Food prices affect food access and choices, so they are hugely important to the food system. Prices change in response to supply and demand, especially in response to changes in policies, new technologies, and food industry structure. Market models simulate how supply and demand generate feedback for prices and quantities marketed. Some of these models have been adapted to predict not only price and food quantity effects but also likely greenhouse gas emissions due to land-use change. Two such computable general equilibrium models that simulate international trade and market effects are GTAP (Global Trade Analysis Project) and IMPACT (International Model for Policy Analysis of Agricultural Commodities and Trade), both included in Appendix B, Table B-4. The Forest and Agricultural Sector Optimization Model (FASOM) (Schneider et al., 2007) is a computable partial equilibrium model that simulates the agricultural and forest sector in greater detail than the other two, but it does not model feedbacks with the nonagricultural parts of the world economy. The Food and Agricultural Policy Research Institute maintains a proprietary econometric partial equilibrium simulation model that is used to generate detailed price and market forecasts based on current policy and market conditions (Meyers et al., 2010).

Standards of Evidence

Randomized controlled trials (RCTs) are limited in research on the social and economic effects of the food system. Nearly all social science research uses observational study designs, although in some instances, cluster randomized trials are used to explore differences by settings (e.g., schools). Because observational and even quasi-experimental studies are more the norm, social science scholars have posed questions about finding reliable evidence on a program or intervention, and about what the standard of evidence should be (Boruch and Rui, 2008; Flay et al., 2005). Over the past 2 years, a number of organizations have been created to develop an evidence grading scheme across various social science disciplines, including the Society for Prevention Research Committee on Standards and the What Works Clearinghouse of the U.S. Department of Education (Boruch and Rui, 2008).

The Campbell Collaboration was created in 2000 as "the younger sibling" to the Cochrane Collaboration, which was created in 1993 to review studies on the effectiveness of health and health care interventions

(Boruch and Rui, 2008). The Campbell Collaboration focuses on reviews from the social sciences. Unlike the Cochrane Collaboration, which tends to include RCTs, the Campbell Collaboration importantly admits quasi-experimental studies in its evidence standards. This presents an opportunity for additional reviews of the social science literature on relevant areas of the food system. Currently, reviews of the evidence on the role of farmer's wealth and food security, land property rights, and water and sanitation are included in the Campbell Collaboration database (Campbell Collaboration, 2014).

Opportunities for Improvement

Many valuable and widely used national datasets are being eliminated or modified, or are at risk for being eliminated, because of funding limitations. Although a full description of these databases and the extent of the cuts is beyond the scope of this section, several databases that include important metrics for assessing agriculture and food systems are being reduced in length, changing methodology for sampling, or increasing time between data collection, all as part of cost-saving measures. Several reasons support maintaining these databases, including the tremendous benefits of surveillance. Surveillance data allow for monitoring of trends over time, determining changes in risks and outcomes to inform priority setting, developing targeted policies and programs, and evaluating interventions. Efforts to enhance funding to sustain these important national data systems should emphasize the value and necessity of data for evidence-informed decision making.

SUMMARY

As a substantial contributor to the larger bioeconomy, the U.S. food system carries social and economic effects that are both positive and negative. This chapter briefly describes a selected number of social and economic effects that can be partly attributed to the food system and that are mediated by policy contexts and responses. The effects were categorized into (1) levels of income, wealth, and distributional equity; (2) quality of life; and (3) worker health and well-being. To aid in the design of interventions that minimize negative consequences, approaches that consider these important effects, along with their distributions and interactions, are needed. For example: What are the impacts of a specific policy on overall economic wealth and income and the distribution of wealth and income? What are the impacts on worker well-being? What are the impacts on rural communities? Which subsectors of the food system will gain or lose? How will working conditions and employment opportunities for workers in different sectors of the food system be affected? How will the cost and availability of food for consumers be affected? The analytical framework proposed in Chapter 7 is designed to ensure that the broad implications of these questions can be examined.

REFERENCES

Alaimo, K., C. M. Olson, and E. A. Frongillo. 2001. Food insufficiency and American school-aged children's cognitive, academic, and psychosocial development. *Pediatrics* 108(1):44-53.

Alaimo, K., C. M. Olson, and E. A. Frongillo. 2002. Family food insufficiency, but not low family income, is positively associated with dysthymia and suicide symptoms in adolescents. *Journal of Nutrition* 132(4):719-725.

Alston, J. M., J. M. Beddow, and P. G. Pardey. 2009. Agriculture. Agricultural research, productivity, and food prices in the long run. *Science* 325(5945):1209-1210.

Andorka, R. 1987. Time budgets and their uses. *Annual Review of Sociology* 13:149-164.

Andreyeva, T., M. W. Long, and K. D. Brownell. 2010. The impact of food prices on consumption: A systematic review of research on the price elasticity of demand for food. *American Journal of Public Health* 100(2):216-222.

Artz, G. M. 2012. Immigration and meatpacking in the Midwest. *Choices* 27(2)1-5.

Ashiabi, G. 2005. Household food insecurity and children's school engagement. *Journal of Children and Poverty* 11:1, 3-17.

Badgley, C., J. Moghtader, E. Quintero, E. Zakem, M. J. Chappell, K. Aviles-Vazquez, A. Samulon, and I. Perfecto. 2007. Organic agriculture and the global food supply. *Renewable Agriculture and Food Systems* 22(2):86-108.

Bail, K. M., J. Foster, S. G. Dalmida, U. Kelly, M. Howett, E. P. Ferranti, and J. Wold. 2012. The impact of invisibility on the health of migrant farmworkers in the southeastern United States: A case study from Georgia. *Nursing Research and Practice* 2012:760418.

Banks, V. J. 1986. *Black farmers and their farms*. Rural Development Research Report No. 59. Washington, DC: U.S. Department of Agriculture, Economic Research Service.

Barlett, P. F. 1993. *American dreams, rural realities: Family farms in crisis*. Chapel Hill, NC: University of North Carolina Press.

Becker, G. S. 1965. A theory of the allocation of time. *Economic Journal* 75(299):493-517.

Belasco, W., and P. Scranton. 2002. *Food nations: Selling taste in consumer societies*. New York: Routledge.

BLS (Bureau of Labor Statistics). 2010. Food for thought. *Spotlight on statistics*. November. http://www.bls.gov/spotlight/archive.htm (accessed February 11, 2014).

BLS. 2012. *Consumer expenditure survey. Table 1202. Income before taxes: Annual expenditure means, shares, standard errors, and coefficient of variation*. http://www.bls.gov/cex/2012/combined/income.pdf (accessed November 21, 2014).

BLS. 2013. *Labor force statistics from the Current Population Survey. Table 39: Median weekly earnings of full-time wage and salary workers by detailed occupation and sex*. http://www.bls.gov/cps/cpsaat39.htm (accessed November 24, 2014).

BLS. 2014a. *Consumer expenditure survey. Table 1101. Quintiles of income before taxes: Annual expenditure means, shares, standard errors, and coefficient of variation, Consumer Expenditure Survey, 2012*. http://www.bls.gov/cex/2012/combined/quintile.pdf (accessed November 21, 2014).

BLS. 2014b. *Occupational outlook handbook, 2014-15 edition*. http://www.bls.gov/ooh (accessed February 2, 2014).

BLS. 2014c. Union members–2013. *News Release* USDL-14-0095. http://www.bls.gov/news.release/pdf/union2.pdf (accessed November 21, 2014).

Boruch, R., and N. Rui. 2008. From randomized controlled trials to evidence grading schemes: Current state of evidence-based practice in social sciences. *Journal of Evidence Based Medicine* 1(1):41-49.

Brown, J. L., D. Shepard, T. Martin, and J. Orwat. 2007. *The economic cost of domestic hunger.* Sodexo Foundation. http://www.sodexofoundation.org/newsletter/pdf/economic_cost_of_domestic_hunger.pdf (accessed November 22, 2014).

Calvert, G. M., J. Karnik, L. Mehler, J. Beckman, B. Morrissey, J. Sievert, R. Barrett, M. Lackovic, L. Mabee, A. Schwartz, Y. Mitchell, and S. Moraga-McHaley. 2008. Acute pesticide poisoning among agricultural workers in the United States, 1998-2005. *American Journal of Industrial Medicine* 51(12):883-898.

Campbell Collaboration. 2014. *The Campbell Collaboration library of systematic reviews.* http://www.campbellcollaboration.org/lib (accessed November 22, 2014).

Capps, O., and J. D. Schmitz. 1991. A recognition of health and nutrition factors in food demand analysis. *Western Journal of Agricultural Economics* 16(1):21-35.

Carlson, A., and E. Frazão. 2012. *Are healthy foods really more expensive?: It depends on how you measure the price.* Economic Information Bulletin No. 96. Washington, DC: U.S. Department of Agriculture, Economic Research Service.

Case, A., D. Lubotsky, and C. Paxson. 2002. Economic status and health in childhood: The origins of the gradient. *American Economic Review* 92(5):1308-1334.

CBPP (Center on Budget and Policy Priorities). 2014. *Policy basics: Introduction to SNAP.* http://www.cbpp.org/cms/index.cfm?fa=view&id=2226 (accessed November 15, 2014).

CDC (Centers for Disease Control and Prevention). 2014a. *For food handlers. Norovirus and working with food.* http://www.cdc.gov/norovirus/food-handlers/work-with-food.html (accessed February 11, 2014).

CDC. 2014b. *The National Institute for Occupational Safety and Health (NIOSH).* http://www.cdc.gov/niosh (accessed February 11, 2014).

CDC. 2014c. *Young worker safety and health.* http://www.cdc.gov/niosh/topics/youth (accessed February 11, 2014).

CDC/NIOSH (CDC/National Institute for Occupational Safety and Health). 2014. *Motor vehicle safety.* http://www.cdc.gov/niosh/topics/motorvehicle (accessed November 22, 2014).

Chung, C., and E. Tostao. 2012. Effects of horizontal consolidation under bilateral imperfect competition between processors and retailers. *Applied Economics* 44(26):3379-3389.

Cochrane, W. W. 1993. *The development of American agriculture: A historical analysis*, 2nd ed. Minneapolis, MN: University of Minnesota Press.

Cohen, J. 2013. *Food industries' healthy margins.* http://www.ibisworld.com/media/wp-content/uploads/2013/05/Food-Industries.pdf (accessed November 22, 2014).

Coleman-Jensen, A., M. Nord, and A. Singh. 2013. *Household food security in the United States in 2012.* Economic Research Report No. ERR-155. Washington, DC: U.S. Department of Agriculture, Economic Research Service.

Cone Communications. 2014. *Food issues trend tracker.* http://www.conecomm.com/2014-food-issues (accessed November 22, 2014).

Contento, I. 2010. *Nutrition education: Linking research, theory, and practice*, 2nd ed. Sudbury, MA: Jones and Bartlett.

Creswell, J. W. 2007. *Qualitative inquiry and research design. Choosing among five approaches*, 2nd ed. Thousand Oaks, CA: Sage Publications, Inc.

Cummins, S., and S. Macintyre. 1999. The location of food stores in urban areas: A case study in Glasgow. *British Food Journal* 101:545-553.

Davern, M., H. Rodin, T. J. Beebe, and K. T. Call. 2005. The effect of income question design in health surveys on family income, poverty and eligibility estimates. *Health Services Research* 40(5):1534-1552.

Deaton, A., and C. Paxson. 1998. Economies of scale, household size, and the demand for food. *Journal of Political Economy* 106(5):897-930.

Deaton, A., and C. Paxson. 2001. Mortality, education, income and inequality among American cohorts. NBER Working Paper No. 7140. In *Themes in the economics of aging*, edited by D. A. Wise. Chicago, IL: University of Chicago Press. Pp. 129-165.

Deller, S. C., T. H. Tsai, D. W. Marcouiller, and D. B. K. English. 2001. The role of amenities and quality of life in rural economic growth. *American Journal of Agricultural Economics* 83(2):352-365.

Dimitri, C., and L. Oberholtzer. 2009. *Marketing U.S. organic foods: Recent trends from farms to consumers*. Economic Information Bulletin No. EIB-58. Washington, DC: U.S. Department of Agriculture, Economic Research Service.

Drabenstott, M. 2000. A new structure for agriculture: A revolution for rural America. *Journal of Agribusiness* 18(1):61-70.

Economist Intelligence Unit. 2013. *Global food security index 2013: An annual measure of the state of global food security.* http://foodsecurityindex.eiu.com/Resources (accessed November 18, 2014).

Economist Intelligence Unit. 2014. *Global food security index*. http://foodsecurityindex.eiu.com/ (accessed November 18, 2014).

Edmonson, W. 2004. Economics of the food and fiber system. *Amber Waves*. http://www.ers.usda.gov/amber-waves/2004-february/data-feature.aspx#.VFjiC8lNc3g (accessed November 22, 2014).

EPA (U.S. Environmental Protection Agency). 2014. *Protecting bees and other pollinators from pesticides*. http://www2.epa.gov/pollinator-protection (accessed November 22, 2014).

ERS (Economic Research Service). 1996. *Farmers' use of marketing and production contracts*. Agricultural Economic Report No. (AER-747). http://www.ers.usda.gov/publications/aer-agricultural-economic-report/aer747.aspx (accessed January 6, 2015).

ERS. 2013a. *Ag and food statistics: Charting the essentials*. http://www.ers.usda.gov/publications/ap-administrative-publication/ap062.aspx#.UvoOoPvwv3s (accessed February 11, 2014).

ERS. 2013b. *Farm labor.* Background. http://www.ers.usda.gov/topics/farm-economy/farm-labor/background.aspx#.VEfDWxbYetM (accessed October 22, 2014).

ERS. 2013c. *New products*. http://www.ers.usda.gov/topics/food-markets-prices/processing-marketing/new-products.aspx (accessed November 22, 2014).

ERS. 2014a. *Agricultural productivity in the U.S. Overview*. http://www.ers.usda.gov/data-products/agricultural-productivity-in-the-us.aspx#.U_-SjWPkpQB (accessed November 24, 2014).

ERS. 2014b. *Farm household income (historical)*. http://www.ers.usda.gov/topics/farm-economy/farm-household-well-being/farm-household-income-%28historical%29.aspx#.Uvl3pPvcjTp (accessed February 10, 2014).

ERS. 2014c. Food and beverage manufacturing. http://www.ers.usda.gov/topics/food-markets-prices/processing-marketing/manufacturing.aspx#.VEcFNEtd09c (accessed November 4, 2014).

ERS. 2014d. *Food expenditures*. http://www.ers.usda.gov/data-products/food-expenditures.aspx (accessed November 24, 2014).

ERS. 2014e. *Indicator table*. March 14, 2014. http://www.ers.usda.gov/amber-waves/2014-march/indicator-table.aspx#.VFjoypV0y71 (accessed November 4, 2014).

ERS. 2014f. *Manufacturing*. http://www.ers.usda.gov/topics/food-markets-prices/processing-marketing/manufacturing.aspx#.Uvowa_vwv3t (accessed February 11, 2014).

ERS. 2014g. *Market segments.* http://www.ers.usda.gov/topics/food-markets-prices/food-service-industry/market-segments.aspx#.Uvo36_vwv3t (accessed February 11, 2014).

ERS. 2014h. *Policy issues.* http://www.ers.usda.gov will/topics/food-markets-prices/retailing-wholesaling/policy-issues.aspx#.UvowI_vwv3t (accessed February 11, 2014).

ERS. 2014i. *U.S. and state farm income and wealth statistics.* http://ers.usda.gov/data-products/farm-income-and-wealth-statistics.aspx#.Uvl1r_vcjTo (accessed February 10, 2014).

ERS. 2014j. *Wealth, farm programs, and health insurance.* http://www.ers.usda.gov/topics/farm-economy/farm-household-well-being/wealth,-farm-programs,-and-health-insurance.aspx#.Uvl7ZPvcjTp (accessed February 10, 2014).

FAO (Food and Agriculture Organization of the United Nations). 2013. *The state of food insecurity in the world 2013. The multiple dimensions of food security.* Rome, Italy: FAO.

Farmworker Justice. 2009. *State workers' compensation coverage for agricultural workers.* http://www.farmworkerjustice.org/sites/default/files/documents/6.3.a.1State_Workers_Comp_Information_for_Health_Centers_11-09.pdf (accessed February 10, 2014).

FCWA (Food Chain Workers Alliance). 2012. *The hands that feed us: Challenges and opportunities for workers along the food chain.* Los Angeles, CA: FCWA.

Feeding America. 2013. *Solving hunger together. 2013 annual report summary.* http://www.feedingamerica.org/our-response/about-us/annual-report (accessed October 28, 2014).

Feeding America. 2014a. *About us.* http://feedingamerica.org/how-we-fight-hunger/about-us.aspx (accessed November 23, 2014).

Feeding America. 2014b. *Hunger and poverty fact sheet.* http://www.feedingamerica.org/hunger-in-america/impact-of-hunger/hunger-and-poverty/hunger-and-poverty-fact-sheet.html (accessed November 23, 2014).

Fernandez-Cornejo, J. 2007. *Off-farm income, technology adaptation, and farm income performance.* Economic Research Report No. ERR-36. Washington, DC: U.S. Department of Agriculture, Economic Research Service.

Findeis, J. L., A. M. Vandeman, J. M. Larson, and J. L. Runyan. 2002. *The dynamics of hired farm labour: Constraints and community responses.* New York: CABI Publishing.

Flay, B. R., A. Biglan, R. F. Boruch, F. G. Castro, D. Gottfredson, S. Kellam, E. K. Moscicki, S. Schinke, J. C. Valentine, and P. Ji. 2005. Standards of evidence: Criteria for efficacy, effectiveness and dissemination. *Prevention Science* 6(3):151-175.

Flora, C. B. 1995. Social capital and sustainability: Agriculture and communities in the Great Plains and Corn Belt. *Research in Rural Sociology and Development* 6(6):227-246.

FMI (Food Marketing Institute). 2013. *Grocery store chains net profit—Percent of sales.* http://www.fmi.org/docs/default-source/facts-figures/grocery-store-chains-net-profit_2013.pdf?sfvrsn=2 (accessed November 23, 2014).

Foltz, J., and K. Zeuli. 2005. The role of community and farm characteristics in farm input purchasing patterns. *Review of Agricultural Economics* 27(4):508-525.

Foltz, J. D., D. Jackson-Smith, and L. Chen. 2002. Do purchasing patterns differ between large and small dairy farms? Econometric evidence from three Wisconsin communities? *Agricultural and Resource Economics Review* 31(1):28-38.

Fortune magazine. 2014. *2014 top U.S. companies (Fortune 500 and 100 best companies to work for).* http://money.cnn.com/magazines/fortune/fortune500/2013/full_list/index.html?iid=F500_sp_full (accessed November 23, 2014).

Fraser, C. E., K. B. Smith, F. Judd, J. S. Humphreys, L. J. Fragar, and A. Henderson. 2005. Farming and mental health problems and mental illness. *International Journal of Social Psychiatry* 51(4):340-349.

Free Library, The. 2014. *Ergonomics in the warehouse.* http://www.thefreelibrary.com/Ergonomics+in+the+warehouse%3a+warehouse+workers+face+the+highest+rates...-a092082589 (accessed February 11, 2014).

Freire, C., and S. Koifman. 2013. Pesticides, depression and suicide: A systematic review of the epidemiological evidence. *International Journal of Hygiene and Environmental Health* 216(4):445-460.

Fuglie, K., and P. Heisey. 2007. *Economic returns to public agricultural research.* Economic Brief No. EB-10. Washington, DC: U.S. Department of Agriculture, Economic Research Service.

Fuglie, K., P. Heisey, J. King, and D. Schimmelfennig. 2012. Rising concentration in agricultural input industries influences new farm technologies. *Amber Waves* 10(4):1-6.

Gardner, B. L. 2002. *American agriculture in the twentieth century: How it flourished and what it cost.* Cambridge, MA: Harvard University Press.

Gasson, R., and A. J. Errington. 1993. *The farm family business.* Wallingford, UK: CAB International.

Geiser, K., and B. J. Rosenberg. 2006. The social context of occupational and environmental health. In *Occupational and environmental health: Recognizing and preventing disease and injury*, edited by B. S. Levy, D. H. Wegman, S. L. Baron, and R. K. Sokas. Philadelphia, PA: Lippincott Williams & Wilkins. Pp. 21-39.

Goldschmidt, W. 1978. *As you sow: Three studies in the social consequences of agribusiness.* Montclair, NJ: Allanheld, Osmun, and Co.

Gundersen, C., and B. Kreider. 2009. Bounding the effects of food insecurity on children's health outcomes. *Journal of Health Economics* 28:971-983.

Gundersen, C., B. Kreider, and J. Pepper. 2011. The economics of food insecurity in the United States. *Applied Economic Perspectives and Policy* 33(3):281-303.

Hall, M., and E. Greenman. 2014. The occupational cost of being illegal in the United States: Legal status, job hazards, and compensating differentials. *International Migration Review.* http://onlinelibrary.wiley.com/doi/10.1111/imre.12090/pdf (accessed November 23, 2014).

Hanson, K. 2010. *The Food Assistance National Input-Output Multiplier (FANIOM) model and the stimulus effects of SNAP.* Economic Research Report No. ERR-103. Washington, DC: U.S. Department of Agriculture, Economic Research Service.

Harvard School of Public Health. 2012. *TV watching and "Sit Time."* http://www.hsph.harvard.edu/obesity-prevention-source/obesity-causes/television-and-sedentary-behavior-and-obesity (accessed November 24, 2014).

Henderson, R. 2012. Industry employment and output projections to 2020. *Monthly Labor Review* 135(1):65-83.

HHS (U.S. Department of Health and Human Services). 2014. *Poverty guidelines.* http://aspe.hhs.gov/poverty/14poverty.cfm (accessed March 6, 2014).

Hoppe, R. A., and P. Korb. 2013. *Characteristics of women farm operators and their farms.* Economic Information Bulletin No. 111. Washington, DC: U.S. Department of Agriculture, Economic Research Service.

Hoppe, R., J. MacDonald, and P. Korb. 2010. *Small farms in the United States: Persistence under pressure.* Economic Information Bulletin No. EIB-63. Washington, DC: U.S. Department of Agriculture, Economic Research Service.

HRSA (Health Resources and Services Administration). 2014. *HPSA designation criteria.* http://bhpr.hrsa.gov/shortage/hpsas/designationcriteria/designationcriteria.html (accessed February 10, 2014).

Huang, J., K. M. Mata Oshima, and Y. Kim. 2010. Does household food insecurity affect parenting and children's behaviors? Evidence from the Panel Study of Income Dynamics (PSID). *Social Service Review* 84(3):381-401.

Huang, K. S., and R. C. Haidacher. 1983. Estimation of a composite food demand system for the United States. *Journal of Business and Economic Statistics* 1(4):285-291.

IFIC (International Food Information Council Foundation). 2013. *2013 Food and Health Survey. Consumer attitudes toward food safety, nutrition and health*. http://www.foodinsight.org/articles/2013-food-and-health-survey (accessed November 24, 2014).

IFIC. 2014a. *2014 Food and Health Survey. Consumer attitudes toward food safety, nutrition and health*. http://www.foodinsight.org/articles/2014-food-and-health-survey (accessed November 24, 2014).

IFIC. 2014b. *2014 IFIC consumer perceptions of Food Technology Survey*. http://www.foodinsight.org/2014-foodtechsurvey (accessed November 24, 2014).

IOM (Institute of Medicine). 2013. *Supplemental Nutrition Assistance Program: Examining the evidence to define benefit adequacy*. Washington, DC: The National Academies Press.

Isserman, A. M., E. Feser, and D. E. Warren. 2009. Why some rural places prosper and others do not. *International Regional Science Review* 32(3):300-342.

Jones, C., T. Parker, M. Ahearn, A. Mishra, and J. Variyam. 2009a. *Health status and health-care access of farm and rural populations*. Economic Information Bulletin No. EIB-57. Washington, DC: U.S. Department of Agriculture, Economic Research Service.

Jones, C., T. Parker, and M. Ahearn. 2009b. Taking the pulse of rural health care. *Amber Waves* September 1.

Just, D. 2013. Consumer preferences and marketing as drivers of the food system. Paper presented at the Institute of Medicine/National Research Council Committee on a Framework for Assessing the Health, Environmental, and Social Effects of the Food System Meeting, Washington, DC, September 16.

Just, D. R., and C. R. Payne. 2009. Obesity: Can behavioral economics help? *Annals of Behavioral Medicine* 38(Suppl 1):S47-S55.

Just, D. R., and B. Wansink. 2009. Smarter lunchrooms: Using behavioral economics to improve meal selection. *Choices* 24(3):1-7.

Juster, F. T., and J. P. Smith. 1997. Improving the quality of economic data: Lessons from the HRS and AHEAD. *Journal of the American Statistical Association* 92(440):1268-1278.

Kahneman, D., and A. Tversky. 1979. Prospect theory—Analysis of decision under risk. *Econometrica* 47(2):263-291.

Kandel, W. 2008. *Profile of hired farmworkers. A 2008 update*. Economic Research Report No. ERR-60. Washington, DC: U.S. Department of Agriculture, Economic Research Service.

Kelly, M., H. Lang, G. Bhandal, and C. Electris. 2012. *Worker and social equity in food and agriculture. Practices at the 100 largest and most influential U.S. companies*. Boston, MA: Tellus Institute and Sustainalytics.

Key, N., and W. D. McBride. 2007. *The changing economics of U.S. hog production*. Economic Research Report ERR-52. Washington, DC: U.S. Department of Agriculture, Economic Research Service.

Khoury, C. K., A. D. Bjorkman, H. Dempewolf, J. Ramirez-Villegas, L. Guarino, A. Jarvis, L. H. Rieseberg, and P. C. Struik. 2014. Increasing homogeneity in global food supplies and the implications for food security. *Proceedings of the National Academy of Sciences of the United States of America* 111(11):4001-4006.

Kilkenny, M. 2010. Urban/regional economics and rural development. *Journal of Regional Science* 50(1):449-470.

King, R. P., M. Anderson, G. DiGiacomo, D. Mulla, and D. Wallinga. 2012. *State level food system indicators*. http://foodindustrycenter.umn.edu/Research/foodsystemindicators/index.htm (accessed November 24, 2014).

Kinsey, J. 1983. Working wives and the marginal propensity to consume food away from home. *American Journal of Agricultural Economics* 65(1):10-19.

Kinsey, J. 2013. Expectations and realities of the food system. In *U.S. programs affecting food and agricultural marketing*, edited by W. J. Armbruster and R. Knutson. New York: Springer Science + Business Media. Pp. 11-42.
Kirkpatrick, S., L. McIntyre, and M. L. Potestio. 2010. Child hunger and long-term adverse consequences for health. *Archives of Pediatric and Adolescent Medicine* 164(8):754-762.
Kuchler, F., and H. Stewart. 2008. *Price trends are similar for fruits, vegetables, and snack foods*. Economic Research Report No. ERR-55. Washington, DC: U.S. Department of Agriculture, Economic Research Service.
Kuhn, M. E. 2014. Salaries back on track. *Food Technology* 68(2):22-30.
Labao, L., and C.W. Stofferahn. 2008. The community effects of industrialized farming: Social science research and challenges to corporate farming laws. *Agriculture and Human Values* 25:219-240.
Lambert, D., T. Wojan, and P. Sullivan. 2009. Farm business and household expenditure patterns and local communities: Evidence from a national farm survey. *Review of Agricultural Economics* 31(3):604-626.
LaVeist, T. A. 2005. Disentangling race and socioeconomic status: A key to understanding health inequalities. *Journal of Urban Health* 82(2 Suppl 3):iii26-iii34.
LaVeist, T., K. Pollack, R. Thorpe, Jr., R. Fesahazion, and D. Gaskin. 2011. Place, not race: Disparities dissipate in southwest Baltimore when Blacks and whites live under similar conditions. *Health Affairs (Millwood)* 30(10):1880-1887.
Lawrence, J. D. 2010. Hog marketing practices and competition. *Choices* 25(2):1-11.
Lee, H. 2012. The role of local food availability in explaining obesity risk among young school-aged children. *Social Science and Medicine* 74(8):1-11.
Leonard, C. 2014. *The meat racket*. New York: Simon & Schuster.
Lin, B.-H., and J. Guthrie. 2012. *Nutritional quality of food prepared at home and away from home, 1977-2008*. Economic Information Bulletin No. EIB-105. Washington, DC: U.S. Department of Agriculture, Economic Research Service.
List, J. A. 2004. Neoclassical theory versus prospect theory: Evidence from the marketplace. *Econometrica* 72(2):615-625.
Liu, Y. Y. 2012. *Good food + good jobs for all. Challenges and opportunities to advance racial and economic equity in the food system*. New York: Applied Research Center.
Low, S. A., and S. Vogel. 2011. *Direct and intermediated marketing of local foods in the United States*. Economic Research Report No. ERR-128. Washington, DC: U.S. Department of Agriculture, Economic Research Service.
Lowenstein, G. 2013. Behavioral economics: Implications for the food environment and choices. In *Sustainable diets: Food for healthy people in a healthy planet: Workshop summary*. Washington, DC: The National Academies Press. Pp. 108-116.
Ludwig, D. S., and H. A. Pollack. 2009. Obesity and the economy: From crisis to opportunity. *Journal of the American Medical Association* 301(5):533-535.
Lyson, T. 2004. *Civic agriculture: Reconnecting farm, food, and community*. Medford, MA: Tufts University Press.
Ma, C. T., L. Gee, and M. B. Kushel. 2008. Associations between housing instability and food insecurity with health care access in low-income children. *Ambulatory Pediatrics* 8(1):50-57.
MacDonald, J. M. 2008. *The economic organization of U.S. broiler production*. Economic Information Bulletin No. EIB-38. Washington, DC: U.S. Department of Agriculture, Economic Research Service.
MacDonald, J. M., and P. Korb. 2008. *Agricultural contracting update, 2005*. Economic Information Bulletin No. EIB-35. Washington, DC: U.S. Department of Agriculture, Economic Research Service.

MacDonald, J. M., and P. Korb. 2011. *Agricultural contracting update: Contracts in 2008.* Economic Information Bulletin No. EIB-72. Washington, DC: U.S. Department of Agriculture, Economic Research Service.
MacDonald, J. M., and W. D. McBride. 2009. *The transformation of U.S. livestock agriculture: Scale, efficiency, and risks.* Economic Information Bulletin No. EIB-43. Washington, DC: U.S. Department of Agriculture, Economic Research Service.
Maltsoglou, I., D. Dawe, and L. Tasciotti. 2010. *Household level impacts of increasing food prices in Cambodia.* Rome, Italy: The Bioenergy and Food Security Project, FAO.
Marion, B. W. 1986. *The organization and performance of the U.S. food system.* Lexington, MA: D.C. Heath.
Marion, B., and F. E. Geithman. 1995. Concentration-price relations in regional fed cattle markets. *Review of Industrial Organization* 10:1-19.
Marmot, M. 2002. The influence of income on health: Views of an epidemiologist. *Health Affairs* 21(2):31-46.
Martin, P. 2009. *Importing poverty?: Immigration and the changing face of rural America.* New Haven, CT: Yale University Press.
Martin, P. 2013. Immigration and farm labor: Policy options and consequences. *American Journal of Agricultural Economics* 95(2):470-475.
Martin, P., and D. Jackson-Smith. 2013. Immigration and farm labor in the U.S. *National Agricultural and Rural Development Policy Center Policy Brief* 4. http://www.nardep.info/uploads/Brief_FarmWorker.pdf (accessed November 24, 2014).
Martinez, S., M. S. Hand, M. Da Pra, S. Pollack, K. Ralston, T. Smith, S. Vogel, S. Clark, L. Tauer, L. Lohr, S. A. Low, and C. Newman. 2010. *Local food systems: Concepts, impacts, and issues.* Economic Research Report No. ERR-97. Washington, DC: U.S. Department of Agriculture, Economic Research Service.
McCurdy, S. A., and D. J. Carroll. 2000. Agricultural injury. *American Journal of Industrial Medicine* 38(4):463-480.
McEowen, R. A., P. C. Carstensen, and N. E. Harl. 2002. The 2002 Senate farm bill: The ban on packer ownership of livestock. *Drake Journal of Agricultural Law* 7:267-304.
McGranahan, D., and P. Sullivan. 2005. Farm programs, natural amenities and rural development. *Amber Waves.* http://www.ers.usda.gov/amber-waves/2005-february/farm-programs,-natural-amenities,-and-rural-development.aspx#.VKvZCXtWeT9 (accessed January 6, 2015).
Meyers, W. H., P. Westhoff, J. F. Fabiosa, and D. J. Hayes. 2010. The FAPRI global modeling system and outlook process. *Journal of International Agricultural Trade and Development* 6(1):1-20.
Miles, M. B., and A. M. Huberman. 1994. *Qualitative data analysis: An expanded sourcebook*, 2nd ed. Thousand Oaks, CA: Sage Publications, Inc.
Murray, C. J., S. C. Kulkarni, C. Michaud, N. Tomijima, M. T. Bulzacchelli, T. J. Iandiorio, and M. Ezzati. 2006. Eight Americas: Investigating mortality disparities across races, counties, and race-counties in the United States. *PLoS Medicine* 3(9):1513-1524.
Myers, R. J., R. J. Sexton, and W. G. Tomek. 2010. A century of research on agricultural markets. *American Journal of Agricultural Economics* 92(2):376-402.
NCFH (National Center for Farmworker Health). 2012. *Facts about farmworkers.* http://www.ncfh.org/docs/fs-Facts%20about%20Farmworkers.pdf (accessed November 24, 2014).
Nelson, J. A. 1994. Estimation of food demand elasticities using Hicksian composite commodity assumptions. *Quarterly Journal of Business and Economics* 33(3):51-68.
Nelson, K., W. Cunningham, R. Andersen, G. Harrison, and L. Gelberg. 2001. Is food insufficiency associated with health status and health care utilization among adults with diabetes? *Journal of General Internal Medicine* 16:404-411.

NIH/EPA/NIOSH (National Institutes of Health/Environmental Protection Agency/National Institute for Occupational Safety and Health). 2014. *Agricultural health study*. http://aghealth.nih.gov (accessed November 24, 2014).

NIH/HHS. 2014. *NIH health disparities strategic plan and budget, fiscal years 2009-2013*. http://www.nimhd.nih.gov/documents/NIH%20Health%20Disparities%20Strategic%20Plan%20and%20Budget%202009-2013.pdf (accessed April 30, 2014).

NILC (National Immigration Law Center). 2014. *Affordable Care Act*. http://www.nilc.org/immigrantshcr.html (accessed February 10, 2014).

NIOSH. 2010. *Worker safety on the farm*. DHHS (NIOSH) Publication No. 2010-137. http://www.cdc.gov/niosh/docs/2010-137 (accessed January 5, 2015).

NIOSH. 2011. *NIOSH pesticide poisoning monitoring program protects farmworkers*. DHHS (NIOSH) Publication No. 2012-108. http://www.cdc.gov/niosh/docs/2012-108 (accessed January 5, 2015).

NIOSH. 2014. *Commercial fishing safety*. http://www.cdc.gov/niosh/topics/fishing (accessed October 25, 2014).

Nord, M. 2009. *Food insecurity in households with children: Prevalence, severity, and household characteristics*. Economic Information Bulletin No. EIB-56. Washington, DC: U.S. Department of Agriculture, Economic Research Service.

Nord, M., A. Coleman-Jensen, and C. Gregory. 2014. *Prevalence of U.S. food insecurity is related to changes in unemployment, inflation, and the price of food*. Economic Research Report No. ERR-167. Washington, DC: U.S. Department of Agriculture, Economic Research Service.

O'Donoghue, E. J., R. A. Hoppe, D. E. Banker, R. Ebel, K. Fuglie, P. Korb, M. Livingston, C. J. Nickerson, and C. Sandretto. 2011. *The changing organization of U.S. farming*. Economic Information Bulletin No. EIB-88. Washington, DC: U.S. Department of Agriculture, Economic Research Service.

OSHA (Occupational Safety and Health Administration). 2014. *Meat packing industry*. https://www.osha.gov/SLTC/meatpacking/index.html (accessed February 11, 2014).

OTA (Organic Trade Association). 2011. *Seventy-eight percent of U.S. families say they purchase organic food*. http://www.organicnewsroom.com/2011/11/seventyeight_percent_of_us_fam.html (accessed November 24, 2014).

OTA. 2014. *American appetite for organic products breaks through $35 billion mark*. http://www.organicnewsroom.com/2014/05/american_appetite_for_organic.html (accessed November 24, 2014).

Pena, A. A. 2010. Poverty, legal status, and pay basis: The case of U.S. agriculture. *Industrial Relations* 49(3):429-456.

Phillips, K. S., and D. W. Price. 1982. A comparative theoretical analysis of the impact of the Food Stamp Program as opposed to cash transfers on the demand for food. *Western Journal of Agricultural Economics* 7(1):53-66.

Powell, L., J. Harris, and T. Fox. 2013. Food marketing expenditures aimed at youth. *American Journal of Preventive Medicine* 45(4):453-461.

Probst, J. C., S. B. Laditka, J. Y. Wang, and A. O. Johnson. 2007. Effects of residence and race on burden of travel for care: Cross sectional analysis of the 2001 U.S. National Household Travel Survey. *BMC Health Services Research* 7:40-53.

Reardon, T., and C. P. Timmer. 2012. The economics of the food system revolution. *Annual Review of Resource Economics* 4:224-263.

Reed, A. J., and J. W. Levedahl. 2010. Food Stamps and the market demand for food. *American Journal of Agricultural Economics* 92(5):1392-1400.

Reed, A. J., J. W. Levedahl, and C. Hallahan. 2005. The generalized composite commodity theorem and food demand estimation. *American Journal of Agricultural Economics* 87(1):28-37.

Reinhardt, N., and P. Barlett. 1989. The persistence of family farms in United States agriculture. *Sociologia Ruralis* 29(3-4):203-225.

Richards, L., and J. Morse. 2012. *README FIRST for a user's guide to qualitative research*, 3rd ed. Thousand Oaks, CA: Sage Publications, Inc.

Richards, T. J., and L. Padilla. 2009. Promotion and fast food demand. *American Journal of Agricultural Economics* 91(1):168-183.

Riedl, A. 2010. Behavioral and experimental economics do inform public policy. *Finanzarchiv* 66(1):65-95.

Roberts, S. E., B. Jaremin, and K. Lloyd. 2013. High-risk occupations for suicide. *Psychological Medicine* 43(6):1231-1240.

Rocha, C. 2007. Food insecurity as market failure: A contribution from economics. *Journal of Hunger and Environmental Nutrition* 1(4):5-22.

RWJF (Robert Wood Johnson Foundation). 2013. *Why does education matter so much to health?* http://www.rwjf.org/content/dam/farm/reports/issue_briefs/2012/rwjf403347 (accessed November 24, 2014).

Santelmann, M. V., D. White, K. Freemark, J. I. Nassauer, J. M. Eilers, K. B. Vache, B. J. Danielson, R. C. Corry, M. E. Clark, S. Polasky, R. M. Cruse, J. Sifneos, H. Rustigian, C. Coiner, J. Wu, and D. Debinski. 2004. Assessing alternative futures for agriculture in Iowa, USA. *Landscape Ecology* 19(4):357-374.

Schimmelpfennig, D., and R. Ebel. 2011. *On the doorstep of the information age*. Economic Information Bulletin No. EIB-80. Washington, DC: U.S. Department of Agriculture, Economic Research Service.

Schneider, U. A., B. A. McCarl, and E. Schmid. 2007. Agricultural sector analysis on greenhouse gas mitigation in U.S. agriculture and forestry. *Agricultural Systems* 94(2):128-140.

Schnepf, R. 2013. *Farm-to-food price dynamics*. Washington, DC: Congressional Research Service.

Seattle Global Justice. 2014. *United States farmworker fact sheet*. http://www.seattleglobaljustice.org/wp-content/uploads/fwfactsheet.pdf (accessed November 24, 2014).

Seligman, H. K., A. B. Bindman, E. Vittinghoff, A. M. Kanaya, and M. B. Kushel. 2007. Food insecurity is associated with diabetes mellitus: Results from the National Health and Nutrition Examination Survey (NHANES) 1999-2002. *Journal of General Internal Medicine* 22(7):1018-1023.

Seligman, H. K., B. A. Laraia, and M. B. Kushel. 2010. Food insecurity is associated with chronic disease among low-income NHANES participants. *Journal of Nutrition* 140(2):304-310.

Seligman, H. K., E. A. Jacobs, A. Lopez, J. Tschann, and A. Fernandez. 2012. Food insecurity and glycemic control among low-income patients with type 2 diabetes. *Diabetes Care* 35(2):233-238.

Seufert, V., N. Ramankutty, and J. Foley. 2012. Comparing the yields of organic and conventional agriculture. *Nature* 458:229-232.

Sexton, R. J. 2000. Industrialization and consolidation in the U.S. food sector: Implications for competition and welfare. *American Journal of Agricultural Economics* 82(5):1087-1104.

Sexton, R. J. 2013. Market power, misconceptions, and modern agricultural markets. *American Journal of Agricultural Economics* 95(2):209-219.

Sfiligoj, E. 2012. *Ag retail consolidation trending up*. http://www.croplife.com/special-reports/state-of-the-industry/ag-retail-consolidation-trending-up (accessed November 24, 2014).

Share Our Strength. 2012. *It's dinner time: A report on low income families efforts to plan, shop and cook healthy meals*. http://www.nokidhungry.org/cmstudy (accessed November 24, 2014).

Shiv, B., and A. Fedorikhin. 1999. Heart and mind in conflict: The interplay of affect and cognition in consumer decision making. *Journal of Consumer Research* 26:278-292.

Smith, J. P. 1999. Healthy bodies and thick wallets: The dual relationship between health and socioeconomic status. *Journal of Economic Perspectives* 13(2):145-166.

Smith, L. P., S. W. Ng, and B. M. Popkin. 2013. Trends in U.S. home food preparation and consumption: Analysis of national nutrition surveys and time use studies from 1965-1966 to 2007-2008. *Nutrition Journal* 12:45.

Smith, V. L. 1985. Experimental economics—Reply. *American Economic Review* 75(1):265-272.

Sommers, D., and J. C. Franklin. 2012. Overview of projections to 2020. *Monthly Labor Review* 135(1):3-20.

Stevens-Garmon, J., C. L. Huang, and B.-H. Lin. 2007. Organic demand: A profile of consumers in the fresh produce market. *Choices* 22(2):109-116.

Stofferahn, C. 2006. *Industrialized farming and its relationship to community well-being: An update of a 2000 report by Linda Lobao*. Prepared for the state of North Dakota, Office of the Attorney General. http://www.und.edu/org/ndrural/Lobao%20&%20Stofferahn.pdf (accessed November 24, 2014).

Stull, D. D., M. J. Broadway, and D. Griffith. 1995. *Any way you cut it: Meat processing and small-town America*. Lawrence, KS: University of Kansas Press.

Syed, S. T., B. S. Gerber, and L. K. Sharp. 2013. Traveling towards disease: Transportation barriers to health care access. *Journal of Community Health* 38(5):976-993.

Talukdar, D., and C. Lindsey. 2013. To buy or not to buy: Consumers' demand response patterns for healthy versus unhealthy food. *Journal of Marketing* 77(2):124-138.

TFIC (The Food Industry Center). 2014. *Indicator data*. http://foodindustrycenter.umn.edu/Research/foodsystemindicators/indicatordata/index.htm (accessed February 10, 2014).

Tropp, D. 2014. *Why local food matters: The rising importance of locally-grown food in the United States food system—A national perspective*. USDA Agricultural Marketing Service. http://www.ams.usda.gov/AMSv1.0/getfile?dDocName=STELPRDC5105706 (accessed November 24, 2014).

Tuomisto, H., I. Hodge, P. Riordan, and D. MacDonald. 2012. Does organic farming reduce environmental impacts? A meta-analysis of European research. *Journal of Environmental Management* 112:309-320.

Umberger, W. J., and D. M. Feuz. 2004. The usefulness of experimental auctions in determining consumers' willingness-to-pay for quality-differentiated products. *Review of Agricultural Economics* 26(2):170-185.

Unnevehr, L., J. Eales, H. Jensen, J. Lusk, J. McCluskey, and J. Kinsey. 2010. Food and consumer economics. *American Journal of Agricultural Economics* 92(2):506-521.

U.S. Census Bureau. 2014. *Enterprise statistics. Table 7. Summary statistics for enterprises by industry: 2011*. http://www.census.gov/econ/esp (accessed November 17, 2014).

U.S. Fish and Wildlife Service. 2014. *Environmental quality. Pesticides and wildlife*. http://www.fws.gov/contaminants/Issues/Pesticides.cfm (accessed November 24, 2014).

U.S. GAO (U.S. Government Accountability Office). 2009. *Concentration in agriculture*. GAO-09-746R. http://www.gao.gov/new.items/d09746r.pdf (accessed November 24, 2014).

USDA (U.S. Department of Agriculture). 2009. *2007 Census volume 1, Chapter 1: U.S. national level data. Table 1*. http://www.agcensus.usda.gov/Publications/2007/Full_Report/Volume_1,_Chapter_1_US (accessed February 10, 2014).

USDA. 2013. *SNAP Food Security In-Depth Interview Study*. http://www.fns.usda.gov/snap-food-security-depth-interview-study (accessed November 24, 2014).

USDA. 2014a. *Cooperative directory and data*. http://www.rurdev.usda.gov/BCP_Coop_DirectoryAndData.html (accessed February 11, 2014).

USDA. 2014b. *2012 Census of agriculture. United States*. http://www.agcensus.usda.gov/Publications/2012 (accessed February 11, 2014).

USDA. 2014c. *Definitions of food security*. http://www.ers.usda.gov/topics/food-nutrition-assistance/food-security-in-the-us/definitions-of-food-security.aspx (accessed October 29, 2014).

USDOL (U.S. Department of Labor). 2005. *A demographic and employment profile of United States farm workers. Findings from the National Agricultural Workers Survey (NAWS) 2001-2002*. Research Report No. 9. U.S. Department of Labor. http://www.doleta.gov/agworker/report9/toc.cfm (accessed January 6, 2015).

VanDeCruze, D., and M. Wiggins. 2008. *Poverty and injustice in the food system. A report for Oxfam America*. Durham, NC: Student Action with Farmworkers. http://ducis.jhfc.duke.edu/wp-content/uploads/2010/06/Poverty-and-Injustice-in-the-Food-System.pdf (accessed February 11, 2014).

Ver Ploeg, M., V. Breneman, T. Farrigan, K. Hamrick, D. Hopkins, P. Kaufman, B-H. Lin, M. Nord, T.A. Smith, R. Williams, K. Kinnison, C. Olander, A. Singh, and E. Tuckermanty. 2009. *Access to affordable and nutritious food measuring and understanding food deserts and their consequences: Report to Congress*. Washington, DC: U.S. Department of Agriculture, Economic Research Service.

Volpe, R. 2013. Price inflation for food outpacing many other spending categories. *Amber Waves*. http://www.ers.usda.gov/amber-waves/2013-august/price-inflation-for-food-outpacing-many-other-spending-categories.aspx#.VKvOxntWeT9 (accessed January 6, 2015).

Volpe, R., and A. Okrent. 2012. *Assessing the healthfulness of consumers' grocery purchases*. Economic Information Bulletin No. EIB-102. Washington, DC: U.S. Department of Agriculture, Economic Research Service.

Wainer, A. 2011. Farm workers and immigration policy. *Briefing paper* 12. http://www.bread.org/institute/papers/farm-workers-and-immigration.pdf (accessed November 24, 2014).

Wang, S. L., and E. Ball. 2014. Agricultural productivity growth in the United States: 1948-2011. *Amber Waves* January/February. http://www.ers.usda.gov/amber-waves/2014-januaryfebruary/agricultural-productivity-growth-in-the-united-states-1948-2011.aspx#.VKvaLHtWeT- (accessed January 6, 2015).

Wansink, B. 2006. *Mindless eating*. New York: Bantam Books.

Wansink, B., and J. Sobal. 2007. Mindless eating: The 200 daily food decisions we overlook. *Environment and Behavior* 39(1):106-123.

Ward, C. E. 2007. *Feedlot and packer pricing behavior: Implications for competition research*. Paper presented at Western Agricultural Economics Association annual meeting, Portland, OR, July 29 to August 1, 2007. http://ageconsearch.umn.edu/bitstream/7365/2/sp07wa01.pdf (accessed November 24, 2014).

Wendt, M., and J. Todd. 2011. *Effect of food and beverage prices on children's weights*. Economic Research Report No. ERR-118. Washington, DC: U.S. Department of Agriculture, Economic Research Service.

Whitaker, J. B. 2009. The varying impacts of agricultural support programs on US farm household consumption. *American Journal of Agricultural Economics* 91(3):569-580.

Whitaker, R. C., S. M. Phillips, and S. M. Orzol. 2006. Food insecurity and the risks of depression and anxiety in mothers and behavior problems in their preschool-aged children. *Pediatrics* 118(3):e859-e868.

White, K., J. S. Haas, and D. R. Williams. 2012. Elucidating the role of place in health care disparities: The example of racial/ethnic residential segregation. *Health Services Research* 47(3 Pt 2):1278-1299.

Williams, D. R., and C. Collins. 2001. Racial residential segregation: A fundamental cause of racial disparities in health. *Public Health Reports* 116(5):404-416.

Wood, S., and J. Gilbert. 2000. Returning African American farmers to the land: Recent trends and a policy rationale. *The Review of Black Political Economy* 27(4):43-64.

Yen, H. 2014. The new face of food stamps: Working-age Americans. *AP: The Big Story*, January 27.

PART III

The Framework

6

The U.S. Food and Agriculture System as a Complex Adaptive System

The U.S. food system has many features characteristic of a *complex adaptive system*, both in its structure (see Chapter 2) and in its effects (see Chapters 3-5). The complex systems perspective can offer important insights for understanding the dynamics of both the current configuration of the food system and the potential alternative configurations of the food system. This chapter begins by describing the properties of a complex adaptive system (CAS), illustrated with examples specific to the food system and with references to other chapters in the report as appropriate. The chapter then reviews the implications of these properties for the development of a sufficiently rich and comprehensive framework, including consideration of how specific factors shape the complex dynamics of the food system with regard to health, environmental, social, and economic outcomes.

COMPLEX ADAPTIVE SYSTEMS

A CAS is a system composed of many heterogeneous pieces whose interactions drive system behavior in ways that cannot easily be understood from considering the components separately. Such systems, whether they are social, physical, or biological, tend to share a set of specific properties (Hammond, 2009; Holland, 1992; Miller and Page, 2007). Consideration of these properties and their implications from many scientific and policy perspectives have yielded important insights into system behavior. These perspectives include social science (Axelrod, 1997; Axtell et al., 2002; Epstein, 2002, 2007; Schelling, 1978; Tesfatsion and Judd,

2006), public health (Auchincloss and Roux, 2008; Diez Roux, 2007; Epstein, 2009; Eubank et al., 2004; Homer and Hirsch, 2006; Huang and Glass, 2008; IOM, 2012; Longini et al., 2005; Luke and Stamatakis, 2012; Mabry et al., 2008, 2010), biology (Axelrod et al., 2006; Segovia-Juarez et al., 2004), business (Sterman, 2000), and land/ecosystem management (Parker et al., 2003; Schluter and Pahl-Wostl, 2007). Each of the following sections describes one important general property of CAS and then illustrates its applicability to the U.S. food and agriculture system with specific examples.

Individuality and Adaptation

Complex systems generally contain a variety of autonomous actors. These may vary considerably in local context, motivation, exposure to information or environmental signals, or level of scale. The decentralized interaction of actors is often a key driver of system behavior. At the same time, the actors themselves often adapt through time in response to other actors or to changes in the system state. Adaptation can occur at different speeds and take different forms across individuals. A variety of actors and processes of adaptation can be found within the U.S. food and agriculture system. Human actors in the system include consumers, farmers, laborers, food processors and manufacturers, distributors, food service providers, and researchers. At a higher level of aggregation, multinational firms, governments, regulatory agencies, and universities may act as unified actors that play important roles. At lower levels of scale, pathogenic bacteria, agricultural pests, and even genetic material (e.g., in the resistome[1]) represent distinct actors.

In modern industrialized societies, a vast array of human actors and aggregate institutional actors play important roles in shaping the structure and dynamics of the food system. Individual decisions that shape food system outcomes are made daily by farmers, crop field workers, bankers, crop consultants, grain elevator operators, meat packers, corporate product developers, advertisers, grocery store managers, truck drivers, chefs, waiters, home food gatekeepers, nutritionists, garbage collectors, antihunger and environmental activists, state and federal legislators, government employees, researchers, and physicians (to name a few). Consumer decisions on what, where, when, and how to buy and eat are fundamental drivers of the food supply chain in most countries. These decisions likewise drive ancillary outcomes for health, environmental, social, and economic effects of the food system because they shape what foods are produced,

[1] Resistome refers to the collection of antibiotic resistance genes and their precursors in both pathogenic and nonpathogenic bacteria.

how they are produced, how they are made available, and how our bodies respond to what we eat (or do not eat). Individuals make decisions within organizational and institutional contexts that shape their choice sets and alter the costs and benefits of different options. Leaders of large agricultural input companies, food processing and distribution firms, retail grocery and restaurant chains, and institutional food buyers (like schools and hospitals) are themselves actors—whose business decisions affect the choices of individuals who work for or buy from these firms. Market research guides advertising to influence consumer choices in ways that benefit the marketers. Politicians and public agency leaders develop tax, regulatory, trade, and research policies to respond to shifts in societal values and political power, which in turn constrain the behaviors of economic firms and individual actors.

Processes of adaptation by individual actors in the food system are varied, ranging from changing consumer preferences to changing farming practices to evolution of drug resistance. Changes to the food system thus have impacts across the component subsystems of the food supply chain, and also across space, that go beyond simply "ripples"—because interventions can trigger adaptive responses. Not all actors will adapt to any specific system change, and not all adaptations have "beneficial" (or discernible) effects. Considering the full set of adaptive responses (by multiple types of actors) that is triggered by any change can be important for sufficient understanding of likely system effects. For example, the introduction of herbicide tolerant crops (e.g., Roundup Ready™ soybeans) not only reduced tillage and soil erosion but also reduced labor and energy use per acre, induced land conversion to crop use, and fostered the evolution of herbicide-resistant weeds (Barrows et al., 2014).

Feedback and Interdependence

Just as complex systems usually contain a variety of distinct (but interacting) actors, they tend also to contain several distinct (but potentially linked) mechanisms or pathways. These may cross multiple levels of the system (e.g., the hedonic reward pathway driving some eating behavior, which involves micro-level biological processes within a human, the physical environments surrounding them, the social or market-level processes connecting them), and they often interact with each other, creating interdependence of factors in the system. Obesity is a classic example of a phenomenon driven by multiple interdependent factors (see Chapter 3). A central hallmark of complex systems is the presence of feedback between actors or factors in the system. Feedback describes a dynamic process in which change in one part of a system affects another component, which, in turn, affects the original component again (often with a time lag). Within a complex system, feedback may cross different levels of scale (e.g., within an organism and in the environment surrounding it), sectors (e.g., economic, health, and social), or spatial boundaries (e.g., U.S. consumers and South American agriculture). Feedback can be positive (reinforcing) or negative (balancing).

Numerous examples of feedback and interdependence can be found in the U.S. food and agriculture system. As illustrated in Figure 6-1, the food system can be conceptualized as a transformation process that both depends on and creates important feedbacks for natural resources and human society. Natural resources like air, soil, water, and biota (pollinators, natural enemies of food pests) are essential for agricultural production, as well as the manufacture of many foods like bread, cheese, and wine. Yet depletion and effluents from the food system influence the future status of natural resources. In Figure 6-1, these changes occur from time 0 to time 1. Likewise, the food system depends on a host of human systems that govern our health, markets, policy, and general well-being. These human systems provide the labor, entrepreneurship, capital, and technology needed to produce and distribute food. Once again, the food system generates feedbacks that influence human systems at a future period.

Another prominent feedback example of widespread concern is the evolution of pesticide and antibiotic resistance by insects, pests, weeds, and plant and animal pathogens, which now incurs multibillion-dollar costs each year. These costs reflect the prevalence of inadequate and ineffective strategies for limiting the strength of the selection pressures for resistance created by chemical controls that initially are efficacious. Given the limited availability of new chemistries for controlling pests and pathogens and the ability of resistant organisms to move and transmit genetic material, this form of feedback and interdependence may greatly affect future management options in food, agriculture, and health systems.

Certain grazing practices also can shift rangeland systems to a less productive regime by reducing vegetation cover, setting in motion a feedback relationship that decreases nutrient and water accumulation (Gordon et al., 2008). Similarly, policy efforts to increase animal welfare by promoting free-range housing for hens have in some cases adversely affected the health of the animals by increasing exposure to pathogens through the soil and cannibalistic pecking (see Chapter 7, Annex 5).

Complex feedbacks occur also in the socioeconomic aspects of the food system. Market supply and demand relationships shape prices that act as incentives on the behavior of producers and consumers. Many food grains have well-developed futures markets as well as current markets, allowing prices to adjust based on expectations of future supply and demand. At times markets can reveal surprising indirect effects, as when a U.S. biofuel mandate contributed to higher global corn prices that, in turn, shifted more land into agricultural use (Hayes et al., 2009; Searchinger et al., 2008).

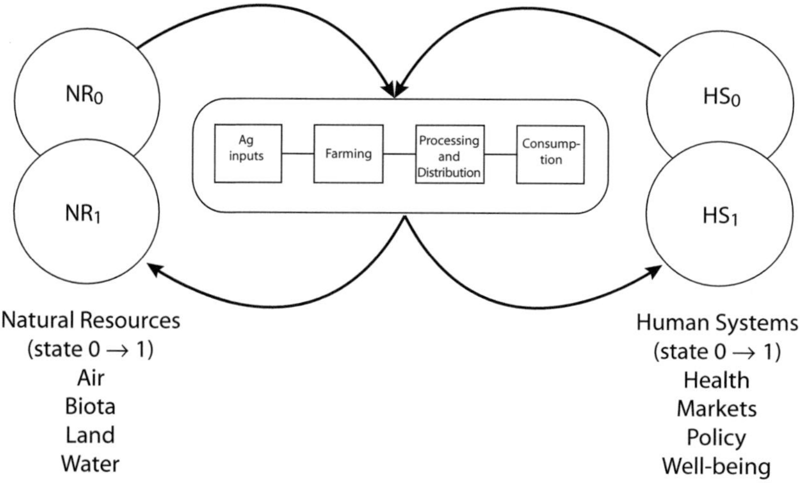

FIGURE 6-1 Food system as a dynamic process transforming the state of natural resources and human systems from one period to the next.

Indeed, this example highlights the fact that market effects are not limited to price feedbacks that communicate incentives to buyers and sellers. Markets also create repercussions for the availability of goods and services that lack clear property rights. Climate stability, a global ecosystem service, is a clear example where a lack of property rights makes markets fail to regulate greenhouse gas emissions (like those from indirect land use), so policy interventions are needed. The political feedback mechanisms that shape policy design represent another layer of complexity in the food system.

Heterogeneity

Actors and processes in a CAS often exhibit substantial *heterogeneity*—they differ from each other in ways that can strongly shape local dynamics in parts of the system. For example, actors within the system may have different goals, different decision-making procedures, different information, different local environmental exposures, or different constraints on their actions. These differences can shape divergent adaptation or responses to changes in the system. Heterogeneity very often occurs across types of actors (as described above). For example, multinational corporations are likely to have very different information and constraints than those faced by individual consumers, and crop insect pests have different behavioral repertoires than pathogenic bacteria do. There also may be substantial heterogeneity *within* a particular type of actor. For example, consumers may vary in income, health status, or preferences; food service operators may face different regulatory regimes in different places; and farms certainly vary in the composition of their soil and in size and sales volume (see Chapter 5).

A good case study example of heterogeneity in types of distinct actors in the food system can be found in fruit and vegetable intake (see Chapter 7, Annex 3). Changing the intake levels of fruits and vegetables is likely to involve farmers, farm workers, food manufacturers, retailers, marketers, restaurants, school food service workers, and household food gatekeepers, each with different incentives and facing different information sets, which must be considered in assessing the likely impact of an intervention in this area.

Socioeconomic, spatial, and cultural heterogeneity also can lead the impacts of food system changes to differ significantly for different subgroups (see Chapter 5). This is an important consideration in the case of cage-free eggs. Because cage-free chickens are more expensive to maintain than those that are confined, switching to such methods could involve a substantial increase in market price. Demand for eggs is relatively inelastic, so most of the impact of that price increase would fall on lower-income families that rely on eggs as an inexpensive source of protein. Ignoring differences among consumers would mask the distributional consequences of such a shift.

Population heterogeneity also is a major consideration for the health effects of the food system (see Chapter 3), where risk factors, exposures, and disease outcomes may all differ substantially.

Spatial Complexity

Complex systems often contain spatial organization that strongly shapes dynamics within them. These spatial properties can govern the interaction of actors, existence and speed of feedback, and heterogeneity across the system. Physical geography (whether naturally occurring or built) and networks (whether representing contacts, flows of materials or information, or relationships among groups such as species) are examples of spatial organization. Within the food and agriculture system, elements of spatial organization include supply chains, market segmentation, the patchwork of geographically specific regulations across states and counties, international borders, and ecosystems and food webs. Spatial structure can matter by directly shaping the local context experienced by actors, but it also can shape impacts at a distance, govern changes in environment over time (e.g., spatial displacement as in environmental effects like pollution; see Chapter 4), and create indirect and possibly unintended effects (e.g., resurgence of target pests or antibiotic resistance through the resistome; see Chapter 7, Box 7-7).

Because of the broad spatial extent of arable cropland, pastures, and rangelands in many regions of the United States, agricultural production systems can have marked effects on water quality and quantity and on wildlife habitat and population densities. A key factor determining the impacts of agricultural production systems on water, wildlife, and other natural resources is the spatial organization of system components. For example, connectivity of strips of non-crop vegetation across a landscape dominated by crops can foster migration corridors for birds of conservation concern. Strips of trees, shrubs, and grasses can dramatically reduce the quantity of soil sediment moving from croplands to adjacent streams. Spatial concentration of livestock production, meanwhile, can magnify environmental effects (see Chapter 4). Spatial structure also is an important driver of consumer behavior (see Chapter 5) and health effects (see Chapter 3). For example, obesity outcomes can be strongly shaped by geography (e.g., the availability and convenience of food or the presence of advertising) as well as by "social" spatial structures (e.g., peer networks) (see Chapter 3). The importance of spatial structure in chronic disease is easily observed in the spatial patterns of incidence that emerge (see Chapter 3).

Dynamic Complexity

The presence of feedback, interdependence, and adaptation in a complex system can produce dynamics with characteristic properties. These often include substantial nonlinearity or "tipping points," path dependence, and system behaviors that appear to be "emergent," that is, system-level behaviors that differ from what might be expected from the sum of behaviors of individual components of the system. Nonlinearity can yield large effects from relatively small changes in system configuration. Examples in the food system include the relationship between arable cropland conversion to conservation buffer strips composed of reconstructed prairie and the consequent reduction in the export of soil sediments from watersheds (see Chapter 4), or the metabolic changes that result from weight gain and loss (see Chapter 3). The coupling of social and ecological systems (each with their own nonlinear processes) within the food system can lead to even stronger nonlinearities in the response of the overall system to changes (see Chapter 5).

Path dependence refers to phenomena whose later dynamics are strongly shaped by the sequence of early events. Examples in the food system include the relative importance of early life nutrition experience in shaping later habits, behaviors, and chronic disease risk (see Chapter 3).

Management of fish stocks is an important (and canonical) example of dynamic complexity at work (see Chapter 7, Annex 1). Overfishing often results in sudden and dramatic collapses in fish stocks if not carefully monitored and managed. This type of phase transition can occur because overfishing both depletes the existing stock of fish and reduces the rate at which fish populations are replenished through breeding. Globally, 90 percent of fisheries are considered fully exploited or overly so. Increasing demand for fish and the effects of climate change threaten to tip many fisheries toward collapse. In many cases, transitioning to aquaculture does not relieve the pressure on natural fisheries because wild stocks of herring, anchovies, and sardines are still sometimes used as feed sources for aquaculture production.

Given the importance of feedbacks in a complex system, another dynamic system characteristic of special interest (as noted in the discussion of environmental effects in Chapter 4) is the degree of resilience the system manifests when stressed by physical and biotic factors. Resilience also is relevant in the context of social and economic stress factors. For all types of stressors, resilience can be viewed as an ability to bounce back from sudden shocks and long-term stressors. For agricultural systems, temperature extremes, droughts, floods, and pests are recurrent, though unpredictable, biophysical stresses. Similarly, rapid increases in input costs, sharp declines in market values of crops and livestock, and regulations form part of the matrix of socioeconomic stress factors acting on agricultural systems. Often, farmers can take actions that minimize risks and susceptibilities to stress factors (e.g., adding irrigation systems to make up for precipitation deficits, purchasing crop insurance to cover lost revenue), but these risk reduction measures can incur significant costs. Other approaches, such as diversifying cropping systems to include crops with different planting and harvest dates, and contrasting vulnerabilities to pests, may incur little or no additional cost. In some cases, as in the case of federally subsidized crop insurance, costs for increasing resilience may be distributed to society at large.

IMPLICATIONS FOR A FRAMEWORK TO ASSESS FOOD SYSTEM EFFECTS

The U.S. food and agriculture system has many of the characteristics of a CAS. It has diverse and adaptive individual actors, with substantial feedback and interdependence among them, and it includes both spatial and temporal heterogeneity as well as an adaptive change dynamic. Recognition of the food system as a CAS has important implications for efforts to assess its effects, and thus for the framework presented in the next chapter (Chapter 7). The complex systems perspective highlights key systemic features that a framework should address and argues for consideration of approaches and methodologies that can appropriately capture these features. Although no one method or approach is likely able to capture all elements of the system at once, the discussion of key aspects of complexity above is intended to guide consideration of what to include in (and what may be left out of) any analysis. In Chapter 7, the committee lays out a framework designed to inform assessments of the food system with a complex system perspective in mind, considering complexity in four distinct ways across six distinct steps. Chapter 7 also discusses specific methods that are well suited to capturing key aspects of complex dynamics, recognizing, however, that not all analyses can (or should) address all of the elements of the complex food system.

REFERENCES

Auchincloss, A. H., and A. V. D. Roux. 2008. A new tool for epidemiology: The usefulness of dynamic-agent models in understanding place effects on health. *American Journal of Epidemiology* 168(1):1-9.

Axelrod, R. 1997. *The complexity of cooperation: Agent-based models of competition and collaboration*. Princeton, NJ: Princeton University Press.

Axelrod, R., D. Axelrod, and K. J. Pienta. 2006. Evolution of cooperation among tumor cells. *Proceedings of the National Academy of Sciences of the United States of America* 103(36):13474-13479.

Axtell, R. L., J. M. Epstein, J. S. Dean, G. J. Gumerman, A. C. Swedlund, J. Harburger, S. Chakravarty, R. Hammond, J. Parker, and M. Parker. 2002. Population growth and collapse in a multiagent model of the Kayenta Anasazi in Long House Valley. *Proceedings of the National Academy of Sciences of the United States of America* 99(Suppl 3):7275-7279.

Barrows, G., S. Sexton, and D. Zilberman. 2014. Agricultural biotechnology: The promise and prospects of genetically modified crops. *Journal of Economic Perspectives* 28(1):99-120.

Diez Roux, A. V. 2007. Integrating social and biologic factors in health research: A systems view. *Annals of Epidemiology* 17(7):569-574.

Epstein, J. 2002. Modeling civil violence: An agent-based computational approach. *Proceedings of the National Academy of Sciences of the United States of America* 99(3):7243-7250.

Epstein, J. M. 2007. *Generative social science*. Princeton, NJ: Princeton University Press.

Epstein, J. 2009. Modeling to contain pandemics. *Nature* 460:687.

Eubank, S., H. Guclu, V. S. Kumar, M. V. Marathe, A. Srinivasan, Z. Toroczkai, and N. Wang. 2004. Modelling disease outbreaks in realistic urban social networks. *Nature* 429(6988):180-184.

Gordon, L. J., G. D. Peterson, and E. M. Bennett. 2008. Agricultural modifications of hydrological flows create ecological surprises. *Trends in Ecology & Evolution* 23(4):211-219.

Hammond, R. 2009. Complex systems modeling for obesity research. *Preventing Chronic Disease* 6:1-10.

Hayes, D., B. Babcock, J. Fabiosa, S. Tokgoz, A. Elobeid, T.-H. Yu, F. Dong, C. Hart, E. Chavez, S. Pan, M. Carriquiry, and J. Dumortier. 2009. Biofuels: Potential production capacity, effects on grain and livestock sectors, and implications for food prices and consumers. *Journal of Agricultural and Applied Economics* 41(2):465-491.

Holland, J. H. 1992. *Adaptation in natural and artificial systems*. Cambridge, MA: MIT Press.

Homer, J. B., and G. Hirsch. 2006. System dynamics modeling for public health: Background and opportunities. *American Journal of Public Health* 96:452-458.

Huang, T. T., and T. A. Glass. 2008. Transforming research strategies for understanding and preventing obesity. *Journal of the American Medical Association* 300(15):1811-1813.

IOM (Institute of Medicine). 2012. *Accelerating progress in obesity prevention: Solving the weight of the nation*. Washington, DC: The National Academies Press.

Longini, I. M., Jr., A. Nizam, S. Xu, K. Ungchusak, W. Hanshaoworakul, D. A. Cummings, and M. E. Halloran. 2005. Containing pandemic influenza at the source. *Science* 309(5737):1083-1087.

Luke, D. A., and K. A. Stamatakis. 2012. Systems science methods in public health: Dynamics, networks, and agents. *Annual Review of Public Health* 33:357-376.

Mabry, P. L., D. H. Olster, G. D. Morgan, and D. B. Abrams. 2008. Interdisciplinarity and systems science to improve population health: A view from the NIH Office of Behavioral and Social Sciences Research. *American Journal of Preventive Medicine* 35(2 Suppl):S211-S224.

Mabry, P. L., S. E. Marcus, P. I. Clark, S. J. Leischow, and D. Mendez. 2010. Systems science: A revolution in public health policy research. *American Journal of Public Health* 100(7):1161-1163.

Miller, J. H., and S. E. Page. 2007. *Complex adaptive systems: An introduction to computational models of social life*. Princeton, NJ: Princeton University Press.

Parker, D. C., S. M. Manson, M. A. Janssen, M. J. Hoffmann, and P. Deadman. 2003. Multi-agent systems for the simulation of land-use and land-cover change: A review. *Annals of the Association of American Geographers* 93(2):314-337.

Schelling, T. C. 1978. *Micromotives and macrobehavior*. New York: W.W. Norton and Co.

Schluter, M., and C. Pahl-Wostl. 2007. Mechanisms of resilience in common-pool resource management systems: An agent-based model of water use in a river basin. *Ecology and Society* 12(2):4.

Searchinger, T., R. Heimlich, R. A. Houghton, F. X. Dong, A. Elobeid, J. Fabiosa, S. Tokgoz, D. Hayes, and T. H. Yu. 2008. Use of U.S. croplands for biofuels increases greenhouse gases through emissions from land-use change. *Science* 319(5867):1238-1240.

Segovia-Juarez, J. L., S. Ganguli, and D. Kirschner. 2004. Identifying control mechanisms of granuloma formation during m. Tuberculosis infection using an agent-based model. *Journal of Theoretical Biology* 231(3):357-376.

Sterman, J. D. 2000. *Business dynamics: Systems thinking and modeling for a complex world*. Boston, MA: Irwin McGraw-Hill.

Tesfatsion, L., and K. J. Judd. 2006. *Handbook of computational economics, Vol. 2: Agent-based computational economics*. Amsterdam, The Netherlands: North-Holland.

7

A Framework for Assessing the Food System and Its Effects

As the other chapters in this report make clear, the U.S. food system has evolved into a highly complex one, where changes due to new policies, products, or technologies can have diverse and sometimes unanticipated repercussions. A robust framework for assessing the health, environmental, social, and economic effects of the food system should recognize the system's complexity while offering a tractable way forward.

This chapter proposes such a framework, including key principles, important food system traits, and specific steps for developing an assessment. The chapter also reviews specific approaches for communicating findings, along with ways to engage key stakeholders and conduct a thoughtful analysis of a complex system within a budget. In this sense, not all steps or methods will apply equally, depending on the scope and topic chosen by a researcher. The committee recognizes that discrete questions might not require a full systemic analysis, although assessors still need to recognize boundaries and implications (i.e., potential relevant effects, actors, interactions that are left out of the analysis) so that others may conduct complementary research. In other cases, there may be a lot of data already on some discrete questions. In such cases, a systematic review of the literature for the relevant questions would need to be conducted to synthesize the results and identify future data or analyses needed.

FRAMEWORKS FOR ASSESSMENT

A framework for assessment provides a conceptual and empirical structure to guide an evaluation. A good framework identifies best practices to facilitate well-informed decisions, given the resources available and the goals of those conducting the assessment. The main users of an assessment framework for the food system will be researchers and decision makers (e.g., at government agencies, private firms, or advocacy groups). Other stakeholders might not be users per se, but the recipients of reports developed from the assessment. Previous frameworks for assessment have generally identified several key steps to be followed in an iterative manner: identify the problem, define the scope, identify the scenario, conduct the analysis, synthesize the findings, and report to stakeholders. These six key steps are part of widely used assessment frameworks, such as environmental assessment (Powers et al., 2012), health impact assessment (with stakeholder engagement throughout the entire assessment process) (NRC, 2011), and risk assessment (NRC, 2009). Our framework for assessment of the food system follows these same six steps for implementing the assessment.

Frameworks for assessment will vary from one area of application to another. The scope and complexity of the application area, along with data and analytical methods, will drive the principles that pertain to a specific assessment framework.

RECOMMENDED FRAMEWORK FOR ASSESSING HEALTH, ENVIRONMENTAL, SOCIAL, AND ECONOMIC EFFECTS OF THE FOOD SYSTEM

The recommended framework for assessing the health, environmental, social, and economic effects of the food system revolves around four key principles (represented by the four quadrants in Figure 7-1). These principles draw on knowledge and evidence from across the various segments of the U.S. and global food systems and the many interactive agents and activities that currently deliver food from seed to table. Because changes in any one segment of the food system result in changes, intended or not, in many other parts of the system, the committee recommends a comprehensive approach that captures the food system holistically and accounts for several types of potential effects. In Figure 7-1, the two upper quadrants illustrate principles associated with the desirable scope of an assessment:

- *Recognize Effects Across the Full Food System* to highlight the connections among different food supply chain sectors and the important role of biophysical, social, economic, and institutional contexts.
- *Consider All Domains and Dimensions of Effects* to ensure that the assessment captures the potential trade-offs across health, envi-

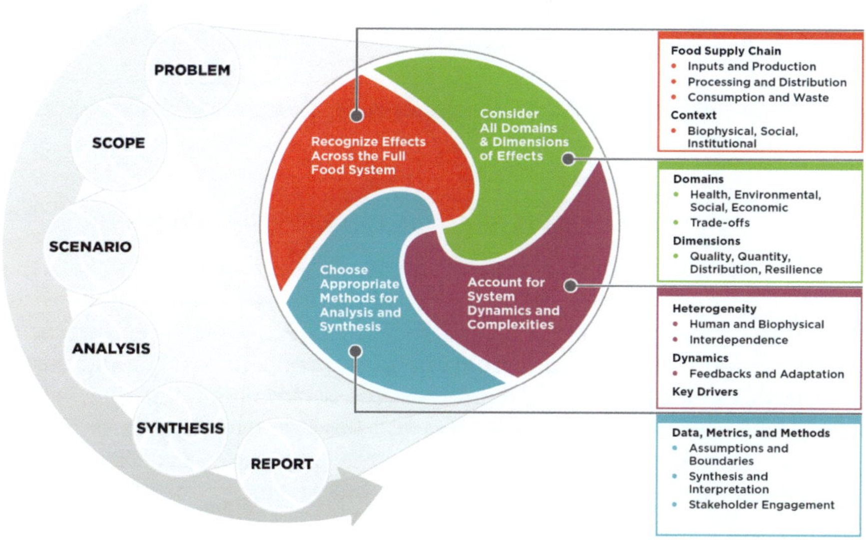

FIGURE 7-1 Conceptual illustration of the analytical framework. The four principles of the framework are represented in the larger circle, the core of the framework. These principles need to be considered throughout the assessment steps, represented in the figure as six small circles.

ronmental, social, and economic outcomes associated with alternative configurations[1] of the food system effects.

The lower quadrants of the figure highlight criteria for choosing analytical methods that can recognize the complex adaptive nature of the food system. Reading clockwise, they are:

- ***Account for System Dynamics and Complexities*** by treating the food system as a dynamic, adaptive system with heterogeneous actors and not necessarily predictable systems-level outcomes.
- ***Choose Appropriate Methods for Analysis and Synthesis,*** including data, metrics, and analytical methods suited to systems analysis, while making explicit any assumptions needed for simplification.

[1] Configurations are elements within the food system, such as policy interventions, technologies, market conditions, or organizational structure of different segments of the food system, that can be modified to achieve a particular goal or to explore how potential drivers (e.g., growth in demand for foods with particular traits) might impact the distribution of health, environmental, social, and economic effects.

In this context, "appropriate" means suited for the purpose and available.

These four key principles and the six framework steps are described in the following sections.

Principle 1: Recognize Effects Across the Full Food System

The first key principle recognizes the food system as a supply chain that is managed by diverse actors with competing interests and goals. Positive and negative health, environmental, social, and economic effects occur all along the food supply chain, from the farm production and input supply sectors through the first line handlers; processing, manufacturing, wholesale, and logistics sectors; retail food and food service sectors; and finally consumption and waste disposal. Along the way, the management of the food system is shaped by changes in natural resources, markets, policies, technologies, organizations, and information. The combination of the food supply chain and its surrounding biophysical and institutional context, introduced in Chapter 2, defines what we mean by a food system, and this should be recognized in any assessment.

Principle 2: Consider All Domains and Dimensions of Effects

The second key principle calls for consideration of all four important domains of food system effects (health, environmental, social, and economic) in any single assessment and directs attention to four specific dimensions of these effects (quantity, quality, distribution, and resilience) within each domain. Not only are all four domains of effect potentially important to accurately assess the system in current or alternative forms; trade-offs among the different effects (within each domain and across them) will often occur and should be evaluated, too.

Within each domain, four dimensions of effects—quantity, quality, distribution, and resilience—provide guidance that can help assessors consider a sufficiently broad range of potential outcomes. All are theoretically important and can serve as distinct components of scientific measures. The relative importance of these dimensions will vary with the specifics of the data underpinning any particular assessment. Even with the same data, individual assessors may disagree about the relative importance of each dimension, but the relevance of these four dimensions to assessing the food system is indisputable.

Quantity, quality, distribution, and resilience measure how much of what the food system provides, where and to whom it goes, and how sustainably it can do so. *Quantity* in the food system often matters relative to a benchmark, because too little or too much can be problematic. Just as hunger and obesity relate to food quantity consumed, so, too, lake sterility and eutrophication relate to insufficient and excess phosphorus runoff. Monitoring quantity characteristics of the food system also can capture depletion, degradation, or protection of natural resources upon which food production depends (e.g., soil), as well as amounts of pollutants delivered from agricultural systems to the environment (e.g., nutrients, pesticides, greenhouse gases).

Quality characterizes an outcome. If the outcome is food produced, then quality might measure nutrition, taste, or safety. If the outcome is diet, then quality might measure dietary components relative to a benchmark, such as the *U.S. Dietary Guidelines for Americans*. Job quality is also considered here and relates to the degree to which compensation and working conditions align with societal, legal, and worker expectations.

Distribution measures where an outcome goes. An important distribution for the study of obesity is incidence across different consumer populations. For food access, a relevant distribution is distance to food retailers. For biodiversity, the spatial dispersion of species numbers is a key distribution.

Resilience measures the food system's ability to bounce back from sudden shocks and long-term pressures (combining Conway's [1987] notions of stability and sustainability). Resilience can refer to how a food system responds to sudden events or to gradual pressures. For example, in response to honeybees dying of disease, resilience measures the food system's ability to continue supplying crops that rely on bee pollination. In response to sudden collapse of a manure retention lagoon, resilience might refer to how well the adjacent river recovers its ecosystem functions. In an illustrative economic context, resilience would refer to the speed and thoroughness by which other retailers meet consumers' food needs after a declaration of bankruptcy by a major supermarket chain.

These four dimensions manifest themselves across health, environmental, social, and economic outcomes of the food system. Table 7-1 illustrates ways in which all four dimensions touch upon the broad effect domains of this report. For example, reading down the Environment domain column, the reader can see examples of four dimensions of measurement. An illustrative measure of quantity is the amount of food produced; an illustration of quality is biodiversity and the aesthetic quality of the natural environment; an illustration of distribution is how agrichemical runoff risk varies across landscapes; and an illustration of resilience is the time needed for agricultural production to recover after a drought or flood. As a practical matter, the four dimensions vary in how they are measured, so they should be benchmarked to assess relative performance changes in the food system.

Assessing the desirability of alternative configurations of the food sys-

TABLE 7-1 Illustrations of How the Four Dimensions Can Measure Food System Effect Domains

Dimensions \ Domains	Health	Environment	Social and Economic
Quantity	Sufficient calories consumed for good health, but not obesity	Plentiful food production from agricultural land and water	Rising disposable income for consumers and/or food system workers
Quality	Safe working conditions and/or availability of food that is safe and meets recommended dietary allowances and dietary guidelines	Biodiversity and quality of natural environment in agricultural setting	Variety of affordable foods across income levels
Distribution	Access to a variety of foods for all groups in population	Distribution of agrochemical run-off risks across diverse landscapes	Cost of meeting dietary needs as share of household income at different income levels
Resilience	Recovery of trusted food safety level after contamination event	Recovery time for agricultural production after drought or flood	Community retains viability after loss of a major employer

NOTE: Many more examples about specific dimensions could be measured within each domain.

tem depends on the goals and values of the evaluator. One cannot identify the "best" of a set of configurations without adopting a particular set of normative judgments. An evaluation framework that seeks to identify a better alternative must make clear how different metrics of performance are being weighted or ranked. Assessors who reject these judgments may reject the entire analysis. A useful evaluation framework provides factual and objective information that can be used by people with different judgments about the relative importance of these dimensions to develop a well-informed ranking of alternatives consistent with their own normative preferences (Nyborg, 2012). Thus, consideration of *all* dimensions remains an important goal.

Principle 3: Account for System Dynamics and Complexities

As discussed in Chapter 6, the food system is complex, dynamic, and adaptive. With these traits in mind, an assessment should account for the heterogeneity of the actors and processes at each step of the food chain. Heterogeneity can apply to people—their tools, resources, relationships, and knowledge. Likewise, diversity abounds in a biophysical setting, including terrain, climate, and other natural resources. These heterogeneous traits are all highly interdependent.

Systems embed dynamic processes by which actors (human and other) can adapt their behavior. Just as farmers react to market price incentives by changing what or when or how they produce food, insect pests respond to repeated use of the same pest control method by evolving modes of resistance. Given the tendency of complex interactions to trigger dynamic repercussions, assessments should always (to the extent feasible) account for those effects across time, space, and heterogeneous populations. Moreover, assessments should acknowledge the potential role of underlying drivers of food system dynamics, such as changes in people's diet preferences and patterns of food consumption, farm and food policy, market prices, food industry structure, technology, natural resource base and climate conditions, to name a few. Other potential drivers of health, environmental, social, and economic effects may come primarily from outside the food system, such as lifestyle changes, heath care policies, energy policies, cross-border atmospheric deposition of nitrogen, or nonfood employment opportunities. Although scope limitations will preclude any specific study from careful consideration of all effects and drivers, it is important for any study to acknowledge the potential role of relevant aspects not included.

Principle 4: Choose Appropriate Methods for Analysis and Synthesis

Assessments are ultimately no better than the data and methods they employ. The careful choice of metrics to measure data and empirical methods to learn from data is fundamental to conducting a meaningful assessment. Within this context, appropriate methods are those that are suited to the purpose and means available. Appropriate methods might include those that:

- Allow consideration of effects across the full food system;
- Capture some information about each domain and dimension of effects;
- Capture system dynamics (e.g., feedbacks, interactions, heterogeneity);

- Capture processes and outcomes at the scales suited to the problem at hand; and
- Are able to address the critical concerns of stakeholders or policy makers.

Prevailing standards of evidence govern the choice of metrics and methods. These standards, in turn, vary across health, environmental, social, and economic effects because of measurement challenges specific to each domain. Assessment methods divide between two broad areas: (1) methods for analyzing and predicting effects of changes in the food system, and (2) methods for synthesizing findings across effects. Major approaches in both areas are summarized in the latter part of this chapter, and the appendix lists selected metrics, analytical methods, databases, and methodologies. The assumptions, limitations, accuracy, sensitivity, and other relevant factors for methods used should be clearly stated in the assessment. This is particularly important when assessments are made in new areas where data or previous research results are lacking.

ASSESSMENT STEPS

With the four key principles in Figure 7-1 guiding the thinking behind an assessment, six specific steps emerge from the broader literature on assessment frameworks. The steps (see Box 7-1) begin with describing the problem of interest, which involves identifying the goal, question, or concern. Next, through scoping, an assessment should characterize the system, including its boundaries, functional units, processes, outcomes, stakeholders, and key interventions and leverage points. As no assessment can be completely comprehensive, the scoping step is the point at which to determine the breadth and depth of the assessment. Third, an assessment

BOX 7-1
Steps for Assessment of Food System and Its Effects

1. PROBLEM: Motivate need with goals and objectives
2. SCOPING: Characterize system boundaries, components, processes, and linkages
3. SCENARIO: Identify baseline (and alternatives, as appropriate)
4. ANALYSIS: Conduct assessment
5. SYNTHESIS: Synthesize and interpret the results
6. REPORT: Communicate findings to key stakeholders

should clearly identify a scenario to be examined, typically a baseline, reference scenario and often one or more alternatives, as appropriate. With these elements in place, the fourth step is to conduct the analysis. The analysis will entail important choices of data (including potential solicitation of stakeholder to fill data gaps), models, and appropriate analytical methods to assess the complex dynamics of the food system across the four key dimensions of quantity, quality, distribution, and resilience. Fifth, results must be synthesized and interpreted, often into recommendations. Finally, the entire assessment should be reported and disseminated to stakeholders by appropriate means.

Throughout the assessment process, stakeholders can play an important role, particularly when they will be expected to act on the results of the analysis. Stakeholders can help identify issues that may not be obvious to researchers; validate choices about methods, metrics, and models; and provide data that are not readily available from other sources. At the same time, stakeholder engagement requires careful attention to representation of a broad diversity of stakeholder perspectives, and scientific assessments also may require a certain distance or buffer from the influence of powerful stakeholders in order to avoid conflicts of interest and create space for objective and independent decisions—whether related to scoping, scenario development, or analysis activities. Additional comments pertaining to considerations for managing stakeholder participation are presented after the assessment steps.

Although the remainder of this chapter discusses all six steps, it elaborates in greatest detail on Steps 4 and 5, analysis and synthesis of the assessment.

Problem: Motivate the Need for Assessment and Define Goals and Objectives

Assessments are motivated by broad problems or concerns. These should be carefully considered and explicitly stated. Development of a problem statement is often based on interactions with stakeholders, formal public health and safety criteria, and reviews of relevant literature about the problem and key findings from past assessments in the area. The problem statement should guide where the assessment is going, including its goals, objectives, and research questions and all future assessment decisions.

Scoping: Characterize System Boundaries, Components, Processes, Actors, and Linkages

Clearly framing the scope of the assessment is an essential step, given the complexity of the food system. A comprehensive analysis of the food system that analyzes the entire food supply chain across all effect domains in all dimensions and accounts fully for dynamics and complexities is a dauntingly ambitious undertaking. Analysts in all but the rarest instances will choose to narrow the scope of analysis. The scoping step considers appropriate boundaries and assumptions to frame the scope of an assessment in the context of the food system as a whole. The scoping step involves the choice of boundaries and assumptions that are part of "Choose Appropriate Methods for Analysis and Synthesis" in Figure 7-1. In doing so, scoping draws on the other three quadrants of the framework in clockwise order.

Determining the scope of an assessment begins with situating the topic for the assessment in the context of the full food system, both in the food supply chain and in the biophysical, social, and institutional contexts. Through what parts of the food system is the assessment topic likely to have significant repercussions? Those parts of the food system should fall within the boundaries of the analysis.

Moving on to the next quadrant, which effect domains are likely to be affected by the study focus? A study focused on dietary changes may have little effect on the environment but a large one on health. Which dimensions are likely to be important? Scale matters. A targeted school diet study may have negligible economic effects, but a large-scale dietary intervention could shift market prices. Effect domains and dimensions that are unlikely to be affected by the study focus can reasonably be left outside the boundary of the study, with the stated assumption that it is exogenous.

Considering system dynamics and complexities is the point at which to ask questions about how dynamics and heterogeneity affect a proposed topic of study: How long are repercussions likely to endure? What (if any) are important feedback processes and interdependencies? Are there key interventions or leverage points that lead to alternative scenarios deserving consideration? Responses to these questions will be based on qualitative generalizations about the system, but they can offer useful *ex ante* justifications for where detailed empirical analysis is merited, and where it is not. More specifically, the answers to these questions will influence the time horizon, the extent of relevant causal relationships, and other boundaries, along with assumptions about what lies outside those boundaries.

The boundaries may enclose a subset of the larger food system, such as the U.S. food system as part of the global system (see Figure 2-3 in Chapter 2), or a particular food commodity as part of a larger crop–livestock complex (see the egg example in Annex 5). They may designate a specific period of time or geographic area. Inside those boundaries, the assessment seeks to describe the interactions and relationships among key actors along the relevant parts of the food supply chain as well as to show the impacts of changes on a range of health, environmental, social, and economic effects.

Outside the boundaries, the assessment may assume constant conditions or exogenous changes, as is often the case with analyses of the U.S. food system that take the rest of the world as given. Boundaries for the system under analysis can be shaped by the nature of the problem, and they often depend on input from stakeholders, but they also may be determined by budget limitations (discussed on p. 268).

Within the defined boundaries, the characterization of the system should expand to identify the endogenous (or internally determined) processes and pathways that produce the outcomes of interest (Collins et al., 2011). For example, the nitrogen case study in Annex 4 focuses on the subsystem of crop production using nitrogen fertilizer; it does not consider aspects outside the defined system boundary, such as crop and livestock production, that do not directly involve nitrogen. Nor does it consider consumers and total food output. The processes and pathways that are endogenous, or inside the system boundary, involve nitrogen, the people who apply it, where it goes, how it affects crops, and how it affects climate, water, and other environmental fates. Identification of stakeholders to include in the assessment process is particularly useful at the scoping stage, because they can help identify potential sources of data or information to fill in any data gaps that may be present.

The choice of an appropriate time horizon for the assessment shapes the types of health, environmental, social, and economic effects that can be considered. Options range along a continuum from immediate to long-term cumulative impacts. Health effects may be acute or chronic, ranging from food poisoning to obesity and heart disease. The same is true of environmental effects, which range from sudden storms that washed previously applied phosphorus fertilizers into Lake Erie and may have triggered the algal blooms of 2011 and 2014 (Michalak et al., 2013) to incremental emissions of agricultural greenhouse gases that contribute to gradual climate change (Robertson, 2004). Social and economic effects associated with rapid change in the short run may be different from long-run impacts, which capture the dynamic adaptive responses of key actors. The time horizon should match the research goals and system boundaries because, in effect, the time period is an additional boundary.

Some studies may be narrow in scope, focusing on one or a few stages in the food supply chain or one domain of effects (e.g., health outcomes). In such cases, the committee recommends that any assessment at least acknowledge the existence of the potentially important effects of drivers that are outside the scope of the specific assessment. Although it is preferable to incorporate as many domains and dimensions of effects as possible, explicit assumptions that acknowledge what is beyond the scope of study can help to balance the importance of being comprehensive while focusing on a tractable assessment area.

Scenario: Identify the Baseline (and Alternatives, as Appropriate)

Assessments characterize how a system performs. Most assessments compare system performance to a baseline scenario and sometimes to one or more alternative scenarios. Alternative scenarios typically specify potential changes in a system to reflect an intervention, such as a new policy or a new technology. Any assessment of health, environmental, social, and economic effects of the food system should be explicit about each intervention being considered, including when, where, and how the intervention occurs. Stakeholder input can help identify and define a set of realistic scenario options.

It can be tempting to identify one state of the system simply as the "status quo" or "conventional" state without further characterization. But because the food system is constantly evolving (see Chapter 2), such descriptors lose meaning over time if they fail to define explicitly the system state in a baseline scenario. Descriptions of changed interventions need to be equally explicit so that what is changing and what is held constant are clear.

Analysis: Conduct the Assessment

Given the intended scope, an analysis draws on suitable methodologies to interpret data and build models to assess the likely health, environmental, social, and economic effects associated with alternative food system scenarios. The goal is to provide a scientifically valid basis for public and private decision making. The next major section will summarize common assessment methodologies in more detail.

Synthesis: Synthesize and Interpret Results

Analyses of food systems should be designed to clarify the likely outcomes—and their magnitudes—and the trade-offs associated with different alternatives. Often outcomes include both beneficial and harmful effects and, as noted above, the results of a scientific assessment may not by themselves provide clear guidance about which scenario is "the best." Therefore, a synthesis and interpretation of the outcomes are needed to help integrate disparate results into a clear message and potential interventions. Ultimately, value judgments of stakeholders and decision makers are required to determine how to weigh the various outcomes. Approaches to synthesis, interpretation, and evaluation of trade-offs also are discussed below following the section on analytical methodologies.

Report: Communicate Findings to Stakeholders

Reporting involves communicating the assessment and recommendations to key stakeholders, broadly defined as the end-user of the assessment in affected communities, and also the general public. The reporting step typically involves creating a report that documents the assessment methods; the data sources and analytical tools, including the assumptions; interactions with stakeholders; findings; and recommendations. Ensuring that the report is clearly written, is easily understood, and is transparent are also important considerations. Although a single report may be created, additional summary documents may be tailored to the various audiences. As a matter of best practice, a succinct executive summary should also accompany the longer text.

Related to reporting is dissemination, which aims to inform a wide range of stakeholders of the assessment's purpose, approach, findings, and recommendations. For any assessment, a variety of processes and media may be used, including public forums, presentations, and policy briefs. For example, risk analysis methodology typically includes risk communication as a separate activity from risk assessment (the scientific element) and risk management (the policy element) in order to ensure that the messaging is structured to effectively communicate to distinct audiences that may interpret the information in different ways. During dissemination, stakeholders can help to ensure that reports are written in a manner appropriate for the intended audiences and reach these key audiences as well as help to gain buy-in from key decision makers.

ANALYSIS: METHODS FOR ANALYZING FOOD SYSTEM EFFECTS

The right empirical or modeling method for a food system assessment depends on the specific problem, its scope, and the scenarios defined for the study. The relevant analytical methods divide importantly between two broad types of assessment scenarios: (1) a specific current food system configuration (e.g., a policy or a practice), and (2) potential alternative configurations. A study of a current system configuration can measure observable effects of the system; by contrast, a study into alternative system configurations is by its nature a "counterfactual" study—one that seeks to understand what would happen if matters were different. In counterfactual studies, it is inherently difficult to learn solely by observation of the current system, so other approaches are needed. The challenges of counterfactual studies compared to factual ones are analogous to the challenges of *ex ante* versus *ex post* impact evaluations (Alston et al., 1998).

The four dimensions of measurement—quantity, quality, distribution, and resilience—interact closely with the purpose of the assessment in determining the most relevant methods to use. Quantity and quality are dimensions where overall average effects may suffice, whether for food produced and consumed or regarding health, environmental, social, and economic effects of the food system. The next dimension—distribution—requires consideration of the heterogeneity of system effects, including variation across geography, time, and population. Finally, the dimension of resilience requires measures of how the system performs over time, including how it responds to stresses and shocks that could undermine its sustainability.

Measuring Quantity and Quality Dimensions in the Current Food System

Assessing quantity and quality effects in the current food system centers on (1) describing the system and (2) explaining what causes it to function as it does. Understanding causation is challenging because underlying causes can be easily confused with correlated effects that are not true causes. A correlation may exist because the underlying relationship is mischaracterized or because of measurement error. The rise of obesity in America is clearly related to food, but it may also be related to growing levels of inactivity, as well as social and economic factors (Hammond, 2009). An assessment that ignores nonfood determinants of obesity may reach biased results. This illustrates a first requirement for understanding what causes food system effects: construction of a conceptual model containing all possible causes of the relevant effects. Such a conceptual model offers two benefits. First, it can reduce the risk that an assessor is blind to causes outside of a target set. Second, it can reduce the odds of confusing cause and effect. These benefits only occur if the conceptual model is informed by reliable metrics measuring the current food system.

A second requirement for understanding what causes food system effects is to use good metrics. Metrics can be divided into three types: (1) directly measured data, (2) indicator data that serve as indirect measures, and (3) simulation models that provide artificial data ("pseudo-data") that represent projections or inferences about the real world.

Directly measured data are the gold standard, but in many circumstances, direct measurement is either too costly (consider all water pollutants in U.S. lakes) or infeasible (consider nitrous oxide emissions from fertilizer on commercial farms). Moreover, all measurements—even direct measurements—are subject to error (see Box 7-2).

Indirect measurement through indicators is sometimes more cost-effective than direct measurement is—especially for spatially diffused effects. Water quality may be measured by the population of *Daphnia*, a water flea that serves as a sentinel species for waterborne ecotoxins. Likewise, remote sensing technologies make it possible to use indicators like reflectance of

BOX 7-2
Measurement Error in Directly Measured Data, Indicators, and Models

All metrics are subject to measurement error. In the words of two eminent statisticians, "essentially, all models are wrong, but some are useful" (Box and Draper, 1987, p. 424). Even in directly measured data, the measured value and the true value are almost never the same because the act of measurement is never perfectly consistent. The difference between measured and true values is called measurement error. In this case, "error" does not refer to a mistake, but rather to the diverse factors that can cause a measurement to depart from a true value.

Measurement error includes both random error and systematic error (also known as bias). Random error can be dealt with by averaging repeated measurements, so it is the less troubling of the two. Systematic error is more problematic, because it may cause consistent overestimates or underestimates of the true effects. Selection bias is one form of systematic error that occurs when sampled individuals do not represent the population of interest. For example, gathering data by interviewing daytime food shoppers at a supermarket excludes individuals who are unable to shop in person or unable to shop during the day. Social science research has used a variety of methods for minimizing confounding, ranging from randomized controlled trials (Moffitt, 2004) to cluster randomized trials for community-based interventions (Cornfield, 1978; Donner and Klar, 2000) to special statistical methods and research designs to control for the effects of selection bias (Barrett and Carter, 2010; Deaton, 2010; Heckman et al., 1998).

Indicator data can be an imperfect measure of the underlying phenomenon or concept they are meant to capture. For example, satellites record spectral reflectance from the Earth's surface. Those measures of reflected light correlate highly with different plant species, enabling the U.S. Department of Agriculture to produce maps annually of U.S. cropland using light reflectance as an indicator of crop location. But maps of U.S. cropland based on remote sensing indicator data show less land area under crops than was reported in the nearest agricultural Census (Johnson, 2013), presumably because of translational error in associating the sensed wavelengths of light with real crops planted on the ground.

Simulation models also can contain errors that lead to misleading conclusions. Errors of omission or specification may occur in their equations or algorithms as well as in the numerical parameters that shape those equations. Reliable models have undergone procedures of verification, validation, calibration, and sensitivity analysis to catch mistakes and refine predictive power (Arnand et al., 2007; Howitt, 1995). However, even well-validated models never predict perfectly.

All three kinds of metrics (directly measured data, indicator data, and pseudo-data coming out of simulation models) experience measurement error. In all cases, systematic error is to be avoided. Random error, while it reduces accuracy, can be averaged out in repeated measures. Although indicator data and model pseudo-data may seem less desirable than directly measured data, they are used when direct measurements are so costly that it would mean not measuring at all—or only doing so in a handful of scientific studies.

BOX 7-3
Testing for Statistical Effects

Statistical analysis can answer important questions about the food system. But measurement error can obscure the answer. How big must an effect be to be meaningful? To separate ordinary random variability from meaningful effects, statisticians commonly start by assuming there is no effect. Under this "null" hypothesis, one would assume that an outcome Y is not affected by cause X, with the alternative hypothesis that X does affect Y. Tests of statistical significance aim to contain the probability of a Type I error, which occurs if the null hypothesis is rejected when the null hypothesis was true—there in fact was no effect (Mendenhall et al., 1986). This approach is entirely appropriate when the consequence of wrongly rejecting the null hypothesis is serious and costly. To illustrate with a stylized example, suppose that a company is developing a new process to inactivate foodborne pathogens, and it wishes to test how the process compares to the existing inactivation process. Assume that Y is inactivation achieved by the current process and X is inactivation achieved with the new process. Because inactivation kinetics for different pathogens may vary when different methods are applied, multiple regression models are used to examine inactivation of various foodborne pathogens in relation to X. Before the firm developing the new inactivation process would want to begin steps toward commercialization, it would want very compelling evidence that X inactivates foodborne pathogens at least as effectively as Y. A low significance threshold (5 or 1 percent) would sharply limit the probability of wrongly concluding that X is at least as effective as Y for inactivation of foodborne pathogens.

However, for many important food system effects where costs are low but benefits are high, a very demanding-level statistical significance is unnecessary and may be undesirable. The reason is that requiring a high significance increases the odds of failing to reject the null hypothesis when it is false (Type II error). Consider the case where Y is improvement in lake water quality when farmers use low-cost conservation practice X, and the null hypothesis is: X has no effect on Y. Consider a multiple regression analysis that includes many factors that potentially affect lake water quality, including practice X. A significance level set at 5 percent probability of Type I error would require strong evidence that the conservation practice was effective. But if the practice is not costly and the value of better water quality is substantial, then a higher significance threshold of 20 percent (meaning the observed improvement would have occurred 20 percent of the time without the practice) would be appropriate.

light wavelengths (albedo) to identify vegetation or to use audio sensing to identify wildlife in a place where no human observer is present.

Statistical methods are well suited to describing effects from the current food system. Multiple regression models (see Box 7-3), if properly designed, can identify correlates of important food system effects. A key to proper design is to include among the explanatory variables only those that are exogenous, or determined outside the system, with respect to the outcome variable (in order to avoid confounding correlation with causation) (Intriligator, 1978). In interpreting the results of a multiple regression model, the appropriate significance level to use will depend on the type of statistical error that is most relevant for the study at hand.

The U.S. government maintains a variety of major datasets that can be useful for assessing the health, environmental, social, and economic effects of the food system. Several of these are listed in Appendix B, Table B-3, with additional notable datasets discussed in the earlier chapters on health, environmental, social, and economic effects of the food system.

An important point to remember is that data sources should be carefully evaluated to determine whether they are appropriate to the question being examined and to identify any limitations. If existing resources are insufficient to appropriately address the question being examined, the researcher should consider collecting new data.

Measuring Quantity and Quality Dimensions in Alternative Food System Configurations

Alternative food system configurations differ from the predominant current system either because they do not exist (yet) or because they currently exist only on a different (often smaller) scale. As a result, direct measurement and indicator measures typically are either not feasible or not sufficient to anticipate their effects on a large scale. Given that the food system is a complex adaptive system, simulation modeling may be the best tool to predict certain effects of the food system (van Wijk et al., 2012). Simulation models (see Box 7-4) can be used to run "experiments" in which each alternative system is tested under the same conditions.

Although simulations may not be fully accurate representations of reality, such experiments have certain advantages. In the real world, an alternative food system configuration may exist only in a limited area or under special market or policy conditions. As a result, making real-world comparisons between the dominant food system and a smaller alternative may raise problems of selection bias—meaning that findings from the smaller alternative may not be scaled up reliably. For example, the price premium for organically grown foods sold in relatively small quantities may result from purchases by customers who are willing and able to pay high prices. For the same organic foods to be sold in greater volume, the price premium would likely have to shrink to accommodate customers who were not willing or able to pay the full, current premium.

Simulation models are best used with virtual versions of an experimental research design, like those used for laboratory experiments in the real world. The experimental treatments may take the form of scenarios,

BOX 7-4
Types of Simulation Models

Simulation models come in several types, all of which can help to measure one or another of the quantity, quality, distribution, and resilience dimensions of food system assessment analyses. They can be broadly classified as descriptive, predictive, postdictive, and prescriptive (Schoemaker, 1982). Descriptive models help to understand systems by describing their components and processes. Predictive models forecast future system performance. Postdictive models help to diagnose past system performance. Prescriptive models make recommendations for actions to achieve desired outcomes. Models can further be organized based on time horizon, spatial extent, and number of actors. Statistical models are often used for descriptive and postdictive purposes to understand a system. Statistical models can often be improved by supplementing data with knowledge from scientific theory, as is done in the subfields of biometrics and econometrics. Several important models of the food system use statistics to understand basic relationships or to extrapolate to the future from recent experience. Examples of basic relationships are children's rates of growth in response to nutrients and changes in consumer purchases in response to changes in price and income (price and income elasticity of demand). Microbiological growth and inactivation models also are available to predict behavior of foodborne pathogens in foods.

Certain important research questions involve predicting the distant future or analyzing unprecedented shocks to the food system that cannot be analyzed statistically. Climate change is one example. For such questions, dynamic simulation models can generate useful predictions. These models are built from data, variables, parameters, and equations that describe how the state of the system responds as components of the model evolve over time (Dent and Blackie, 1979; Law and Kelton, 1991; Van Dyne and Abramsky, 1975).

such as scenarios for alternative policy treatments in the face of a set of different climate change projections. The simplest approach to simulation experiments is to compare treatments under average conditions. Results from such "deterministic" models can be treated as most likely outcomes under the alternative scenarios. More sophisticated experiments compare probability distributions of simulated outcomes from different scenarios, which exemplify the distribution and resiliency dimensions of assessment.

Simulation models can be particularly useful for assessing multiple outcome effects from scenarios describing possible conditions that cannot currently be observed (e.g., changed climate). Depending on the nature and complexity of the model(s), a variety of outcome effects can be simulated and compared. For example, a comprehensive literature review on possible climate change effects on farm households included a wide variety of simulation model types. The review examined model outcome effects,

A simulation approach often used to study complex systems is agent-based computational modeling (ABM). In an ABM, complex dynamics are modeled by representing individual actors ("agents") in the system, each with specified initial conditions and a set of adaptive rules that govern their interaction with each other and with their environment. In this way, the computer simulation of individual decision making and decentralized interactions "grows" dynamics and patterns (at both the individual and aggregate levels) from the bottom up (Hammond, 2009). ABMs offer certain advantages for modeling complex systems. Because every individual is explicitly modeled in an ABM, substantial heterogeneity can be captured in both the types of actors and the distributions of individual characteristics within actor types. Thus, ABMs can incorporate "bounded rationality" or insights from behavioral economics. ABMs also can incorporate spatial complexity (e.g., of geography or social networks), interactions among actors, and adaptation through time. The ABM approach has been used to study a wide variety of topics in social science and public health, including some work focused on the food system.

Prescriptive models are appropriate when the research question dwells on identifying an optimal strategy. Mathematical programming models identify optimal solutions to a specified objective function. These are often used for economic purposes, such as minimizing the cost of meeting nutritional needs. Computable general equilibrium models represent one important class of math programming models of the food system that capture market feedbacks for prices and quantities in response to some system change (e.g., due to policy or technology). Dynamic programming models optimize over a fixed time horizon, although they can be adapted to a moving time horizon (Chen et al., 2014).

including profit, food self-sufficiency, food security, risk, and altered climate change (van Wijk et al., 2012). These outcomes span health, environmental, social, and economic effects. Although the authors found a trend toward integration of multiple models in order to simulate more diverse effects, they called for further advances in coordinated modeling—even at the agricultural production scope of their study. Box 7-5 illustrates integrated modeling of economic and environmental effects from biofuel market and policy analysis.

Measuring Distribution and Resiliency Dimensions

The distribution dimension of assessment measures helps to capture the heterogeneity in our world. People, food, weather, and landscapes all exhibit enormous diversity. Some individuals may be particularly vulner-

BOX 7-5
Integrated Models to Predict Feedbacks and Multiple Effects: Biofuel Policy Analysis

The complexity of food systems makes it particularly important to conduct assessments from a system-wide perspective. Simulation models that are connected across domains of the food system can capture feedbacks between human choices in policy and markets and associated repercussions for environmental and health effects. The best developed category of such linked human-biophysical models is composed of "bioeconomic" models that link economic behavior with biophysical processes. Recently, linked bioeconomic models have been used to evaluate how bioenergy policy affects food and energy supplies along with environmental effects. For example, the BEPAM computable general equilibrium model has been linked to the GREET greenhouse gas model to forecast U.S. national biofuel policy outcomes for prices in food and fuel markets as well as associated climate change consequences (Chen et al., 2014). Similar biofuel policy analysis at the regional scale has linked an economic optimization model to the EPIC biophysical model to simulate water quality, soil quality, and climate effects from profit-maximizing farmers in the face of rising prices for energy biomass with other prices assumed to remain constant (e.g., Egbendewe-Mondzozo et al., 2011).

able to bad outcomes (e.g., poor people are vulnerable to food price spikes, residents living over shallow aquifers may have greater exposure to nitrate contamination of groundwater from fertilizers, and people with immune-depressed systems are more vulnerable to foodborne illness). Understanding the distribution of food system effects over a range of possible conditions as well as resilience (the food system's ability to bounce back after unusual pressures) matters for good assessments.

Distribution and resilience are more difficult to measure than are average quantity and quality effects because they refer to the range of possible effects over space and time. It is possible to measure the range of many outcomes from the current food system because we can observe it. But we cannot observe "what if" scenarios—potential realities that might happen or might have happened; instead we can only observe what actually did happen. Some of the variability (both in what happened and in what might have happened) is driven by underlying processes that are understood, but other parts of that variability are random and less understood. If the underlying processes are changing, it may not even be possible to understand the true distribution of effects from the current food system by studying historical data. For example, if the climate is changing due to rising greenhouse gas levels, then the likely range of possible weather conditions next year is not what it was 30 years ago. The same evolving processes also make it difficult to measure resilience because the system's past ability to bounce back after unusual pressure may not be a good measure of its ability to do so in the future.

Some important food system effects occur under extreme conditions. For example, properly managed pesticides can still cause a consumer health hazard if sudden hard rain after spraying washes the unabsorbed pesticide into a drinking water supply. Appropriately capturing these uncommon situations will require a focus not just on average quantity or quality effects but rather on measuring the probability that any given effect exceeds a threshold level. Exceeding certain threshold levels can trigger extreme outcomes with irreversible consequences that matter not just in a distributional sense but, more importantly, because they can alter the resilience of a system. Information on the probability of extreme effects can be used to evaluate the appropriate margin of safety to reduce the probability of undesirable outcomes, such as rain-generated spikes in soluble phosphorus that can cause lakes to become eutrophic (Langseth and Brown, 2011). Margins of safety based on such thresholds are the basis of existing upper bound reference doses (RfDs) established by the Environmental Protection Agency (EPA) for a variety of toxic substances, including pesticide residues and food contaminants (NRC, 2009). Understanding the nature of thresholds and associated regulatory reference values is important in estimating or simulating the probability of extreme effects. For example, EPA's RfD approach, discussed in the example in Annex 1A, is built on RfDs below which there is a high probability of no observable adverse effect. Comprehensive measurement or modeling of extreme effects (e.g., exposure–response relationships for toxic substances) should focus on the entire probability distribution of outcomes, not truncating measurement at regulatory thresholds (Cohen et al., 2005).

Once well-validated simulation models have been developed, they can be used to generate a large number of experimental replications with input data representing the full range of potential real conditions (Law and Kelton, 1991). Stochastic simulations produce a range of outcomes in response to random inputs like weather; they may explicitly incorporate measurement error associated with key variables and equations. Outputs from these simulations can be ordered into empirical probability distributions of key outcomes. These, in turn, can be compared across treatments to reach conclusions about resilience and vulnerability under extreme situations, as well as to inform decision making given differing tolerances for risk (Arrow, 1971; Hadar and Russell, 1969; Pratt, 1964). Stochastic simulation that integrates multiple models can generate probability distributions of outcomes on multiple effects of interest for risk analysis (van Wijk et al., 2012). For example, Rabotyagov (2010) was interested in policies to limit the risk of soil carbon loss. Using a soil and crop model, he ran stochastic simulations to compare how two policies (land retirement versus conservation tillage) would affect soil carbon sequestration over time and space in one Iowa watershed. He then linked the soil environmental effect simulated data to randomly drawn cost data from the U.S. Department of Agriculture and used an economic optimization model to evaluate which policy would generate the best margin of safety against soil carbon loss (Rabotyagov, 2010).

With simulation models, as with datasets, the assessment team must decide whether to build a new one or to draw on an existing model. The most compelling argument for building a new simulation model is that the model can be tailored to the specific research question of interest. A variety of simulation modeling methods exist, along with methods for evaluating the validity of the model (Anderson, 1974; Hanks and Ritchie, 1991; Van Dyne and Abramsky, 1975). However, using an existing simulation model can be desirable if a suitable model exists. Key criteria for determining whether a model is suitable are: it has passed scientific peer review, it has been well validated through testing in multiple settings, and it is well suited to the time horizon, spatial extent, and key component interactions of interest. Preexisting simulation models are best used in collaboration with knowledgeable modelers, because the models often need some adaptive programming to address new research questions. For many agricultural, economic, and environmental purposes, good models do exist (see Appendix B, Table B-4).

Developing or adapting reliable simulation models to measure distributional and resilience effects can be costly. At least for monetary measures of income or expenditures, a less costly approach than simulating a probability distribution is to calculate conditions needed to reach a threshold of price or quantity under an alternative scenario that would match a baseline case (e.g., when an alternative food system configuration would match the current system). Breakeven analysis is a tool for calculating such a threshold, typically applied to breakeven price or quantity levels (Dillon, 1993; Tyner, 2010).

SYNTHESIS: INTERPRETATION, SYNTHESIS, AND TRADE-OFFS

A comprehensive assessment that covers all four effect areas will have results related to health, environment, society, and economics. Even a single one of those areas can have different results for different population groups or over different time horizons. Consider an assessment that finds that a policy change would improve child nutrition, deplete aquifers, reduce farm income, improve retail food affordability, and reduce rural employment. Should the policy change be enacted? To reach a conclusion requires synthesis of these diverse effects.

How to synthesize results to reach appropriate conclusions or recommendations is a major challenge for comprehensive assessments that account for effects on multiple domains across multiple measurement dimensions. Especially when alternative scenarios are evaluated, assessors are often called on to identify which is "best" by one or more criteria. Yet when outcomes have multiple attributes and involve trade-offs, a definitive answer may not be possible. In the case of the food system, quantity, quality, distribution, and resilience represent four important dimensions—but attributes within each of these dimensions may be of concern to some people and not others, and they may vary by place (different communities) and time (different seasons or years).

For evaluating preferences across outcomes, it may be sufficient to consider only the *differences* between the outcomes rather than the actual levels of the attributes. For example, in comparing two outcomes that differ on food prices, it may be sufficient to know only the difference in prices (of various foods) rather than the absolute prices of foods under each outcome. For other attributes, the absolute levels are also important. For nutrients, the benefit of increased intake is much greater if dietary intake is insufficient; increased intake may even be harmful if dietary intake exceeds requirements.

Evaluation methods differ in the extent to which they aggregate across multiple attributes. At one extreme, synthesis can include the levels of each relevant attribute under each of the outcomes (alternatively, the differences in each attribute from one of the outcomes, i.e., the base case). This information can be presented in many formats. For example, it can be presented as a table, with each column corresponding to a relevant attribute and each row displaying the attribute levels for a particular outcome. It also can be presented as a radar or spiderweb diagram (see Figure 7-2), where each attribute is represented by a ray from the origin (center) of the diagram and the length of the ray shows the level of the attribute for a particular outcome. Radar diagrams can be used to compare the pattern of attributes from one scenario to another.

Alternatively, some or all of the attributes may be aggregated into an index. A very simple (probably nonsensical) index could be obtained by adding the attribute levels together; a potentially more useful index might be the total benefits minus costs of an outcome (compared with a reference outcome).

Each method (indexing versus disaggregating measures) has advantages and disadvantages. A disaggregate approach, like a table or radar diagram, can present a large amount of information, but it relies on the

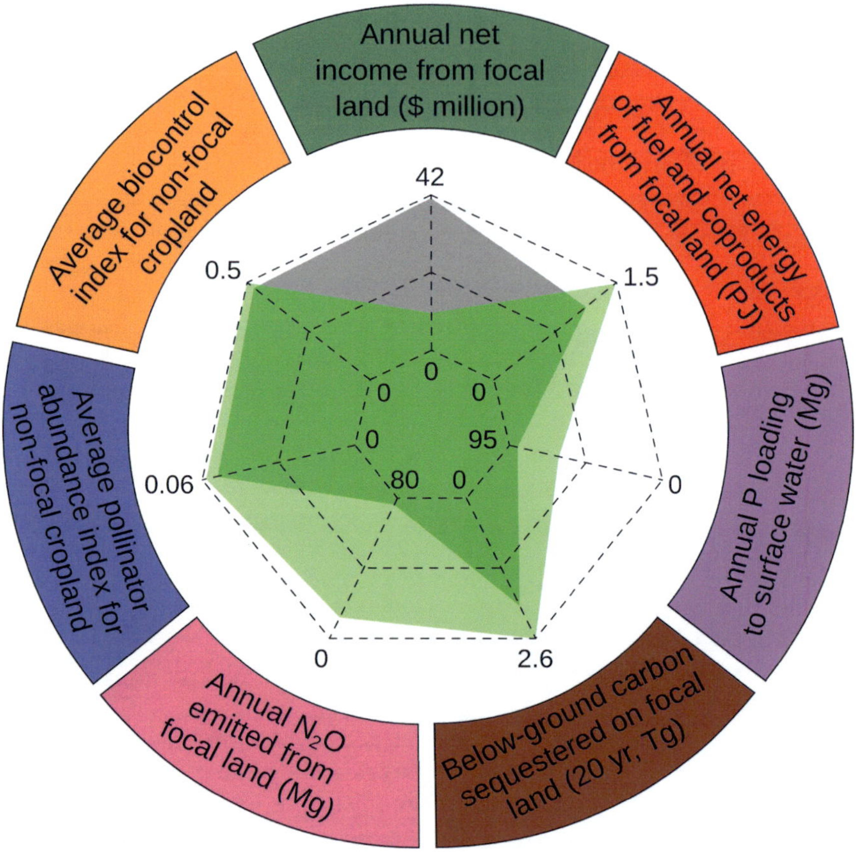

FIGURE 7-2 Radar diagram illustrating multidimensional trade-offs among ecosystem services associated with continuous corn (gray) versus bioenergy crops (green) (Meehan et al., 2013). As indicated by numbers on the axes, greater distance from origin is desirable for some dimensions (e.g., income), while less distance is desirable for others (e.g., less P or N_2O pollution). Units of measure are described in the outer circle.

reader to aggregate across attributes, typically by holistic judgment. Moreover, even if analysts choose not to aggregate across attributes, they must still choose which attributes to report. Different readers may be interested in different attributes; so, in principle, analysts need to include all of the attributes that any reader would judge relevant, potentially producing a table or radar diagram that provides so much information it is unwieldy to evaluate. Such a presentation also must consider the issue of units of measure. For a table, the choice of units can make the level of an attribute look large or small relative to other attributes; for a radar diagram, the attributes that extend farthest from the origin will tend to appear most salient. Interpretation is easier if all of the attributes can be described by measures for which an increase is beneficial; it is difficult for a reader to synthesize disaggregated information when an increase is beneficial for some attributes (or for some levels of an attribute) but otherwise harmful (as illustrated by Figure 7-2).

Some evidence suggests that evaluation using holistic judgment tends to be less accurate than evaluation using the competing approach of aggregating attributes using a mathematical formula (Dawes et al., 1989; Sunstein, 2000). Because it is difficult for humans to consider more than a handful of attributes at the same time, a few attributes may receive undue weight in a judgmental evaluation.

The attribute levels can be combined into an index in many ways. One theoretical approach is to construct a social utility function that includes weights of each of the effects (or attributes) that people care about, including health, environmental, social, economic, and other attributes. A social utility function assigns a larger number to a societally more preferred outcome. Such a function can (sometimes) be created by considering how society should trade off among different attributes (Keeney and Raiffa, 1976). However, when individuals rank the outcomes differently, the Arrow impossibility theorem (Keeney and Raiffa, 1976; Stokey and Zeckhauser, 1978) shows there is no best way to reconcile these differences.

Benefit–cost analysis (BCA) and cost-effectiveness analysis (CEA) are often used to help evaluate social outcomes. BCA attempts to estimate the net monetary benefits of an outcome compared with a reference outcome. These are defined as the benefits to the individuals who gain from the move to a new outcome minus the costs to individuals who are harmed by that move. Benefits and costs to individuals are defined as the monetary compensation that provides the same change in well-being as the change in outcome. Use of BCA requires that these monetary amounts can be estimated for all of the (important) changes in attribute levels. CEA is similar to BCA except that changes in one of the attributes are measured in some non-monetary unit, often a physical unit (like tons of corn produced or cases of cancer avoided), or a unit that aggregates changes in a subset of attributes (like quality-adjusted life years, or QALYs, that combine fatal and nonfatal health effects into a measure of healthy time lost to death or illness). CEA can be used to compare the cost (in terms of all of the attributes measured in monetary terms) per unit gain in the effect (the attribute measured in nonmonetary terms), but the question of whether that cost is justified by the gain must be answered independently of the CEA. (For further reading on BCA, see Boardman et al., 2010; Freeman, 1993; Layard and Glaister, 1994; Stokey and Zeckhauser, 1978; for further reading on CEA, see Drummond et al., 2005; Gold et al., 1996.)

Social welfare functions (SWFs) provide an alternative method for creating an index, one which attempts to account for concerns about the distribution of well-being in a society (Adler, 2012). The utilitarian SWF adds the well-being of everyone in society. Under this SWF, a gain of one unit of utility counts the same regardless of who receives it. In contrast, a prioritarian SWF adjusts each person's well-being by a concave function, then adds these transformed well-being levels across people. The concave function has the effect of counting a gain in well-being more heavily if it is received by someone with an initially low well-being than by someone who is better off. An important limitation of SWFs is that they require agreement on some method to measure (summarize) individuals' well-being in a way that can be compared between individuals (i.e., so that one can say which of two individuals gains more from a specified change). A second limitation is that one must specify which SWF is appropriate, including specification of numerical parameters that characterize the degree of aversion to inequality and other features of the SWF. Although these functions have strength in theory, they have rarely been applied in practice.

One advantage of methods that aggregate the attributes (effects) into an index is that the aggregation formula is explicit. This promotes transparency, in comparison with reporting disaggregated attributes. On the other hand, individuals who disagree with the weighting of attributes in an index may find the index invalid. An advantage of reporting individual attributes separately (as in the radar diagrams) is that stakeholders can discuss and debate trade-offs among the attributes.

BUDGETARY CONSIDERATIONS

The complexity and dynamics of the food system make truly comprehensive approaches to assessing its health, environmental, social, and economic effects ambitious and costly. But quality assessments of focused problems can be done at lower cost, with acknowledged limitations.

Simplified, lower-cost assessment approaches should explicitly recognize how simplification is likely to affect results. Simplification calls for assumptions that narrow the validity and/or the potential to extrapolate general lessons from the results. Plans for how to simplify assessments should start by considering the food system as a whole. First, they should explicitly identify what assumptions are necessary to make the simplification(s) under consideration useful and appropriate. One common simplifying assumption

BOX 7-6
Checklist for Implied Simplifying Assumptions

1. Does it encompass the full food supply chain?
2. Does it address all four domains and dimensions of effects?
3. Does it account for interactions and dynamic feedback processes?
4. Does it account for heterogeneity in the human population and environmental setting?

of *ceteris paribus* holds that everything outside the model is held constant. Another is to restrict focus to only certain effects of the food system (often because budgets limit the range of expertise among the assessors). Assessment teams should be explicit about potential effects of narrowing the range of assessors' domains of expertise, which can include biases from their own professions or scientific disciplines. Second, for each simplifying assumption, assessors should evaluate the likelihood of conditions occurring that would invalidate the assumptions. If such a condition is likely to occur, then the assumption is inappropriate.

One useful way to present a simplified assessment protocol is to list explicitly the domains and dimensions of the food system, indicating how each one is addressed and what the associated assumptions are. Explicit acknowledgment of the assumptions behind the scope of a study is rare, and we know of no assessment to date that clearly documents assumptions along these lines. One assessment protocol that moves in this direction describes for each step in the assessment what is "basic" information (cheaper to collect, but implicitly with more limiting assumptions) versus "extended" information (more costly, but freer of assumptions). This listing is applied to multi-domain assessment of the impacts of integrated pest management (Swinton and Norton, 2009).

All studies make some simplifying assumptions. To inventory relevant assumptions, a checklist can be a useful point of departure. Box 7-6 offers a series of questions to help test for implied assumptions about several dimensions of complexity that are especially prone to simplification. Whether these assumptions are valid deserves attention at the time of the initial scoping exercise. Specifically, what major interactions are omitted? Are dynamic feedbacks omitted or reduced? What level of heterogeneity is captured in human populations? What about heterogeneity in the environmental setting (e.g., land, water, air, biodiversity)?

ENGAGING STAKEHOLDERS

Similar to the guidance provided in the National Academy of Sciences reports on risk assessment, science and decision making, and health impact assessment, this committee views stakeholder[2] engagement and participation as important components of the proposed framework. The early and central role of stakeholder identification and participation has been described in these aforementioned reports, as well as by the Presidential/Congressional Commission on Risk Assessment and Risk Management (1997), and this approach also is supported here. Stakeholders have the potential to make valuable contributions at each stage of the assessment process. For example, information collected from stakeholders can help to illuminate important issues, focus the scope, provide local knowledge on the problem of interest and potential impacts, offer suggestions for alternatives that might be acceptable to the public, share perspectives on the recommendations, identify ways to disseminate the findings, and allow for representative participation from those with a stake in the problem bring addressed by the assessment (NRC, 2008, 2011). Stakeholder involvement during the assessment step can be especially important when data are lacking.

Techniques for active stakeholder engagement vary, but they should address and respond to the specific barriers and challenges identified for engaging each stakeholder group relevant to any given assessment. Prior assessments have engaged stakeholders using open community meetings, public hearings, more structured focus groups, surveys, webinars, interactive technologies, and open written comment periods (NAS, 2003; NRC, 2008, 2009, 2011). Further guidance on the best practices to engage stakeholders can be found in several documents, including the Stakeholder Participation Working Group of the 2010 HIA (Health Impact Assessment) in the Americas Workshop (2011), NRC (2008), Israel and colleagues (1998), and a classic paper by Arnstein (1969).

The committee also recognizes that stakeholder participation can present many challenges, and teams conducting food system assessments should become familiar with potential pitfalls and consult with other groups that are experienced at addressing them. Reported experiences from previous impact assessments (e.g., environmental impact assessment [EIA], health impact assessment [HIA]) show that participatory processes can sometimes favor those who have more resources and expertise and exclude those with fewer resources (NRC, 2008, 2009, 2011). In addition to representation of

---

[2] Stakeholders are community groups, industry, consumers, advocacy organizations, and workers who are not part of the technical assessment team and are often detached from the assessment process (NRC, 2009, 2011).

diverse interests, careful consideration should be made about whether key leaders or formal groups are authorized or in a position to "represent" the class of stakeholders or the broader public, such as in the case of a union leader speaking on behalf of his or her union membership, or industry executives representing the interests of consumers or workers. Thus, using a participatory process requires careful thought about both who is involved in the process and who is omitted from the process. Stakeholders inevitably have biases in their perspectives, and effective engagement processes use mechanisms to make these biases transparent. Other challenges to effective stakeholder engagement may include limited resources or expertise among the assessors in participatory engagement methods; the public's distrust of scientists, research, or public processes; and practical considerations, such as language or literacy barriers (NAS, 2003; NRC, 2011). Finally, it is important to note that applying the framework to a highly polarized and controversial topic may require that the scientific assessment process maintain a certain distance or buffer from the influence of powerful stakeholders in order to create space for objective and independent decisions related to scoping, scenario development, and analysis activities.

USING THE FRAMEWORK

The framework provides a set of design considerations for planning an assessment of the food system across the domains of health, environmental, social, and economic effects. It invites the user to think explicitly about system boundaries, dynamics, heterogeneity across space and populations, and the range of driving forces that shape food system outcomes. The framework is necessarily very general, as specifics for any particular study will depend on the problem being examined. Most existing studies, regardless of methodology, define rather narrow boundaries to construct a model, find or collect suitable data, and interpret the results in a way useful to their purpose. Inevitably, many of these studies make the assumption that "all else remains equal/unchanged" except the perturbations in their study. What this framework suggests is that all else does not remain equal and that any meaningful assessment must consider the likely and unintended consequences of proposed change or of the status quo when its performance is in question. An illustrative, brief example on antibiotic resistance (see Box 7-7) is provided to demonstrate how the various steps of the framework might be applied. Five additional detailed examples are presented in the annexes to this chapter.

BOX 7-7
Illustrative Example: Antibiotic Resistance

The recent rise in antibiotic resistance (AR) among pathogenic bacteria has become a global public health crisis and is now recognized as one of the top health challenges facing the world in the 21st century (CDC, 2013; Marshall and Levy, 2011; Smith et al., 2002; Woolhouse and Ward, 2013). Growing resistance may lead within decades to ineffectiveness of entire classes of antibiotics that are currently central to clinical treatment of humans (Wellington et al., 2013) as well as agricultural production (Teuber, 2001).

The problem of antibiotic resistance provides an excellent example to motivate and illustrate the framework presented in this report. Below, we walk through the six key framework steps, discussing key considerations for potential assessments of the problem of AR and highlighting the importance of all four crosscutting framework themes. As will become clear, the problem of AR involves all four domains of effects, substantial complexity and dynamics across the entire food system, and important potential trade-offs between food system or policy configurations.

Steps for Applying the Framework

The text below does not represent an implemented assessment of AR, but rather is intended to highlight the features of the problem and potential decisions that would be important to consider in undertaking each step of any such assessment. It follows the six central steps of the framework: (1) Problem and Question; (2) Scope; (3) Scenario; (4) Analysis; (5) Synthesis; and (6) Reporting.

Identify the Problem

Assessment should begin by defining the key elements of the problem under consideration, including historical and food system context. Antibiotic resistance is a naturally occurring and ancient phenomenon, but its extent has likely been affected in recent history by increased use of antibiotics by humans for two purposes: medical care and food system use (CDC, 2013; Gustafson and Bowen, 1997; Marshall and Levy, 2011; Teuber, 2001; Wellington et al., 2013; Woolhouse and Ward, 2013). Widespread antibiotic use for treatment of bacterial infection in humans began in the early 20th century. More recently, antibiotic use also has become widespread within the food system, in three distinct applications: therapy (veterinary treatment in farm animals or aquaculture); prophylaxis to prevent endemic disease in herds, flocks, or orchards; and use at subtherapeutic levels for increased growth and feed efficiencies (especially in livestock) (Marshall and Levy, 2011; Smith et al., 2002; Teuber, 2001; Woolhouse and Ward, 2013).[a] The use of antibiotics as growth promoters was first advocated in the 1950s and became widespread as the cost of application came down (Gustafson and Bowen, 1997; Marshall and Levy, 2011). Today, estimates vary regarding the relative quantity of antibiotics used in the U.S. food system versus those used in human medicine—and antibiotic use in food production varies substantially throughout the world (CDC, 2013; Marshall and Levy, 2011; Smith et al., 2002; Teuber, 2001; Wellington et al., 2013; Woolhouse and Ward, 2013). However, most experts agree that antibiotic resistance is now widespread in both settings (human and food system) and that both contribute to the rise in AR through multiple, complex pathways (Woolhouse and Ward, 2013).

To proceed with applying the framework, the assessment team should define clearly the specific question to be answered. Several distinct questions are raised by the growing problem of AR, and the relative focus might vary between assessments. For example, one central question is "What is the impact of the current U.S. food system (relative to human medicine) in driving the growth and maintenance of AR?" Other relevant research questions are, "What is the relative importance of the various distinct pathways through which food system dynamics influence AR?" and "What will be the likely impact on future AR of one or more specific shifts in food system structure or policy?" Some assessments may wish to answer more than one of these questions in a linked way. Choices of scenario, data, and analytical method (below) will be driven in part by the choice of question.

Define the Scope and Scenario

The next steps in applying the framework involve defining the scope and scenario under consideration. In these steps, two important themes are central to a good assessment. The first is to "recognize effects across the full food system" and across biophysical, social, economic, and institutional contexts for the system. For an assessment of AR, consideration of the entire supply chain is likely to be important—including chemical manufacture of antibiotics as inputs, use for treatment or growth promotion (e.g., in animal husbandry, aquaculture, or fruit production), use for medical purposes by food workers, and the potential exposure of consumers to resistant bacteria through food or environment (Marshall and Levy, 2011; Smith et al., 2005; Teuber, 2001; Wellington et al., 2013; Woolhouse and Ward, 2013). Multiple contexts also will be important, including environmental transfer of resistance genes among co-located bacteria, the food production and processing workplaces, and even patterns of global flow in water, human contact, and animal migration (Allen et al., 2010; Marshall and Levy, 2011).

A second key theme is to "consider all domains and dimensions of effects." In the case of AR, existing evidence already suggests multiple effects in all four major domains considered in this report. Economic effects include benefits of antibiotic use, such as enhanced production of food at decreased cost and the prevention of costly epidemics, but also economic costs, such as excess medical spending due to AR (CDC, 2013; Gustafson and Bowen, 1997). Health benefits include reduction in zoonotic disease and bacteria and parasites entering the food chain; health costs include decreased ability to effectively treat some diseases due to resistance and movement to more toxic or less effective medicines due to AR (CDC, 2013; Marshall and Levy, 2011; Wellington et al., 2013). Antibiotic resistance developed in the food system can affect human health via two pathways, direct contact with animals by way of food consumption and contact with bacteria in the environment. Environmental effects extend beyond growth in the soil and water "resistome" within ecosystems to impacts on nonhuman, nonfood species

continued

BOX 7-7 Continued

through the buildup of antibiotics (many of which are not very biodegradable) (Wellington et al., 2013).

The choice of a scenario (specific food system configuration) for assessment should be driven primarily by the specific question chosen in Step 1. For questions about the relative contribution of the food system and human medicine to current AR, historical and/or current configurations of the system will be appropriate to consider. For questions about the potential impact on future AR of changes to the status quo, appropriately modified configurations may be more relevant.

Conduct the Analyses

Choice of data metrics and analytical method also will be driven, in part, by the specific question chosen. However, features of the topic (here, antibiotic resistance) will likely also provide important guidance. In applying the framework, two key themes for analysis are critical.

First, analysis should "account for system dynamics and complexities." This is especially important in the case of AR, as the evidence suggests that each of the characteristics of a complex system (see Chapter 6) is both present and important. *Adaptation* is central to AR—evolution of resistance is an adaptive response by bacteria species over time (Allen et al., 2010; Smith et al., 2005). The emergence and spread of AR within and between species is a *complex and dynamic* process involving selection pressure, population dynamics, and evolution (Marshall and Levy, 2011; Smith et al., 2005; Wellington et al., 2013); sufficiently rich representation of this process can be critical to accurate assessment of changes in AR. Some evidence suggests that timing and sequence of any interventions into the system can matter enormously, and that the dynamics of AR spread may be highly nonlinear (Marshall and Levy, 2011; Smith et al., 2002). Also important is *interdependence* between factors within (and outside of) the food system. For example, genetic selection for resistance can be driven by the interaction of the total amount of antibiotics used in the system and how many individual animals are consuming them (Marshall and Levy, 2011). Similarly, the impact of use within the food system may depend on interaction with transmission dynamics outside of the system (e.g., within human health care) (Smith et al., 2005). *Feedback* between prophylactic and treatment use within the food system, as well as feedback among classes of antibiotic drugs used in food production and in human medicine, are well documented (Marshall and Levy, 2011; Phillips et al., 2004). Finally, *spatial complexity* plays an important role in AR. Population structure and movement (both of humans and animals) shape the dynamics of its spread, and antibiotics themselves (as well as resistance genes) move through space via wind, dust, watershed, insects, and soil (Allen et al., 2010).

A second theme for analysis is to choose appropriate methods and metrics for the topic. In the case of AR, data challenges loom large. The spread of AR bacteria and resistance genes are intrinsically difficult to measure, given the multiple pathways at work and the potentially long chain from origin to destination (Smith et al., 2005). Moreover, data are in short supply. Data on antibiotic use are not systemically collected in the United States; in much of the world, the use of antibiotics for growth promotion is unregulated and no data are collected at all (Marshall and Levy, 2011; WHO, 2014). Widely varying empirical estimates can be found for many questions. For example, attempts to estimate the relative *amount* of antibiotics used in human medicine and in the food system reach conclusions ranging from roughly comparable amounts in both contexts to much higher levels of use in the food system than in medicine (Phillips et al., 2004; Smith et al., 2005). Within the food system, comparisons of the amount of antibiotic use for growth-promotion versus therapeutic treatment range from roughly equal to an order of magnitude higher (Phillips et al., 2004; Smith et al., 2005). Similarly, attempts to interpret the impact of the "natural experiment" created by the European ban of nontherapeutic antibiotic use vary, with some studies finding significant reduction in use and resistance (Marshall and Levy, 2011), but others finding concomitant (and offsetting) increase in therapeutic use (Phillips et al., 2004). New methods for measurement, including genome sequencing and advanced molecular detection technology, offer the potential to address some of these gaps (Marshall and Levy, 2011; Woolhouse and Ward, 2013), but they are unlikely to fully address the limitations of empirical analysis in this arena.

Partly for this reason, and partly because of their ability to capture dynamic complexity, mathematical and computational models are promising tools for the study of AR (Smith et al., 2002, 2005; Wellington et al., 2013). They offer the potential to directly represent the biological mechanisms at work (many of which are well understood) and to simulate dynamics across populations and space (Singer and Williams-Nguyen, 2014; Verraes et al., 2013). Such models can sometimes help to anticipate the potential consequences of policy choices and to guide timing and implementation of interventions (Singer and Williams-Nguyen, 2014; Smith et al., 2002, 2005; Wellington et al., 2013).

Synthesize and Report

The final steps in applying the assessment framework involve synthesizing and interpreting results from the analysis, and then reporting the outcomes to multiple audiences.

In the context of rising AR, the absence of definitive data (and the limited amount of modeling completed to date) has led to a debate over what to do (Marshall and Levy, 2011; Woolhouse and Ward, 2013). The "precautionary principle" has led the European Union and the U.S. Food and Drug Administration (FDA) to err on the side of caution and limit antibiotic use (FDA, 2014; Smith et al., 2005). The Centers for Disease Control and Prevention has argued that the use of antibiotics for growth promotion in the food system, for example, "is not necessary and should be phased out" (CDC, 2013). FDA proposes a voluntary plan with industry to phase out the use of certain antibiotics in food production. On the other side of the debate, many have argued that appropriate risk assessments have not yet been carried out, and that limiting antibiotic use in the food system is likely to have costly, known (and perhaps unanticipated) consequences (Phillips et

continued

BOX 7-7 Continued

al., 2004). This helps to illustrate an important aspect of many assessments—the results may offer no certainty or definitive guidance, leaving an important role for judgment. Indeed, the assessment may uncover unavoidable trade-offs. An assessment should aim to present results in a balanced and accurate manner that neither over- nor underinterprets, recognizing that different audiences may draw different conclusions from the report about "what to do."

The framework also stresses the need to address (and include) many stakeholders as audiences to whom the results are reported. In the AR case, potential stakeholders include regulatory bodies, livestock and aquaculture producers, food safety groups, physicians and hospitals, insurance companies, drug manufacturers, environmental safety agencies, and consumers.

---

[a] Use of antibiotics for growth promotion in aquaculture has been phased out in North America (although imported seafood may have been treated in this way); therapeutic treatment of fish en masse by including antibiotics in fish food continues (Marshall and Levy, 2011).

SUMMARY

This chapter provides the committee's recommendation for an analytical framework that can be used by decision makers, researchers, and other stakeholders to examine the possible impacts of interventions and collectively evaluate the outcomes of specific food system configurations in terms of the health, environmental, social, and economic domains. The committee recognizes that a systemic analysis will be an expensive endeavor, and guidance is provided for situations where analytical and financial resources may limit the scope of an assessment. Therefore, not all steps or methods will apply equally, depending on the scope and topic chosen by the assessor(s). Also, although boundaries and implications should be recognized, discrete questions might not require a full systemic analysis. In other instances, a systematic review of the literature for the relevant questions might be warranted rather than a full systemic analysis.

The goal of the framework is to guide the evaluations and the decision-making processes in the area of food and agriculture. However, any analysis is simply one input into the actual decision making, and many other factors come into play, such as judgments, that are beyond the scope of the report. This framework would be useful for (1) identifying and potentially preventing unintended effects of an intervention; (2) promoting transparency among stakeholders about decisions; (3) improving communication and providing a better understanding of values and perspectives among scientists, policy makers, and other stakeholders; and (4) decreasing the likelihood of misinterpretation of results.

The framework is based on four principles that are associated with a desirable scope of an assessment. A good assessment should:

1. Recognize effects across the full food system;
2. Consider all domains and dimensions of effects;
3. Account for system dynamics and complexities; and
4. Choose appropriate methods for analysis and synthesis.

The assessment framework calls for considering four dimensions of effects—quantity, quality, distribution, and resilience—that measure how much of what the food system provides, where and to whom it goes, and how sustainably it can do so.

An assessment follows six implementation steps, including problem definition (determining the need for assessment and defining goals and objectives), scoping (characterizing system boundaries, components, processes, actors, and linkages), scenario definition (identifying baseline and alternatives, as appropriate), analysis (conducting the assessment), synthesis (synthesizing and interpreting results), and reporting (communicating findings to stakeholders).

The chapter discusses in detail the steps outlined and considers the variety of analytical methods that might be used in an assessment as well as how to engage stakeholders throughout the assessment process.

REFERENCES

Adler, M. 2012. *Well-being and fair distribution. Beyond cost distribution.* New York: Oxford University Press.

Allen, H. K., J. Donato, H. H. Wang, K. A. Cloud-Hansen, J. Davies, and J. Handelsman. 2010. Call of the wild: Antibiotic resistance genes in natural environments. *Nature Reviews Microbiology* 8(4):251-259.

Alston, J. M., G. W. Norton, and P. G. Pardey. 1998. *Science under scarcity: Principles and practice for agricultural research evaluation and priority setting.* New York: CAB International.

Anderson, J. R. 1974. Simulation: Methodology and application in agricultural economics. *Review of Marketing and Agricultural Economics* 42(1):3-55.

Arnand, S., K. R. Mankin, K. A. McVay, K. A. Janssen, P. L. Barnes, and G. M. Pierzynski. 2007. Calibration and validation of ADAPT and SWAT for field-scale runoff prediction. *Journal of the American Water Resources Association* 43(4):899-910.

Arnstein, S. R. 1969. Ladder of citizen participation. *Journal of the American Institute of Planners* 35(4):216-224.

Arrow, K. J. 1971. *Essays in the theory of risk bearing.* Chicago, IL: Markham Publishing Co.

Barrett, C. B., and M. R. Carter. 2010. The power and pitfalls of experiments in development economics: Some non-random reflections. *Applied Economic Perspectives and Policy* 32(4):515-548.

Boardman, A., D. Greenberg, A. Vining, and D. Weimer. 2010. *Cost–benefit analysis*. The Pearson Series in Economics. Upper Saddle River, NJ: Prentice Hall.

Box, G. E. P., and N. R. Draper. 1987. *Empirical model building and response surfaces*. New York: Wiley.

CDC (Centers for Disease Control and Prevention). 2013. *Antibiotic resistance threats in the United States*. http://www.cdc.gov/drugresistance/threat-report-2013 (accessed January 6, 2015).

Chen, X., H. Huang, M. Khanna, and H. Onal. 2014. Alternative transportation fuel standards: Economic effects and climate benefits. *Journal of Environmental Economics and Management* 67(3):241-257.

Cohen, J. T., D. Bellinger, W. E. Connor, P. M. Kris-Etherton, R. S. Lawrence, D. S. Savitz, B. Shaywitz, S. M. Teutsch, and G. Gray. 2005. A quantitative risk–benefit analysis of changes in population fish consumption. *American Journal of Preventive Medicine* 29:325-334.

Collins, S. L., S. R. Carpenter, S. M. Swinton, D. Ornstein, D. L. Childers, T. L. Gragson, N. B. Grimm, J. M. Grove, S. L. Harlan, K. Knapp, G. P. Kofinas, J. J. Magnuson, W. H. McDowell, J. M. Melack, L. A. Ogden, G. P. Robertson, M. D. Smith, and A. C. Whitmer. 2011. An integrated conceptual framework for social–ecological research. *Frontiers in Ecology and the Environment* 9(6):351-357.

Conway, G. R. 1987. The properties of agroecosystems. *Agricultural Systems* 24:95-117.

Cornfield, J. 1978. Randomization by group: A formal analysis. *American Journal of Epidemiology* 108(2):100-102.

Dawes, R. M., D. Faust, and P. Meehl. 1989. Clinical versus actuarial judgment. *Science* 243:1668-1674.

Deaton, A. 2010. Instruments, randomization, and learning about development. *Journal of Economic Literature* 48(2):424-455.

Dent, J. B., and M. J. Blackie. 1979. *Systems simulation in agriculture*. London, UK: Applied Science.

Dillon, C. R. 1993. Advanced breakeven analysis of agricultural enterprise budgets. *Agricultural Economics* 9(2):127-143.

Donner, A., and N. Klar. 2000. *Design and analysis of cluster randomisation trials in health research*. London, UK: Arnold.

Drummond, M. F., M. J. Sculpher, G. W. Torrance, B. J. O'Brien, and G. L. Stoddart. 2005. *Methods for the economic evaluation of health care programmes*. Oxford, UK: Oxford University Press.

Egbendewe-Mondzozo, A., S. M. Swinton, R. C. Izaurralde, D. H. Manowitz, and X. Zhang. 2011. Biomass supply from alternative cellulosic crops and crop residues: A spatially explicit bioeconomic modeling approach. *Biomass & Bioenergy* 35:4636-4647.

FDA (Food and Drug Administration). 2014. *Judicious use of antimicrobials*. http://www.fda.gov/AnimalVeterinary/SafetyHealth/AntimicrobialResistance/JudiciousUseofAntimicrobials (accessed January 6, 2015).

Freeman, A. M. 1993. *The measurement of environmental and resource values: Theory and methods*. Washington, DC: Resources for the Future.

Gold, M. R., J. E. Siegel, L. B. Russell, and M. C. Weinstein. 1996. *Cost-effectiveness in health and medicine*. Oxford, UK: Oxford University Press.

Gustafson, R. H., and R. E. Bowen. 1997. Antibiotic use in animal agriculture. *Journal of Applied Microbiology* 83:531-541.

Hadar, J., and W. R. Russell. 1969. Rules for ordering uncertain prospects. *American Economic Review* 59:25-34.

Hammond, R. A. 2009. Complex systems modeling for obesity research. *Preventing Chronic Disease* 6(3):A97.

Hanks, J., and J. T. Ritchie. 1991. *Modeling plant and soil systems*. Madison, WI: Society of Agronomy, Crop Science Society of America, and Soil Science Society of America.

Heckman, J., H. Ichimura, J. Smith, and P. Todd. 1998. Characterizing selection bias using experimental data. *Econometrica* 66(5):1017-1098.

Howitt, R. E. 1995. Positive mathematical programming. *American Journal of Agricultural Economics* 77:329-342.

Intriligator, M. D. 1978. *Econometric models, techniques and applications*. Englewood Cliffs, NJ: Prentice-Hall.

Israel, B. A., A. J. Schulz, E. A. Parker, and A. B. Becker. 1998. Review of community-based research: Assessing partnership approaches to improving public health. *Annual Review of Public Health* 19:173-202.

Johnson, D. M. 2013. An assessment of pre- and within-season remotely sensed variables for forecasting corn and soybean yields in the United States. *Remote Sensing of the Environment* 141:116-128.

Keeney, R. L., and H. Raiffa. 1976. *Decisions with multiple objectives: Preferences and value tradeoffs*. New York: Wiley.

Langseth, D., and N. Brown. 2011. Risk-based margins of safety for phosphorus TMDLs in lakes. *Journal of Water Resources Planning and Management* 137(3):276-283.

Law, A. M., and W. D. Kelton. 1991. *Simulation modeling and analysis*. New York: McGraw-Hill.

Layard, R., and S. Glaister. 1994. *Cost-benefit analysis*, 2nd ed. Cambridge, UK: Cambridge University Press.

Marshall, B.M., and S. B. Levy. 2011. Food animals and antimicrobials. *Clinical Microbiology Reviews* 24(4):718.

Meehan, T. D., C. Gratton, E. Diehl, N. D. Hunt, D. F. Mooney, S. J. Ventura, B. L. Barham, and R. D. Jackson. 2013. Ecosystem-service tradeoffs associated with switching from annual to perennial energy crops in riparian zones of the US Midwest. *PLoS ONE* 8(11):e80093.

Mendenhall, W., R. L. Scheaffer, and D. D. Wackerly. 1986. *Mathematical statistics with applications*. Boston, MA: Duxbury.

Michalak, A. M., E. J. Anderson, D. Beletsky, S. Boland, N. S. Bosch, T. B. Bridgeman, J. D. Chaffin, K. Cho, R. Confesor, I. Dalo lu, J. V. DePinto, M. A. Evans, G. L. Fahnenstiel, L. He, J. C. Ho, L. Jenkins, T. H. Johengen, K. C. Kuo, E. LaPorte, X. Liu, M. R. McWilliams, M. R. Moore, D. J. Posselt, R. P. Richards, D. Scavia, A. L. Steiner, E. Verhamme, D. M. Wright, and M. A. Zagorski. 2013. Record-setting algal bloom in Lake Erie caused by agricultural and meteorological trends consistent with expected future conditions. *Proceedings of the National Academy of Sciences of the United States of America* 110(16):6448-6452.

Moffitt, R. A. 2004. The role of randomized field trials in social science research—a perspective from evaluations of reforms of social welfare programs. *American Behavioral Scientist* 47(5):506-540.

NAS (National Academy of Sciences). 2003. *Understanding risk. Informing decisions in a democratic society*. Washington, DC: The National Academies Press.

NRC (National Research Council). 2008. *Public participation in environmental assessment and decision making*. Washington, DC: The National Academies Press.

NRC. 2009. *Science and decisions: Advancing risk assessment*. Washington, DC: The National Academies Press.

NRC. 2011. *Improving health in the United States: The role of health impact assessment.* Washington, DC: The National Academies Press.

Nyborg, K. 2012. *The ethics and politics of environmental cost–benefit analysis.* Abingdon, Oxon, UK: Routledge.

Phillips, I., M. Casewell, T. Cox, B. De Groot, C. Friis, R. Jones, C. Nightingale, R. Preston, and J. Waddell. 2004. Does the use of antibiotics in food animals pose a risk to human health? A critical review of published data. *Journal of Antimicrobial Chemotherapy* 53(1):28-52.

Powers, C. M., G. Dana, P. Gillespie, M. R. Gwinn, C. O. Hendren, T. C. Long, A. Wang, and J. M. Davis. 2012. Comprehensive environmental assessment: A meta-assessment approach. *Environmental Science & Technology* 46(17):9202-9208.

Pratt, J. W. 1964. Risk aversion in the small and in the large. *Econometrica* 32:12-36.

Presidential/Congressional Commission on Risk Assessment and Risk Management. 1997. *Framework for environmental health risk management.* Washington, DC: RiskWorld.

Rabotyagov, S. S. 2010. Ecosystem services under benefit and cost uncertainty: An application to soil carbon sequestration. *Land Economics* 86(4):668-686.

Robertson, G. P. 2004. Abatement of nitrous oxide, methane and other non-CO_2 greenhouse gases: The need for a systems approach. In *The global carbon cycle*, edited by C. B. Field and M. R. Rapauch. Washington, DC: Island Press. Pp. 493-506.

Schoemaker, P. J. H. 1982. The expected utility model: Its variants, purposes, evidence and limitations. *Journal of Economic Literature* 20(2):529-563.

Singer, R. S. and J. Williams-Nguyen. 2014. Human health impacts of antibiotic use in agriculture: A push for improved causal inference. *Current Opinion in Microbiology* 19:1-8.

Smith, D. L., A. D. Harris, J. A. Johnson, E. K. Silbergeld, and J. G. Morris, Jr. 2002. Animal antibiotic use has an early but important impact on the emergence of antibiotic resistance in human commensal bacteria. *Proceedings of the National Academy of Sciences of the United States of America* 99(9):6434-6439.

Smith, D. L., J. Dushoff, and J. G. Morris. 2005. Agricultural antibiotics and human health. *PLoS Medicine* 2(8):e232.

Stakeholder Participation Working Group of the 2010 HIA in the Americas Workshop. 2011. *Best practices for stakeholder participation in health impact assessment.* Oakland, CA. October 2011. http://www.hiasociety.org/documents/guide-for-stakeholder-participation.pdf (accessed January 6, 2015).

Stokey, E., and R. J. Zeckhauser. 1978. *A primer for policy analysis.* New York: Norton.

Sunstein, R. 2000. Cognition and benefit–cost analysis. *Journal of Legal Studies* 29(2):1059-1103.

Swinton, S. M., and G. W. Norton. 2009. Economic impacts of IPM. In *Integrated Pest Management*, edited by E. B. Radcliffe, W. D. Hutchison, and R. E. Cancelado. Cambridge, UK: Cambridge University Press. Pp. 14-24.

Teuber, M. 2001. Veterinary use and antibiotic resistance. *Current Opinion in Microbiology* 4:493-499.

Tyner, W. E. 2010. The integration of energy and agricultural markets. *Agricultural Economics* 41:193-201.

Van Dyne, G. M., and Z. Abramsky. 1975. Agricultural systems models and modelling: An overview. In *Study of agricultural systems*, edited by G. E. Dalton. London, UK: Applied Science Publishers. Pp. 23-106.

van Wijk, M. T., M. C. Rufina, D. Enahoro, D. Parsons, S. Silvestri, R. O. Valdivia, and M. Herrero. 2012. *A review on farm household modelling with a focus on climate change adaptation and mitigation.* Working Paper No. 20. Copenhagen, Denmark: CGIAR Research Program on Climate Change, Agriculture and Food Security.

Verraes, C., S. Van Boxstael, E. Van Meervenne, E. Van Coillie, P. Butaye, B. Catry, M. A. de Schaetzen, X. Van Huffel, H. Imberechts, K. Dierick, G. Daube, C. Saegerman, J. De Block, J. Dewulf, and L. Herman. 2013. Antimicrobial resistance in the food chain: A review. *International Journal of Environmental Research and Public Health* 10(7):2643-2669.

Wellington, E. M., A. B. Boxall, P. Cross, E. J. Feil, W. H. Gaze, P. M. Hawkey, A. S. Johnson-Rollings, D. L. Jones, N. M. Lee, W. Otten, C. M. Thomas, and A. P. Williams. 2013. The role of the natural environment in the emergence of antibiotic resistance in gram-negative bacteria. *Lancet Infectious Diseases* 13(2):155-165.

WHO (World Health Organization). 2014. *Antimicrobial resistance—global report on surveillance*. Geneva, Switzerland: WHO.

Woolhouse, M. E. J., and M. J. Ward. 2013. Sources of antimicrobial resistance. *Science* 341:1460.

7-A

Annexes: Examples to Illustrate the Framework

In the process of developing this report, the committee found several instances where a change in a configuration (in policy or practice) or recommendation within the food system could lead to unintended and unexpected consequences in multiple domains beyond its immediate objective. These various instances demonstrate how an analytical framework that includes health, environmental, social, and economic domains is necessary for conducting more accurate assessments of any potential change to the food system.

The committee chose six examples (see Box 7-A-1) from different parts of the food system to illustrate how its proposed analytical framework would be applied. The framework could assess the effects of a change in a food system configuration (e.g., a policy or practice) either on its own or in comparison with a different scenario. Each example below illustrates how the lack of consideration in areas beyond the immediate desired outcome can result in wide-ranging and unexpected effects, and how a comprehensive approach is needed to incorporate possible ripple effects, interdependencies, interactions, and feedbacks. An illustrative, brief example on antibiotic resistance (see Box 7-7) is provided to demonstrate how the various steps of the framework might be applied. Five additional detailed examples are presented in these Annexes.

The examples were selected because they address current questions or concerns that have had or could have important consequences, whether those consequences are positive, negative, or unintended. Each example takes the framework and follows the steps prescribed within it (see Box 7-1)

BOX 7-A-1
Examples of Food System Configurations Selected to Illustrate the Application of the Framework

The use of antibiotics in agriculture (see Chapter 7, Box 7-7). The wide use of antibiotics in agriculture may contribute to the development of antibiotic-resistant organisms with implications for human and animal health. Analysis of historical and/or current configurations of the system may yield insights about the relative contributions of the food system and of human medicine to current growth in antibiotic resistance.

Recommendations for fish consumption and health (see Annex 1). Consumption guidelines for fish have not considered the availability of enough fish to meet them and the potential environmental impacts. Several alternative scenarios could entail a change in dietary recommendations or the application of new technologies (e.g., sustainable farming production methods).

Policies mandating biofuel blending in gasoline supplies (see Annex 2). Biofuel policies intended to increase the country's energy independence and decrease greenhouse gas emissions compared to fossil fuel were implemented without consideration of wider environmental effects and effects on domestic and global food prices.

Recommendations to increase fruit and vegetable consumption (see Annex 3). The purpose of this assessment could be to understand the barriers and inducements to fruit and vegetable consumption so that better interventions to increase consumption can be implemented.

Nitrogen dynamics and management in agroecosystems (see Annex 4). The use of high levels of nitrogen fertilizer to increase crop yields has environmental, health, and economic consequences that go beyond immediate concerns with crop yields. A baseline scenario could be one that is mostly reliant on mineral fertilizers without the use of methods to increase nitrogen uptake and retention. For comparison, an alternative cropping system could be less reliant on mineral nitrogen fertilizer and emphasize biological nitrogen fixation, manure and organic matter, amendments, cover crops, and perennial crops.

Policies on hen housing practices (see Annex 5). This case study presents an assessment that is currently being conducted to analyze the implications for productivity, food safety, and workers' health of changing egg production practices. Data for the assessment are currently being collected on three types of hen management systems.

to show how it could be used. However, any analysis, synthesis, and reporting on those examples are excluded from this report as those steps go beyond the committee's Statement of Task. Also, even though the scoping step is critical for identifying important dynamics of the system, the committee was unable to carry out that step in a thorough manner (it did not include a systematic review of topic areas) due to time and resource limitations. Instead, the committee selected the most salient effects and identified relevant scientific papers. For the analysis step, the committee reflected on needs in the area of data collection and general methods, but it did not deliberate on the best data or methods for a particular scenario. In addition to the time and resource limitations mentioned, a thorough assessment needs to carefully select the assessment team and level of stakeholder participation based on the initial questions. The committee was not constituted with the goal of performing an analysis in any of the particular questions, a step that was clearly outside of the Statement of Task and would need an assessment team with expertise in areas relevant to the particular question(s) to be addressed. Likely, the details of performing the synthesis (e.g., whether to aggregate the traits into an index or to do a cost–benefit analysis) and the reporting (e.g., who are the stakeholders) would be the prerogative of the assessment team. Therefore, readers should not take any of the specific analyses or configurations as recommendations, but rather as examples for future consideration.

Each of the examples below conveys how different aspects and principles of the framework need to be applied. For instance, the example on fruits and vegetables focuses on the number and diversity of actors that drive the system, whereas the nitrogen example highlights the need for intense data collection over time and geographical locations. It should also be noted that the example on policies on animal welfare dealing with commercial egg production is the only example for which a team of assessors is currently conducting an assessment. This example is of particular interest because the methodical approach taken to answer the questions happens to closely coincide with what is proposed for a framework. As recommended in the framework and outlined in the examples, the limitations and boundaries should be noted: for example, if data collection was restricted to one farm, it may not be appropriate to extrapolate such data to other regions or farms where other factors could play a role.

Lastly, for all of the examples, the steps of the framework are followed in a sequential manner: the problem, the scope, the scenario, and the analysis. However, the committee recognizes that in reality the framework might be implemented in a circular, iterative manner where additional questions, description of the scope, reviews of the literature, or analysis of data might be initiated when needed at any point during the process of assessing the system.

ANNEX 1: DIETARY RECOMMENDATIONS FOR FISH CONSUMPTION

The Fish System: A Complex Adaptive System with Diverse Actors

Despite the presence of contaminants such as methyl mercury in fish, the belief of many experts has been that consuming fish is beneficial for health. The *Dietary Guidelines for Americans, 2010* recommends consumption of 8 ounces of seafood per week (USDA and HHS, 2010). An analysis of the impacts of this recommendation constitutes a good example of a policy that, if realized, could have unintended consequences in dimensions beyond health, including environmental, social, and economic effects. The committee's framework could be applied to study how to integrate the health, environmental, social, and economic effects of fish consumption.

The fish example specially illustrates Principle 3 in the committee's framework—account for system dynamics and complexities—because it illustrates a dynamic global system that involves multiple actors at all levels, from fishers to development agencies to nutritionists offering dietary guidance. These actors have different goals and information, and they often disagree among themselves on issues such as the strength of the evidence of effect of eicosapentaenoic acid and docosahexaenoic acid on health. They also may have different views and awareness of food security in the short and long terms, and most have not thought about the effects of changed fishing policies on different populations. For example, in some geographical areas, the fisheries sector might benefit from increased demand while in others it might lead to economic declines and food insecurity. A lack of institutional capacity makes it difficult to include those most directly affected in policy decisions and safety and biodiversity discussions. At the same time, multiple signs of adaptation by various actors to the decline in fish and aquatic stocks are evident. These include the immense growth in aquaculture, especially in Asia; the significant research on environmentally benign production methods; and the distribution of information about fish caught or produced under sustainable conditions. These changes are not consistent around the world or even within the same country. Geographical diversity and spatial complexity are particularly important in the fish example.

continued

The global nature of fish and the particular circumstances of its production and distribution by multiple players along multiple supply chains governing flow among countries, as well as global market signals, produce many unintended effects, including those described above. The geographic distances introduce long lag times into feedback loops between consumption and production. A dearth of research on the effects of current practices, as well as climate change on future capacity, present serious challenges to all of the actors in the system.

A number of the elements of this complex adaptive system have already been assessed. Still, knowledge gaps persist, stakeholders disagree about the extent of the problem, and debates continue among scientists about the validity of research findings and assumptions.

Fish and other types of seafood are an important source of protein worldwide. Globally, they comprise about 6 percent of dietary protein, but for 3 billion people, fish account for up to 20 percent of the average per-capita intake of animal protein (FAO, 2014). Fish and seafood also are sources of other important nutrients, including the long-chain polyunsaturated fatty acids (PUFAs) eicosapentaenoic acid/docosahexaenoic acid (EPA/DHA), which are associated with reduced heart disease risk.

Because of the potential health benefits of fish, the *Dietary Guidelines for Americans, 2010* (DGA) recommend that people consume 8 ounces of seafood per week—especially marine-derived "oily" fish such as salmon, mackerel, sardines, pompano, anchovies, swordfish, trout, and tuna—to provide an average daily consumption of 250 mg of EPA/DHA per day (USDA and HHS, 2010). Other fish provide these fatty acids, but levels are low enough that very large amounts of fish would have to be consumed each day to meet the recommendation. Although another omega-3 fatty acid, alpha linolenic acid (ALA), can be converted into EPA and DHA, the conversion is fairly limited in humans. The DGA also recommend consumption of a variety of types of seafood to reduce the amount of methyl mercury consumed from any one type. Five of the top 10 consumed seafood are low in mercury—shrimp, light tuna, salmon, pollock, and catfish (AHA, 2014).

Fish consumption in the United States is low: 6.8 kg per capita in 2011 (measured by food intake, not availability). Per-capita intake data show the mean seafood intake is approximately 9 g per day, and nearly 50 percent of this is shrimp (Raatz et al., 2013). Of the top 10 seafood consumed,[1] only salmon contains a sufficient amount of EPA/DHA per serving to meet the 250 to 500 mg per day recommended by some groups. Moreover, data from the National Health and Nutrition Examination Survey (NHANES) 2003-2008 food consumption survey show that only 20 percent of seafood consumed was in the high omega-3 group (Papanikolaou et al., 2014). At best, the intake of these PUFAs is about 40 percent of the suggested level.

The amount of fish available per capita in the United States has declined since 2006 from 16.5 to 14.4 pounds in 2012 (NFI, 2013). Studies show that familiarity, price, and freshness most influence consumer decisions to purchase fish (Hall and Amberg, 2013), and the decline has been attributed to fish prices among a number of other factors. Some research suggests one reason for the decline is the fish advisories regarding methyl mercury and other toxicants, as discussed below. An unintended consequence is that instead of choosing seafood with lower mercury levels, many consumers have reduced their intake of fish altogether (Rheinberger and Hammitt, 2012). Given that consumers often do not have access to the facts they need to make fully informed choices, the seafood industry along with restaurants and retailers are key determinants of the amount, type, and form of fish that people consume by affecting cost, availability, and the desirability of different fish (Oken et al., 2012).

Fish consumption is the final link along the supply chain of the fish subsystem, which is connected to natural resources both domestically and globally. Figure 7-A-1 represents a map of this food subsystem with a selection of actors and processes that will be affected if demand is increased.

Identify the Problem

Assessments are typically triggered by a broad problem or concern. The first step, identifying the problem, is often done based on a literature review and consultation with stakeholders. The problem identified in this example is that if consumers were to fully follow the DGA seafood recommendation, significant increases in the supply of fish would be necessary. An assessment team would explore the health, environmental, social, and economic consequences (in the United States and abroad) of following the current DGA's recommendations for fish consumption compared with the current consumption of fish.

[1] The top 10 are shrimp, canned tuna, salmon, tilapia, pollock, pangasius, crab, cod, catfish, and clams.

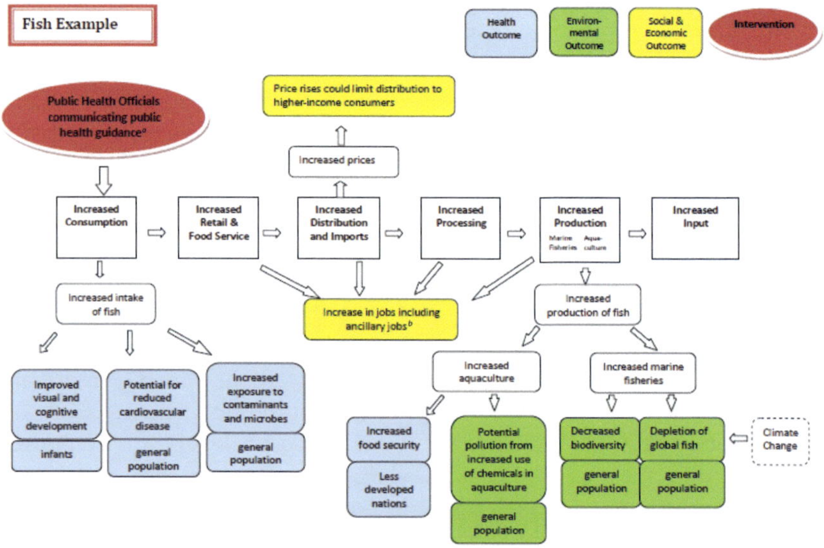

FIGURE 7-A-1 Conceptual model of selected drivers and potential effects of the current U.S. health guidance on fish consumption. The arrows show the potential effects both within the supply chain and in the broader physical and socioeconomic context. The effects noted are based on a review of selected scientific publications, not a systematic review of the literature. Interactions such as feedbacks (e.g., the fact that increased prices might decrease the demand, ameliorating the effects) are not illustrated.

[a] The 2010 *Dietary Guidelines for Americans* (USDA and HHS, 2010) state that Americans should increase the amount of seafood they eat to at least 8 or more ounces (2 to 3 servings) each week. Smaller amounts of seafood are recommended for children. Pregnant and breastfeeding women should eat at least 8 and up to 12 ounces of seafood, from choices that are lower in methyl mercury, each week to boost babies' brain and eye development.

[b] Ancillary jobs include processing, packaging, marketing, distribution, manufacturing of fish processing equipment, net and gear making, ice production, supply, boat construction and maintenance, retail, research, and administration.

Define the Scope of the Problem

After identifying the problem, the second step in an assessment is to establish the boundaries of the analysis and to describe the major drivers and the relevant health, environmental, social, and economic effects (see Figure 7-A-1). This step is critical to defining appropriate dietary recommendations for oily fish consumption that meet multiple goals, because meeting those goals may require trade-offs between the potential health effects of the recommendations and their environmental, social, and economic effects. For this example, the boundary of the system to be modeled is the United States, operating within a global fish system, and we provide a brief literature review to describe these drivers and their mechanisms.

Health Effects

Nutrition In the early 1970s, researchers reported that Greenland Eskimos (Inuits) had very low rates of heart attacks and less heart disease in general compared with their Danish counterparts (Bang et al., 1971). The scientists attributed these health benefits to the consumption of fish and sea mammals containing high levels of the long-chain PUFAs. Over the ensuing decades, thousands of research studies have been conducted to determine the effects of fish and fish oils on human health (O'Keefe and Harris, 2000). The results of this extensive research led to the recommendations for fish consumption in the 2010 DGA. The benefits are primarily considered to be a reduction in risk of coronary heart disease in adults and an improvement in cognitive development in infants and young children. Recently, Fodor et al. (2014) questioned the early studies of Greenland Eskimos, pointing out that subsequent studies showed the incidence of heart disease in the Eskimo population in Greenland and in Alaska and Canada to be similar to that of the non-Eskimo population.

These inconsistencies in results raise the question as to how strong the association is between reduced cardiovascular disease risk and fish intake. Despite this question, experts in many countries offer dietary advice to their populations regarding fish and fish oil intake. At this time, seafood is the primary source of EPA/DHA in human diets (IOM, 2007). Fish do not synthesize these fatty acids; they obtain them through diets consisting of algae and krill or other fish. Most infant formula is now supplemented with DHA that comes from algal sources.

Food safety Some health organizations (e.g., the American Heart Association, the World Health Organization) acknowledge that a number of species of fish contain significant levels of methyl mercury, polychlorinated biphenyls, dioxins, and other environmental contaminants. These contaminants are generally higher in marine mammals and in older, larger fish that are higher on the food chain (i.e., higher trophic-level fish). Mercury is a contaminant of oceans, fresh water lakes and rivers, and soil arising from natural geologic processes or from atmospheric fallout, largely from coal-fired power plants. The mercury concentrates through the fish food chain primarily in the form of methyl mercury, which is a neurotoxin and a possible risk factor for cardiovascular illness (Ginsberg and Toal, 2009). Since the early 1970s, states have provided advisories regarding the safety of fish caught in their waterways and lakes. In 1994, the U.S. Food and Drug Administration (FDA) issued its first national advisory to limit consumption of swordfish. In 2001, it issued its second advisory for commercially harvested and processed fish.[2] FDA was criticized then for ignoring the stronger recommendations of a National Research Council panel, which had concluded that FDA standards were outdated (NRC, 2000). In 2001, the U.S. Environmental Protection Agency (EPA) also issued similar advisories for fish being caught by anglers. In 2004, FDA and EPA published their first joint advisory warning pregnant women, women planning to become pregnant, nursing mothers, and young children to eliminate shark, swordfish, king mackerel, and tilefish from their diets and to limit their consumption of other fish to 12 ounces per week to minimize exposure to methyl mercury (FDA/EPA, 2004). This was a higher amount than recommended by the Dietary Guidelines, demonstrating an inconsistency in consumer advice. In June 2014, FDA and EPA issued a draft of a new advisory suggesting that pregnant women eat at least 8 ounces and as many as 12 ounces per week of fish that are low in mercury. They also recommended limiting consumption of albacore tuna by pregnant women to 6 ounces a week and said that women and children should follow advisories from local officials regarding fish from local bodies of water (FDA/EPA, 2014). This advice was given despite recent research (Karagas et al., 2012) that demonstrated adverse effects of prenatal methyl mercury exposure at doses similar to FDA recommended limits. A recent analysis of blood samples collected during the 2007-2010 NHANES showed that 4.6 percent of adults sampled had blood levels of mercury at or above 5.8 μg mercury/liter, EPA's cut-off point for a level without appreciable lifetime risk of deleterious effects. Blood mercury levels increased significantly as the frequency of consumption of shark and swordfish increased. Blood mercury increased as well when the frequency of salmon and tuna increased, though not as rapidly (Nielsen et al., 2014).

In 2007, the Institute of Medicine (IOM) released a set of recommendations intended to balance the risks and benefits of fish consumption with regard to nutrients and toxicants. In general, the advice was to eat two 3-ounce portions (cooked) of fish per week, and for females who are or may become pregnant or breastfeeding, and for children up to age 12, to avoid higher trophic-level predatory fish (IOM, 2007). All other demographic groups were urged to choose a variety of types of seafood to reduce the risk of exposure to contaminants from a single source. Under the assumption that the potential benefits of fish consumption outweigh the potential health risks, recent research has increased the specificity by quantitatively

[2] The 2001 FDA advisory recommended that pregnant women, nursing mothers, young children, and women who may become pregnant not consume shark, swordfish, king mackerel, and tilefish and that they not consume more than 12 ounces of other fish per week.

analyzing the net risk/benefit of individual fish species based on their methyl mercury and EPA/DHA content (Ginsberg and Toal, 2009). Ginsberg and Toal found that the omega-3 fatty acid benefits outweigh methyl mercury risk for some species (farmed salmon, herring, and trout). The opposite was true for swordfish and shark. Other species were associated with a small net benefit (e.g., canned light tuna) or a small net risk (e.g., albacore canned tuna). In another study, researchers calculated that newborns gained a modest amount of IQ points if their mother complied with the FDA/EPA fish advisory. When health effects where monetized, their model also showed that this gain could be offset by an increase in cardiovascular risk if those older than 40 reduced their fish intake by one monthly meal (Rheinberger and Hammitt, 2012).

Seafood also has well-characterized hazards caused by microbes and naturally occurring toxins (see Chapter 3). In 2007, the U.S. Centers for Disease Control and Prevention (CDC) reported that among 235 outbreaks that could be attributed to a single commodity, seafood was stated as the cause of 24 percent of the total. This means that given its low consumption, seafood is responsible for a disproportionate number of outbreaks (Upton, 2010). In 2013, CDC reported 299 outbreaks in 2010 that could be attributed to a single commodity, and 37 of these were for fish (CDC, 2013).

Environmental Effects

Caught fish To increase the availability and affordability of needed protein-rich foods in the developing world, government efforts to increase fishing capacity were greatly expanded in the 1950s. This was mainly accomplished by developing large industrial fishing operations with the capability of landing a much greater tonnage of fish than before. World fisheries production leveled off in the 1970s when the majority of fish stocks were being fully exploited. Global fish production has increased about 80 times in volume since 1950 and was 158 million metric tons (mmt) in 2012, including capture fish and aquaculture (FAO, 2014). The former has stabilized at about 90 mmt over the past decade and aquaculture contributes more than 40 percent of total production at this point. About 136 mmt (86 percent) of fish production was used as food for people in 2012 at a level of 19.2 kg per capita (FAO, 2014). This is a large increase from the 1980s, when about 70 percent was used for human consumption and the remainder for non-food uses such as fish meal or oil. In 2012, edible fish and shellfish landings from marine waters by U.S. fishers were 4.4 mmt, the third largest producer country behind China and Indonesia (FAO, 2014). The United States also is the second largest importer of fish in the world, importing approximately 90 percent of its fish supply (FAO, 2012).

Customary natural resource management policies have favored the pursuit of maximum yields, which has led to "spectacular resource collapses" (Newman and Dale, 2009). Since the 1970s when concerns about depletion started to increase, fisheries and fish stocks have been studied extensively by different sectors using different metrics—a cause of some of the disagreement about the issue. Demonstrating one example of the heterogeneity in the fish subsystem, conservationists look at extinction risk (defined as species that have declined more than 50 percent within the most recent 10 years or three-generation period). Fisheries[3] estimate biomass trajectories (called stock assessments) and reference points against which to benchmark population status (Davies and Baum, 2012).

Although fisheries management has had some success in the United States, seeing a decline in overfishing and some fisheries' stocks rebuilding to healthy levels, the global situation is less optimistic. In spite of a number of international treaties, illegal fishing is still a problem, and management of fisheries is relatively ineffective in some countries. For example, illegal overfishing of bluefin tuna in the Mediterranean continues to be a problem. Globally, nearly 30 percent of fish stocks are overexploited, and about 60 percent are fully exploited (near their maximum sustainable production level, which is defined as the largest catch that can be taken from the species stock over an indefinite period) (FAO, 2014). Most of the stocks of the top 10 species consumed are fully exploited and will not increase in production (FAO, 2012). In addition to human consumption of fish, another human-derived driver of this subsystem is climate change. Wild fish stocks are expected to decline further with the stresses of climate variability, such as ocean acidification, changes in temperature, nutrient supply, light availability, and many others. Concerns are being raised about the negative effects of climate change on marine ecosystems and habitats, decreased biodiversity, as well as fish stock depletions (Rice and Garcia, 2011). The most recent Intergovernmental Panel on Climate Change Assessment Report (IPCC, 2014) states that the projected impacts of climate change on fish stocks are very negative on a global scale, although some fisheries will increase, and that fishers can adapt by decreasing pollution, changing fishing pressures, increasing aquaculture, and instituting more dynamic management policies. In a review of the literature on impacts on ecosystem productivity, a paper by Hollowed et al. (2013) offered a broad perspective on marine fish and shellfish species' habitat, human communities, and food

[3] In the United States, under the Magnuson-Stevens Fishery Conservation and Management Reauthorization Act of 2006, the National Oceanographic and Atmospheric Administration's Office of Sustainable Fisheries helps manage fisheries (e.g., meeting catch limits and ending overfishing, and increased international cooperation), promoting sustainable fisheries and preventing economic losses. They do their work by providing guidance to the Regional Fishery Management Councils on management of fisheries.

security. The authors emphasized that important questions regarding the effects of physical and biological processes and their incorporation into models remain unanswered. They recognized the many uncertainties in assessing the impacts of climate change. They also pointed to several areas where research is needed, such as collecting physiological measurements as affected by multiple factors; ecological monitoring of the interactions among physical, chemical, and biological components; and estimating the vulnerabilities of countries to detriments in fisheries due to climate change.

Aquaculture As an adaptation to the decline in fish stocks, since 1981 world fish production through aquaculture has expanded at an average annual rate of nearly 9 percent, but it slowed recently to approximately 6 percent growth (FAO, 2014). Inland aquaculture, which generally uses fresh water, has increased from 50 percent of total aquaculture production in 1980 to 63 percent in 2012 (FAO, 2014). Of the top 10 consumed seafoods in the United States, 5 are either primarily or substantially produced by aquaculture (Raatz et al., 2013). U.S. aquaculture production is about 6 percent of U.S. seafood demand, but not all species raised are excellent sources of EPA/DHA. Marine aquaculture is about 20 percent of U.S. aquaculture production (NOAA, 2014), but the production was lower in 2012 in North America than in 2000, mainly due to competition from countries with lower production costs (FAO, 2014).

Aquaculture production is steadily expanding. In fact, in 2011, global farmed fish production exceeded beef production (Larsen and Roney, 2013), and by 2015, aquaculture is projected to surpass capture fisheries (OECD/FAO, 2013). The expansion is bringing increased attention to the environmental damage caused by different production systems, including the pressure on wild fish stocks when they are used as feed sources (especially herring, anchovies, and sardines). These are used to preserve traditional flavors and to provide sources of DHA/EPA to farmed fish. Other problems caused by aquaculture operations include declines in water quality, extensive energy use, antibiotic use, and invasive species (Diana et al., 2013; Oken et al., 2012).

Social and Economic Effects

Fisheries and aquaculture provided livelihoods and income for an estimated 58 million people engaged in the primary sector of fish production in 2012, of which an estimated 7 million were occasional fishers and fish farmers, with 84 percent residing in Asia (FAO, 2014). In 2012, about 19 million people were engaged in aquaculture (in Asia 97 percent of fish-related employment is in fish farming). Employment in the fisheries and aquaculture primary sector has continued to grow faster than has employment in agriculture, so that by 2010 it represented about 4 percent of the 1.3 billion people economically active in the broad agriculture sector worldwide. In the past 5 years, the number of people engaged in fish farming has increased by 5.5 percent per year, compared with only 0.8 percent per year for those in capture fisheries (FAO, 2012).

Fisheries and aquaculture also provide numerous jobs in related activities, such as processing, packaging, marketing and distribution, manufacturing of fish processing equipment, net and gear making, ice production and supply, boat construction and maintenance, research, and administration. All of this employment, together with dependents, is estimated to support the livelihoods of 660 to 820 million people, or about 10 to 12 percent of the world's population (FAO, 2014).

Recognizing the size of the global workforce and the importance of engaging the workforce as the industry develops, researchers are investigating (1) ways to place a greater emphasis on local human capital because better trained and educated workforces will be able to adapt to local conditions and production; (2) the development of risk management systems to enhance security against invasive species, including pathogens; and (3) development of global standards for sustainably produced products from aquaculture (Diana et al., 2013). Another useful tool is social impact assessments (SIAs). In the United States, the National Oceanic and Atmospheric Administration provides guidance on how to conduct and implement the results of assessments that allow fishers and fishing communities to address the social impacts of fishery management alternatives (Pollnac et al., 2006). This research makes clear that the seafood industry, especially fishers, should be more involved in developing research and outreach projects to improve management practices regarding environmental pollution such as feed types (replacing fish-based feed with plant sources) and water quality management.

In the United States, commercial fishing is one of the most hazardous and deadliest occupations. The fatality rate for fishers is 124 per 100,000, which is astronomically higher than the overall rate for all workers of 4 per 100,000 (CDC/NIOSH, 2014). Although the work environments for commercial fishing operations vary significantly by the body of water and type of fish being harvested, fishers generally encounter harsh working conditions, including extreme weather, long work hours, strenuous physical labor, and living in confined quarters (BLS, 2014; CDC/NIOSH, 2014). Leading causes of fatalities among fishers are sinking vessels, falling overboard, and contact with onboard machinery and fishing gear (CDC/NIOSH, 2014; Lincoln et al., 2008). The most hazardous U.S. fisheries, based on fatality rates, are the Northeast multispecies ground fish fishery, the Atlantic scallop fishery, and the West Coast Dungeness crab fishery (CDC/NIOSH, 2014).

Yet another issue is concern about the fact that the combined effect of rising demand and the collapse of local fisheries has led developed countries such as the United States, Japan, and members of the European Union to increasingly import large quantities of seafood from developing countries. The proportion of fish and fish products being traded on the global market is 40 percent versus 5 percent for rice (Jenkins et al., 2009). This demand puts intense pressure on developing countries either to allow access of foreign fishing fleets into their coastal fishing grounds or to export their fish to foreign markets. In either case, the local markets of developing countries where basic nutrition and health are challenges (e.g., nations in West Africa) are deprived of an important source of protein for the sake of the developed world (Jenkins et al., 2009).

Identify the Scenarios

To understand the effects of a new policy (e.g., changed dietary recommendations), or technology (e.g., sustainable farming production methods), or a shock to the system (e.g., accelerated ocean warming in some parts of the world), an assessment of the fishing system would include a step that compares the performance of the current system as described in the scope—the baseline—with one or more alternative scenarios that reflect the proposed change. For this example, the baseline is the current consumption of fish in the United States, and the alternative scenarios would be changes in consumption of seafood by the U.S. population, either increases in consumption of fish to meet the current DGA recommendations or decreases in consumption to meet other goals. The alternative scenarios would consider a variety of factors, such as:

- Different levels of fish recommendations, including the present DGA recommendations and several lower percentages of that;
- Different levels of or changes in methyl mercury levels consumed in fish that might result from compliance with fish advisories by targeted populations;
- Different amounts of wild and farmed salmon produced under different environmental, climate change, and biodiversity conditions; and
- Different levels of fish protein needed in various parts of the world.

Conduct the Analysis

In this step of an assessment, data, metrics, and analysis tools are used to examine the likely health, environmental, social, and economic effects associated with the alternative scenarios. A systemic analysis also would consider any assessments already conducted on the health, environmental, social, and economic dimensions. Based on the framework principles, a seafood analysis would use methods that describe potential key dynamic drivers of the system, such as the increased preferences for fish due to admonitions to consume more fish, the growth in aquaculture, and potential fish stock changes due to climate change. Another important feature is that it would account for the global effects as well as the distribution of effects for different populations.

Previous Analyses

Previous work has examined the effects of increasing seafood consumption on various dimensions, both quantitatively and qualitatively. For example, the IOM report described above analyzed the scientific evidence for the nutritional benefits and safety risks from seafood (IOM, 2007). Also, Ginsberg and Toal (2009) identified a dose–response relationship for methyl mercury and omega-3 fatty acid effects on coronary heart disease and neurodevelopment. Other assessments have considered other dimensions of effects, in addition to health. Jenkins et al. (2009) looked at the evidence base for long-chain PUFA consumption; the decline of fish stocks; the global social and economic effects of the increasing demand for fish; fish farming and aquaculture and the constraints on its growth; contaminants in fish; and alternative sources of EPA and DHA. They concluded that there should be an assessment of the environmental impact of dietary guidelines to consume more fish before the guidance is issued, as is the case for other dietary recommendations. In the most comprehensive treatment of this issue, Oken and her colleagues (2012) concluded that information integrating the health, ecological, and economic impacts of different fish choices is lacking. Rice and Garcia (2011) reviewed projections to 2050 for global population growth and fish production that anticipates climate-related change and effects on biodiversity. They concluded that the projected 50 percent increase in fish production from both capture fisheries and intensive farming would be incompatible with the present proposed interventions to address pressure on marine biodiversity. This supports the need for consideration of the impact of climate change and population growth when providing recommendations about fish consumption and the necessity of putting emphasis on lower-intensity aquaculture systems (Diana et al., 2013).

New Analyses

For this example, an assessment team would select specific data sources, metrics, and methodologies for the analysis. Data sources could include

(1) self-reported NHANES data on consumption of oily fish (assuming it can be disaggregated); (2) monitoring data on methyl mercury from FDA, EPA, and mercury concentration databases in Karimi et al. (2012); (3) global data on wild caught and farmed salmon production from the Food and Agriculture Organization or other sources; and (4) simulated or actual data on biodiversity, climate change, and pollution levels in marine and freshwater systems.

A number of different methods already have been used to measure various effects. One of these is a model to carry out SIAs of fisheries (Pollnac et al., 2006). Another is a model of integrated risk/benefit analyses using dose–response relationships and secondary data analyses from individual studies of methyl mercury and omega-3 fatty acid levels in various kinds of fish (Rheinberger and Hammitt, 2012). Two other modeling schemes that seem particularly well adapted to a dynamic and complex fish system are agent-based modeling (ABM) and system dynamics modeling. ABM constructs artificial societies on computers, with agents placed in a spatial context with specified internal conditions and a set of adaptive rules that govern their interaction with each other and with the environment. There can be substantial diversity among actors (e.g., fishers, distributors, and fish eaters): interactions produce output at both the individual and aggregate system levels. Macro-level patterns and trends can be produced and the patterns (e.g., changes in fish consumption, marine biodiversity/fish stocks, and available fish protein) can be compared with data to calibrate the model. ABMs are particularly useful to explore policy questions (Hammond, 2009).

A system dynamics model uses three core components to examine effects: (1) increases or decreases in fish stocks over time; (2) flows, or the rates of change in the stock; and (3) feedback loops that connect stocks and flows over time and over spatial distances and that can incorporate changes in consumption and in recommended levels (Hammond, 2009).

Consideration of the health, environmental, social, and economic effects of fish recommendations also could lead to additional questions requiring further research and analysis. Some of the questions could include

- What other dietary patterns have or could have similar effects on health outcomes?
- Can the proposed benefits from fish consumption be achieved through supplements of EPA/DHA produced by algae or yeast?
- What amount of fish is needed to meet increased fish demand and still maintain healthy fish stocks?
- What balance of wild caught and aquaculture products would produce the optimal environmental outcomes?

- What are the implications of increased demand for fish, specifically the economic implications for populations of fish-exporting countries?
- What are the food security implications for populations that depend on fish as a major source of protein in the diet?
- How will climate change affect marine biodiversity and the productivity of wild caught and farmed fish stocks?
- How will international institutions mediate and develop policies that will reconcile the differences among multiple competing interests related to this difficult problem?

REFERENCES

AHA (American Heart Association). 2014. *Fish 101.* http://www.heart.org/HEARTORG/GettingHealthy/NutritionCenter/Fish-101_UCM_305986_Article.jsp (accessed December 30, 2014).

Bang, H. O., J. Dyerberg, and A. B. Nielsen. 1971. Plasma lipid and lipoprotein pattern in Greenlandic West-coast Eskimos. *Lancet* 1(7710):1143-1145.

BLS (Bureau of Labor Statistics). 2014. *Occupational outlook handbook, 2014-15 edition, fishers and related workers.* http://www.bls.gov/ooh/farming-fishing-and-forestry/fishers-and-related-fishing-workers.htm (accessed December 30, 2014).

CDC (Centers for Disease Control and Prevention). 2013. Surveillance for foodborne disease outbreaks—United States, 2009-2010. *Morbidity and Mortality Weekly Report* 62(3):41-47.

CDC/NIOSH (CDC/National Institute for Occupational Safety and Health). 2014. *Commercial fishing safety.* http://www.cdc.gov/niosh/topics/fishing/#fishus (accessed December 30, 2014).

Davies, T. D., and J. K. Baum. 2012. Extinction risk and overfishing: Reconciling conservation and fisheries perspectives on the status of marine fishes. *Scientific Reports* 2:561.

Diana, J. S., H. S. Egna, T. Chopin, M. S. Peterson, L. Cao, R. Pomeroy, M. Verdegem, W. T. Slack, M. G. Bondad-Reantaso, and F. Cabello. 2013. Responsible aquaculture in 2050: Valuing local conditions and human innovations will be key to success. *BioScience* 63(4):255-262.

FAO (Food and Agriculture Organization of the United Nations). 2012. *The state of world fisheries and aquaculture 2012.* Rome, Italy: FAO.

FAO. 2014. *The state of world fisheries and aquaculture. Opportunities and challenges.* Rome, Italy: FAO.

FDA/EPA (Food and Drug Administration/Environmental Protection Agency). 2004. *What you need to know about mercury in fish and shellfish.* http://water.epa.gov/scitech/swguidance/fishshellfish/outreach/advice_index.cfm (accessed December 30, 2014).

FDA/EPA. 2014. *FDA and EPA issue updated draft advice for fish consumption/Advice encourages pregnant women and breastfeeding mothers to eat more fish that are lower in mercury.* http://yosemite.epa.gov/opa/admpress.nsf/bd4379a92ceceeac8525735900400c27/b8edc480d8cfe29b85257cf20065f826!OpenDocument (accessed December 30, 2014).

Fodor, G. J., E. Helis, N. Yazdekhasti, and B. Vohnout. 2014. "Fishing" for the origins of the "Eskimos and heart disease" story. Facts or wishful thinking? A review. *Canadian Journal of Cardiology* 30(8):864-868.

Ginsberg, G. L., and B. F. Toal. 2009. Quantitative approach for incorporating methylmercury risks and omega-3 fatty acid benefits in developing species-specific fish consumption advice. *Environmental Health Perspectives* 117(2):267-275.

Hall, T. E., and S. M. Amberg. 2013. Factors influencing consumption of farmed seafood products in the Pacific Northwest. *Appetite* 66:1-9.

Hammond, R. A. 2009. Complex systems modeling for obesity research. *Preventing Chronic Disease* 6(3):A97.

Hollowed, A. B., M. Barange, R. J. Beamish, K. Brander, K. Cochrane, K. Drinkwater, M. G. G. Foreman, J. A. Hare, J. Holt, S. Ito, S. Kim, J. R. King, H. Loeng, B. R. MacKenzie, F. J. Mueter, T. A. Okey, M. A. Peck, V. I. Radchenko, J. C. Rice, M. J. Schirripa, Y. Yamanaka, and A. Yatsu, 2013. Projected impacts of climate change on marine fish and fisheries. *ICES Journal of Marine Science* 70(5):1023-1037.

IOM (Institute of Medicine). 2007. *Seafood choices: Balancing benefits and risks*. Washington, DC: The National Academies Press.

IPCC (Intergovernmental Panel on Climate Change). 2014. *Fifth assessment report 2014. Climate change: Implications for fisheries and aquaculture*. Cambridge, UK: IPCC.

Jenkins, D. J., J. L. Sievenpiper, D. Pauly, U. R. Sumaila, C. W. Kendall, and F. M. Mowat. 2009. Are dietary recommendations for the use of fish oils sustainable? *Canadian Medical Association Journal* 180(6):633-637.

Karagas, M. R., A. L. Choi, E. Oken, M. Horvat, R. Schoeny, E. Kamai, W. Cowell, P. Grandjean, and S. Korrick. 2012. Evidence on the human health effects of low-level methylmercury exposure. *Environmental Health Perspectives* 120(6):799-806.

Karimi, R., T. P. Fitzgerald, and N. S. Fisher. 2012. A quantitative synthesis of mercury in commercial seafood and implications for exposure in the United States. *Environmental Health Perspectives* 120(11):1512-1519.

Larsen, J., and J. M. Roney. 2013. *Farmed fish production overtakes beef*. Earth Policy Institute. http://www.earth-policy.org/plan_b_updates/2013/update114 (accessed December 30, 2014).

Lincoln, J. M., D. L. Lucas, R. W. McKibbin, C. C. Woodward, and J. E. Bevan. 2008. Reducing commercial fishing deck hazards with engineering solutions for winch design. *Journal of Safety Research* 39(2):231-235.

Newman, L., and A. Dale. 2009. Large footprints in a small world: Toward a macroeconomics of scale. *Sustainability: Science, Practice, & Policy* 5(1):9-19.

NFI (National Fisheries Institute). 2013. *National Fisheries Institute*. http://www.aboutseafood.com (accessed December 30, 2014).

Nielsen, S. J., B. K. Kit, Y. Aoki, and C. L. Ogden. 2014. Seafood consumption and blood mercury concentrations in adults aged >=20 y, 2007-2010. *American Journal of Clinical Nutrition* 99(5):1066-1070.

NOAA (National Oceanic and Atmospheric Administration). 2014. *NOAA fisheries: Office of Aquaculture*. http://www.nmfs.noaa.gov/aquaculture (accessed December 30, 2014).

NRC (National Research Council). 2000. *Toxicological effects of methylmercury*. Washington, DC: National Academy Press.

OECD/FAO (Organisation for Economic Co-operation and Development/FAO). 2013. *Agricultural outlook 2013-2022*. Paris, France, and Rome, Italy: OECD/FAO.

O'Keefe, J. H., Jr., and W. S. Harris. 2000. From Inuit to implementation: Omega-3 fatty acids come of age. *Mayo Clinic Proceedings* 75(6):607-614.

Oken, E., A. L. Choi, M. R. Karagas, K. Marien, C. M. Rheinberger, R. Schoeny, E. Sunderland, and S. Korrick. 2012. Which fish should I eat? Perspectives influencing fish consumption choices. *Environmental Health Perspectives* 120(6):790-798.

Papanikolaou, Y., J. Brooks, C. Reider, and V. L. Fulgoni, III. 2014. U.S. adults are not meeting recommended levels for fish and omega-3 fatty acid intake: Results of an analysis using observational data from NHANES 2003-2008. *Nutrition Journal* 13:31.

Pollnac, R. B., S. Abbott-Jamieson, C. Smith, M. L. Miller, P. M. Clay, and B. Oles. 2006. Toward a model for fisheries social impact assessment. *Marine Fisheries Review* 68(1-4):1-18.

Raatz, S. K., J. T. Silverstein, L. Jahns, and M. J. Picklo. 2013. Issues of fish consumption for cardiovascular disease risk reduction. *Nutrients* 5(4):1081-1097.

Rheinberger, C. M., and J. K. Hammitt. 2012. Risk trade-offs in fish consumption: A public health perspective. *Environmental Science and Technology* 46(22):12337-12346.

Rice, J. C., and S. M. Garcia. 2011. Fisheries, food security, climate change, and biodiversity: Characteristics of the sector and perspectives on emerging issues. *ICES Journal of Marine Science* 68:1343-1353.

Upton, H. F. 2010. Seafood safety: Background and issues. *CRS Report for Congress*. http://nationalaglawcenter.org/wp-content/uploads/assets/crs/RS22797.pdf (accessed December 30, 2014).

USDA and HHS (U.S. Department of Agriculture and U.S. Department of Health and Human Services). 2010. *Dietary guidelines for Americans, 2010*. Washington, DC: USDA and HHS.

ANNEX 2: U.S. BIOFUELS POLICY

Biofuels Policy: A Problem That Operates in the Context of Energy Policy But Has Ripple Effects in the Food System

U.S. biofuels policy arose in response to shifting concerns about energy independence, agricultural surpluses, and climate change. Before 2005, when the Renewable Fuel Standard (a production mandate for biofuels), import tariffs, and other measures were enacted into law, little prospective analysis was conducted on how the new policies would affect the food system, much less the environment or health. The goal was to stimulate the production and use of biofuels under the assumption that its use would decrease dependence on foreign oil, result in reduced greenhouse gas emissions, and increase rural incomes (Tyner, 2008).

It did not take long after the new policies went into effect, however, for economists and others to recognize that the linkages between energy markets and the food system created by the policies had unintended consequences. These included increased costs for food producers, upward pressure on globally traded commodity prices, and a public (and a private) outlay of subsidies for ethanol production that has been significantly greater than anticipated.

As corn is a food and feed staple, biofuels policy has had unintended effects on U.S. agricultural production by altering the mix of crops planted. This also has had unintended effects on the global food system, which seeks a predictable, and increasing, supply of food. Moreover, the energy and environmental footprint of corn production calls into question its suitability as a renewable substitute for gasoline. These trade-offs weaken the justification of the current policy on the basis of U.S. energy security, particularly as reliance on imported oil has been reduced recently by increased domestic energy production.

Although some studies have suggested that perennial grasses would provide environmental and energy benefits over corn as an energy feedstock, the production of such crops and their conversion to gasoline-compatible fuel on a commercial scale remain elusive. Consequently, fuel blenders are unable to use cellulosic and other "advanced" biofuels at the levels mandated by the Renewable Fuel Standard. Moreover, the most available biofuel—corn ethanol—has reached a blending threshold that cannot be

continued

overcome without a greatly expanded flex-fuel vehicle fleet and widespread fueling infrastructure for E85 (85 percent ethanol).

U.S. biofuels policy has been criticized both for falling short of its intended goals and for its unintended effects on the environment and food system, but would alternative policies have fewer shortcomings? The potential for the framework to be used to analyze trade-offs and unintended effects in the pursuit of energy and environmental security is illustrated in this annex exploring how the Renewable Fuel Standard might be compared to an alternate policy of eliminating subsidies for fossil fuels. The elimination of such subsidies worldwide is a goal to which numerous international bodies and their member countries, including the United States, have committed, but not yet fulfilled. This policy alternative has potential impacts on U.S. domestic agricultural production and the global food system, but the ways in which those impacts are manifested are likely to be different from the Renewable Fuel Standard, as are its health, environmental, social, and economic implications. Such a comparison would shed light on the merits and shortcomings of different ways to pursue the same goals.

Identify the Problem

As described in the committee's framework, the first step of an assessment is to identify the problem. For this example, the problem is how to achieve the dual goals of reducing transportation-related greenhouse gas (GHG) emissions and decreasing U.S. reliance on foreign oil while avoiding unintended health, environmental, social, and economic consequences, including those related to the food system, in the process.

Transportation is a major component of the U.S. economy and is fundamental to the mobility and livelihood of Americans, who collectively drove nearly 3 trillion miles in 2013 (DOT, 2014). However, as transportation also consumes 70 percent of imported oil (EIA, 2014) and is responsible for 28 percent of all GHG emissions in the United States (EPA, 2012), cleaner sources of transportation fuel under domestic control are needed. Biofuels produced from domestic crop feedstocks represent one such alternative fuel. Corn, soybeans, and their products have historically been a significant part of the U.S. food system, accounting for nearly half of all acreage in crops. U.S. biofuels policy grew out of mounting corn and soybean surpluses and declining supplies of fossil fuels in the late 1970s, at a time when GHG emissions were scarcely a concern. In the face of recurring grain and oilseed surpluses, the United States saw an opportunity to improve its energy independence, and over time it developed extensive biofuels promotion policies that were built around blending mandates, subsidies, and import protections. Between 1980 and 2005, corn-based ethanol use as fuel grew steadily, aided by forgiveness of the excise tax on gasoline and little foreign competition due to a specific-rate tariff on ethyl alcohol imports of 54 cents per gallon, enacted in 1978 (Koplow, 2009). In 1988, "flex fuel" vehicles (FFVs) capable of running on 85 percent ethanol (E85) were granted credits against manufacturers' Corporate Average Fuel Efficiency (CAFE) requirements, but fewer than 10 percent of FFVs actually used E85, undermining the intent of the credits (MacKenzie et al., 2005). The 2004 enactment of the Volumetric Ethanol Excise Tax Credit changed the gas excise tax exemption into a tax credit for ethanol producers, set initially at 51 cents per gallon (Koplow, 2009). Corn-based ethanol also got a boost from state and local financing credits and mandates and from the banning of methyl-tertiary-butyl ether, a groundwater contaminant, as an oxygenate in reformulated gasoline[1] markets. Under the impetus of these incentives, corn-based ethanol usage had reached around 4 to 5 billion gallons per year by 2005 (EIA, 2012).

Food system effects from this level of usage were generally modest. The co-products of corn ethanol production, known as distillers dry grains and solubles (DDGS), became a larger portion of beef and dairy cattle rations. The overall effects on animal production economics were not large in this early period, but some employment and marketing shifts occurred locally. Net employment gains were modest and sometimes temporary, as many plants failed or operated intermittently in this period. More dramatic effects began in 2004 as oil prices started climbing and in 2005 with the passage of the Energy Policy Act (Tyner, 2008). The Act introduced mandated ethanol use under a Renewable Fuel Standard (RFS1), which was to reach 7.5 billion gallons by 2012. In December 2007, Congress passed the Energy Independence and Security Act (EISA), which doubled the corn-based ethanol mandate to 15 billion gallons by 2015 (RFS2) (NRC, 2011) (see Figure S-1 in the summary of the NRC, 2011, report) and created new, non-grain-based ("advanced") biofuels mandates to reach a combined total of 35 billion gallons of ethanol equivalent and 1 billion gallons of biodiesel by 2022. The 2008 Farm Bill added a $1.01 per gallon subsidy for blending cellulosic biofuels (recently extended retroactively through 2014) and created the Biomass Crop Assistance Program (renewed in the 2014 Farm Bill) to incentivize biomass production for fuel. Currently, the blending of

[1] The reformulated gasoline program was mandated by Congress in the 1990 Clean Air Act amendments and the program started in 1995 with the goal of reducing smog-forming and toxic pollutants in the air.

ethanol at 10 percent (E10) no longer accommodates the RFS2 mandate for higher total amounts of ethanol use. To circumvent this "blending wall," the Environmental Protection Agency (EPA) approved 15 percent ethanol (E15) as a blending rate suitable for use in vehicles built since 2001. Some car manufacturers, however, have been unwilling to maintain engine warranties if E15 is used, and few E15 pumps have been installed because fueling stations would have to monitor their pumps to prevent the fuel from being used in older vehicles and in small engines, such as lawn mowers, for which the higher ethanol blend is not approved. Also, E15 cannot be used in the summer in most regions because its evaporative emissions exceed air quality thresholds. As noted earlier, E85 can be used by FFVs, but E85 has limited availability nationally.

In the meantime, EPA has reduced the advanced biofuels mandates each year. At a proposed 17 million gallons for 2014, the mandate is just 1 percent of the 1.7 billion gallons called for by 2014 in EISA 2007. Cellulosic ethanol is not yet produced in significant volumes, for technological as well as economic reasons. To achieve the currently mandated levels of 16.0 billion gallons of cellulosic ethanol (10.7 billion gasoline equivalent) by 2022 would require an investment of $50 billion in capital costs and sustained oil prices of somewhere between $111 and $190 per barrel, depending on the cellulosic material produced, to make its price competitive with gasoline (NRC, 2011).

U.S. biofuels policy operates in the context of an energy and environmental policy, but it has ripple effects on the food system because the primary feedstocks for biofuels are also a source of feed and food. In 2007-2008, a number of simultaneous circumstances affecting crop commodity markets collectively provoked a dramatic spike in food prices globally, the brunt of which was borne by countries dependent on those commodities as primary food sources. Although analyses differ about the contribution of biofuels to the price increase, the use of prime farmland to produce biofuel feedstocks has subsequently been scrutinized critically in light of mounting global food security concerns (Oladosu and Msangi, 2013). The diversion of 40 percent of the U.S. corn crop for ethanol production decreases the supply of corn and other grains on world commodity markets, stimulating grain producers internationally to increase their production. If that increase involves the conversion of pastures or forest into cropland, the GHG emissions that result undermine the environmental underpinnings of U.S. biofuels policy (Searchinger et al., 2008). The mandate has also caused U.S. farmers to shift agricultural production into intensive corn production, which relies heavily on fertilizers and pesticides that are potential sources of pollution. These unintended effects (among others discussed later in this annex) place the dual policy objectives of the Renewable Fuel Standard in conflict with each other.

Define the Scope of the Problem

Once the problem has been identified, the next step is to frame the scope of the assessment. This is done by characterizing the boundaries, components, processes, actors, and linkages involved in evaluating the intended and unintended effects of current biofuels policies relative to an alternative policy configuration. The alternative chosen for comparison may involve additional or different actors and linkages than are associated with the Renewable Fuel Standard. Thus, a discussion about scope has to take place in conjunction with the selection of the appropriate comparator.

Identify the Scenarios

For this example, the problem is whether, in light of the cost of public incentives involved in promoting biofuels and the difficulty in meeting blending mandates, alternative policies could be implemented to achieve the goals of meeting domestic transportation energy needs, reducing GHG emissions, and improving energy security with better consequences (or fewer unintended consequences) for the food system, health, the environment, and society. Although different options for promoting fuels production have been explored, such as biofuels subsidies that embody both a natural security component (based on their energy value relative to gasoline) and an environmental component (based on their reduced GHG footprint relative to gasoline) (Chen et al., 2014; Tyner, 2008), a policy specifically targeting biofuels is not necessarily the only way to approach these goals.

One hypothetical alternative to achieving the same goals might be to eliminate existing public subsidies for domestic fossil fuel production. Fossil fuel subsidies (tax credits and other incentives) in the United States stood at approximately $6 billion in 2011 (OECD, 2012), which is small relative to the value of oil in the U.S. economy, so the impact of unilaterally eliminating subsidies might have only a tiny effect, if any, on the behavior of the fuel market. Because this policy alternative seems to fall short in producing any of the intended effects that an assessment would measure in comparison to the Renewable Fuel Standard, it might be an inappropriate alternative. If, however, such a policy were accompanied by a carbon tax (a tax on the emissions content of fuels), the cost of fossil fuels would rise significantly, creating incentives to move toward fuels with fewer emissions. Moreover, the tax would create a revenue stream that could be used, in part, to invest in energy alternatives (Palmer et al., 2012).

Another policy alternative is to eliminate fossil fuel subsidies globally. Worldwide subsidies of fossil fuel production (to incentivize exploration) and consumption (keeping prices artificially low) amounted to $550 billion in 2013, according to the International Energy Agency, which concluded that the subsidies contribute to wasteful consumption, reduce the competitiveness of cleaner sources of energy, and ultimately contribute to climate change. At a global level, the elimination of subsidies could have a significant effect on fuel markets.

Although it can be reasoned that it is more balanced to limit the scope of analysis to the comparison of one domestic policy to another, it can also be argued that such a limitation places an artificial constraint on the comparison. The two policy alternatives—one, a mandate for specific market outcomes, and the other, an unencumbering of market forces—already represent very different approaches to achieving the same goal. Moreover, based on the growing implications of climate change, achieving reductions in domestic fossil fuel subsidies might be more realistic in the context of international agreements for multilateral reductions in subsidies. The phase-out and elimination of fossil fuel subsidies was called for by President Obama in 2009 at a meeting of the member countries of the G20, which collectively agreed to pursue the elimination of subsidies by 2020, a goal recently reaffirmed in 2014. The phase-out of subsidies worldwide has been called for by international organizations such as the Asia-Pacific Economic Cooperation countries, the International Monetary Fund (IMF, 2013), numerous policy and economic think tanks, and environmental groups, among others.

Whichever scope is chosen for the analysis, the primary actors include fossil fuel and biofuel producers, consumers of fuels in both the transportation sector (including for food transport) and other energy-intensive economic sectors, particularly electricity generation. The analyses also must focus on agricultural producers, suppliers of energy-intensive agricultural inputs (e.g., fertilizer), food processors, and food consumers.

By definition, the removal of subsidies for fossil fuel production and consumption should initially result in higher prices for those fuels, which will set in motion a cascade of responses worldwide. As prices are affected by supply and demand, the responses of oil and gas producers globally and the reaction of energy-consuming sectors of the global economy will both influence energy prices. The outcome of economic models that predict how fossil fuel prices affect supply and demand and the feedbacks that are likely to occur also depends on the pace at which subsidies for fossil fuels would be eliminated by governments worldwide, and on policies related to climate change (e.g., a carbon tax or regulations on pollutants) and the promotion of renewable energy alternatives (electric and fuel), or increasing fuel efficiency (CAFE) standards. Like those policies, an anticipated effect of eliminating fossil fuel subsidies would be to reduce fossil fuel consumption, thus reducing fossil fuel dependence.

The strong linkage between energy costs and food production will result in feedbacks to each sector that also must be estimated in the analysis. Just as biofuels subsidies have had an influence on what crops farmers decide to grow, high fossil fuel prices could alter both crop planting and agronomic practice decisions by agricultural producers. The modeling of the agricultural responses would itself be complex and subject to feedback from energy prices. For example, biofuels made with feedstocks (e.g., perennial grasses) that are less costly to grow than are more energy-intensive crops might become more economically competitive with fossil fuels and receive expanded investment and use. Electric vehicles, a fast-growing segment of the transportation fleet, might become more or less competitive, as electricity generation responds to the removal of subsidies. Just as biofuel mandates have influenced the price of feed and food, higher fossil fuel prices also might increase costs across the value chain of the food system. Like users of energy, patterns of food demand by consumers also may change as they experience price increases in food.

Examine Effects in All Domains

To meet the requirements of the framework, the assessment must not only evaluate impacts on the use of biofuels and fossil fuels as energy sources but also account simultaneously for their direct and indirect health, environmental, social, and economic consequences. A recent review paper on the effects of biofuels found that relatively few publications used interdisciplinary approaches, integrated more than one dimension, or captured the interactions and feedbacks that exist among different effects (Ridley et al., 2012). The authors added that a dearth of research exists on human health, biodiversity, and trade topic areas. Nevertheless, many publications have focused on one or more dimensions of the impact of biofuels and biofuels policy that could be synthesized and augmented with additional studies. With respect to fossil fuels, an existing literature on economic, environmental, and public health effects (NRC, 2010; ORNL and RFF, 1992-1998; Ottinger et al., 1990) could serve as a starting point for exploring the potential effects of the elimination of subsidies for fossil fuels. It is, of course, conceivable that new effects will emerge as different energy-using sectors of the economy respond.

The sections that follow look at the most studied types of effects, which would be relevant in comparing any set of alternatives to the current policy. As will be discussed, impacts in one domain (e.g., environment) are likely to have consequences in others (e.g., health).

Environmental Effects

The comparative analysis should be mindful that environmental effects of either policy alternative might be both positive and negative, occur on many different scales, and take place directly and indirectly. Since 2007, when the Renewable Fuel Standard expanded mandates for blending biofuels into gasoline in the United States, numerous studies have addressed a range of actual and potential environmental effects of biofuels and, by association, policy mandates for biofuels. As policies have stimulated producers in the Midwest to place more land into corn production (Malcolm and Aillery, 2009), higher nitrate levels in the Mississippi River have been observed (Sprague et al., 2011), along with hypoxia in the Gulf of Mexico associated with nitrogen loads in its watershed (Scavia and Liu, 2009). The levels of protein in DDGs now widely fed to food animals were found to lead to greater nitrogen excretion in manure, increasing environmental risks (Stallings, 2009), although its use for animal feed also offsets GHG emissions elsewhere in the biofuels life cycle (Bremer at al., 2010).

In its first triennial report on biofuels policy to Congress in 2011, EPA found that negative effects resulting from the policy were mainly due to the environmental impacts of corn production. The agency added, however, that other feedstocks could have either negative or positive effects, depending on which feedstock is used, processing practices, and land use (EPA, 2011).

Additional studies have explored environmental effects from biofuel feedstock production (and use) on biodiversity, insects, birds, and vegetation (Fletcher et al., 2011; Landis and Werling, 2010; Meehan et al., 2012; Robertson et al., 2011); pesticide use (Schiesari and Grillitsch, 2011); air quality and emissions (EPA, 2011; Liaquat et al., 2010; Wagstrom and Hill, 2012); and water demand, water quality, and soil loss (EPA, 2011; Hill et al., 2006; Khanal et al., 2013).

The environmental effects (positive and negative) of biofuels policy scenarios also have been modeled at different scales, from subregional (Egbendewe-Mondzozo et al., 2013) and regional (EPA, 2011; Georgescu et al., 2009) to global (Frank et al., 2013; Taheripour et al., 2010). The literature around projections of GHG emissions associated with market-mediated effects of biofuels is growing. These include life cycle analyses that incorporate land-use change (Ahlgren and Di Lucia, 2014; Chen et al., 2014; Hertel et al., 2010a,b; NRC, 2011; Searchinger et al., 2008) and so-called rebound effects, in which biofuels ostensibly spur greater fossil fuel use because of their downward influence on oil prices (Smeets et al., 2014).

In contrast to the many environmental aspects that have been examined related to biofuel policy, fewer evaluations have been conducted on the full range of potential environmental impacts of reducing or eliminating fossil fuel subsidies. A review of six major studies exploring the potential environmental and other impacts of reforming fossil fuel subsidies found that reductions in GHGs and carbon dioxide (CO_2) emissions were the most commonly modeled impacts. The studies (published from 1992 through

2009) predicted reductions in carbon dioxide that ranged from 1.1 percent in 2010 to 18 percent by 2050 (Ellis, 2010). More recent estimates place reductions of CO_2 at 10 percent by 2050 (IEA, 2012). Undoubtedly, a range of other local and regional environmental effects of reduced production and consumption of fossil fuels would need to be calculated. Furthermore, as noted earlier, price effects may reduce consumption and influence greater investments in alternative energy sources, or they may catalyze changes in agricultural practices that would have environmental impacts.

Social and Economic Effects

Between 2000 and 2010, the number of ethanol plants in operation in the United States grew from 50 to more than 200 (RFA, 2014). A recent analysis of job growth between 2000 and 2010 in a 12-state region (comparing counties with an ethanol plant to similar counties without a plant) found that the biofuels industry was responsible for increasing employment by 0.9 percent, creating 82 new jobs on average (Brown et al., 2013). In the early 2000s, many of the plants were constructed by local cooperatives, but ownership of the plants has increasingly diversified to include absentee investors, including multinational companies. Somewhat surprisingly, a study of local reactions to ethanol plant ownership suggests that many communities have more support for absentee ownership than for local ownership, with one explanation being that the "deeper pockets" of large corporate owners would allow the plant to withstand the volatility of the ethanol market. Community expectations of the potential traffic, water, air, and other effects of an ethanol plant did not vary based on ownership (Bain et al., 2012).

Today, about 40 percent of U.S. corn production is used for biofuels (27 percent after accounting for DDGs recycled into the animal feed system). Although corn production has expanded in response to ethanol demand, corn prices have, on average, doubled since 2005, when the price hovered near $2.00 per bushel (Schnepf and Yacobucci, 2013). In the United States, biofuels' effects on food prices are limited because the value of corn in food products is small relative to labor, processing, and retailing costs. However, corn is a major component of the cost of producing animal protein. Under some conditions, animal producers can use more forages to feed cattle to reduce the direct impact of feed prices, but others, such as producers of poultry products, are more affected by fluctuating feed costs, which are seen in higher food prices by U.S. consumers many months later. In developing countries, corn often is a staple food, so price changes directly affect household budgets. Estimates of the impact of biofuels production on food prices globally are affected by the time frame examined. Over the long term, corn prices are shaped by production costs as well as demand trends. For example, a 2008 review of 25 studies and reports concluded that higher commodity prices were the result of the depreciation of the U.S. dollar, increasing global demand for agricultural commodities amid sluggish agricultural productivity growth and rapid growth in the production of first generation biofuels (Abbott et al., 2008). These results tended to be associated with long-term analytical approaches, which cite factors such as rising energy costs, a weak dollar, fiscal expansion, and investment fund activity (Babcock, 2011; Babcock and Fabiosa, 2011; Baffes and Haniotis, 2010).

In contrast, research on short-term effects reached very different conclusions, finding that increased biofuels production was the chief driver of grain price spikes (like those in 2008 and 2012), accounting for up to 75 percent of the increases. These analyses (Wise, 2012) also predicted that production will continue to drive prices up as a consequence of escalating usage mandates, with no effective "relief valves," such as the normal ability of high corn prices to reduce demand and ration short supplies across users (Koplow, 2009).

Although the diversion of land to produce biofuels instead of food is especially a concern in developing countries that are less able to absorb higher commodity prices, data from the Food and Agriculture Organization indicates that since 2006, more than 40 million hectares of land have been added to the global cropland base, most of that in developing countries. That means that higher commodity prices may have helped agricultural producers in those countries while harming urban consumers, who face higher food prices (Tyner, 2013).

The social and economic impacts of eliminating fossil fuel subsidies globally would be more far-reaching than U.S. biofuels policy, affecting all industrial sectors, including food production. Socioeconomic consequences are likely to be distributed unevenly, given differences in the types of subsidies in place worldwide. Developed countries like the United States typically use production subsidies, which tend to be direct transfers to fossil fuel producers. According to some analyses, eliminating U.S. production subsidies alone would return $41.4 billion in revenues to the federal government over the next 10 years (Aldy, 2013), with minimal impacts on prices for U.S. consumers (Allaire and Brown, 2009). By contrast, developing countries employ consumer subsidies, which keep prices for fuel artificially low with the goal of alleviating poverty, increasing access to energy, and encouraging growth in local economic sectors. Sharp price increases for essential goods have been associated with large-scale civil unrest, regardless of their specific causes, so eliminating consumption subsidies poses risks. Some studies suggest that incomes in poorer countries decrease when subsidies are removed (Coady et al., 2006), but others suggest that these effects can be mitigated by providing assistance to the poor with savings from expenditure subsidies. A review of empirical and modeling studies of economic effects of fossil-fuel subsidy reform suggest positive overall effects, with increases of up to 0.7 percent in gross domestic product in both developed and developing countries by 2050 (Ellis, 2010).

Health Effects

Scovronick and Wilkinson (2014) identify four major pathways through which biofuels affect health: occupational hazards; water and soil pollution; air pollution (both in biofuels production and use); and food prices. The authors suggest that the biggest health impacts at the population level would be those due to improved air quality (at least in urban environments) and those due to higher food prices (among food-insecure populations). Another study estimated the combined costs of climate change and health effects associated with GHGs and air pollution from the production and use of corn ethanol relative to gasoline and cellulosic biofuels, finding the highest costs associated with corn ethanol. The predicted effects shifted geographically depending on fuel production systems (Hill et al., 2009).

A wide-ranging study monetized the negative externalities of energy production and use. It focused particularly on health damages such as premature mortality and morbidity (chronic bronchitis and asthma) due to particulate matter in air pollution, but it also looked at losses to crops, timber, and recreation. The study estimated the costs in 2005 at approximately $56 billion, with health constituting "the vast majority" of damages (NRC, 2010). The methodologies used by the National Research Council study could be useful in predicting the public health benefits of reduced fossil fuel use, if that occurred, due to subsidy reforms.

Other Issues

Resilience and energy security are two related issues that cut across the domains of health, the environment, and the economy. Resilience, "the ability to prepare and plan for, absorb, recover from, and more successfully adapt to adverse events" (The National Academies, 2012, p. 1) has been used mainly with respect to natural disaster preparedness, but it could apply to examining the risks of disruption of the food and fuel systems, particularly in the biofuel context, where climate, disease, and pests play a role in determining supply. U.S. energy security is related to resilience, as it is viewed as a potential buffer to extreme political or other shocks to international fuel markets. Energy security was a specific rationale for developing the Renewable Fuel Standard. The elimination of U.S. production subsidies would likely reduce domestic oil and gas production, but experts debate by how much (Allaire and Brown, 2009). The extent to which either policy alternative affects both energy security and food security would be an important feature to compare, not only in terms of quantity but also with respect to the distribution of effects.

Conduct the Analysis

In this step of an assessment, data, metrics, and tools are used to examine the likely effects associated with the alternative scenarios. An analysis of how different policy configurations perturb the nexus between the global food and energy systems would be a complex and broad undertaking. Nevertheless, assembling and synthesizing the existing literature would provide a good initial picture of the distinctions between the two policies that could be sufficient to make broad comparisons of their potential and actual effects on the dimensions of interest and provide perspective on how they might operate in combination with other policies (e.g., supporting research into alternative energy production) to meet mutually desirable social goals. A first step would be to create a map of the pathways and connections through which policy has impacts on the dimensions of interest.

Comparing trade-offs inherent in different policy approaches in the context of food production, energy use, and the environment is an active area of research (Sarica and Tyner, 2013), and models that integrate economic activity with some environmental parameters (see Box 7-5) and health (NRC, 2010) have been developed. These efforts are important building blocks for a synthesis of information across the dimensions of interest. Because empirical evidence to account for some effects is not available (e.g., see Annex 4 on Nitrogen), estimates based on surrogate measures will need to be used, and the limits of that accounting must be acknowledged. Because of the necessary reliance on models for predicting policy outcomes, the greatest challenge to interpreting the synthesis of information gathered for this analysis would be to identify and describe the assumptions used by experts in quantifying effects, particularly where experts and models disagree, and to acknowledge gaps, uncertainties, and trade-offs.

REFERENCES

Abbott, P. C., C. A. Hurt, and W. E. Tyner. 2008. *What's driving food prices?* Washington, DC: Farm Foundation.

Ahlgren, S., and L. Di Lucia. 2014. Indirect land use changes of biofuel production—A review of modelling efforts and policy developments in the European Union. *Biotechnology for Biofuels* 7(1):35.

Aldy, J. E. 2013. *Eliminating fossil fuel subsidies. A policy proposal for the Hamilton Project.* Washington, DC: The Brookings Institution.

Allaire, M., and S. Brown. 2009. *Eliminating subsidies for fossil fuel production: Implication for U.S. oil and natural gas markets. Issue brief.* Washington, DC: Resources for the Future.

Babcock, B. 2011. *The impact of US biofuel policies on agricultural price levels and volatility.* International Centre for Trade and Sustainable Development. Issue Paper No. 35. Geneva, Switzerland: International Centre for Trade and Sustainable Development.

Babcock, B. A., and J. F. Fabiosa. 2011. *The impact of ethanol and ethanol subsidies on corn prices: Revisiting history.* CARD Policy Brief No. 11. http://www.card.iastate.edu/publications/synopsis.aspx?id=1155 (accessed December 23, 2014).

Baffes, J., and T. Haniotis. 2010. Placing the recent commodity boom into perspective. In *Food prices and rural poverty.* Washington, DC: The World Bank. Pp. 40-70.

Bain, C., A. Prokos, and H. X. Liu. 2012. Community support of ethanol plants: Does local ownership matter? *Rural sociology* 77(2):143-170.

Bremer, V. R., A. J. Liska, T. J. Klopfenstein, G. E. Erickson, H. S. S. Yang, D. T. Walters, and K. G. Cassman. 2010. Emissions savings in the corn-ethanol life cycle from feeding coproducts to livestock. *Journal of Environmental Quality* 39(2):472-482.

Brown, J., J. G. Weber, and T. Wojan. 2013. *Emerging energy industries and rural growth.* Economic Research Report No. ERR-159. Washington, DC: U.S. Department of Agriculture, Economic Research Service.

Chen, X. G., H. X. Huang, M. Khanna, and H. Onal. 2014. Alternative transportation fuel standards: Welfare effects and climate benefits. *Journal of Environmental Economics and Management* 67(3):241-257.

Coady, D., M. El-Said, R. Gillingham, K. Kpodar, P. Medas, and D. Newhouse. 2006. *The magnitude and distribution of fuel subsidies: Evidence from Bolivia, Ghana, Jordan, Mali and Sri Lanka.* Working paper. Washington, DC: The International Monetary Fund.

DOT (U.S. Department of Transportation). 2014. *Travel monitoring and traffic volume.* http://www.fhwa.dot.gov/policyinformation/travelmonitoring.cfm (accessed December 23, 2014).

Egbendewe-Mondzozo, A., S. M. Swinton, R. C. Izaurralde, D. H. Manowitz, and X. S. Zhang. 2013. Maintaining environmental quality while expanding biomass production: Sub-regional U.S. policy simulations. *Energy Policy* 57:518-531.

EIA (U.S. Energy Information Administration). 2012. *Annual energy outlook 2012.* Washington, DC: U.S. Department of Energy.

EIA. 2014. *Annual energy outlook 2014.* Washington, DC: U.S. Department of Energy.

Ellis, J. 2010. *The effects of fossil-fuels subsidy reform: A review of modelling and empirical studies.* A paper for the Global Subsidies Initiative of the International Institute for Sustainable Development (IISD). Geneva, Switzerland: IISD.

EPA (U.S. Environmental Protection Agency). 2011. *Biofuels and the environment: First triennial report to Congress.* Washington, DC: Office of Research and Development, National Center for Environmental Assessment.

EPA. 2012. *Inventory of U.S. greenhouse gas emissions and sinks: 1990-2012.* Washington, DC: EPA.

Fletcher, R. J., B. A. Robertson, J. Evans, P. J. Doran, J. R. R. Alavalapati, and D. W. Schemske. 2011. Biodiversity conservation in the era of biofuels: Risks and opportunities. *Frontiers in Ecology and the Environment* 9(3):161-168.

Frank, S., H. Bottcher, P. Havlik, H. Valin, A. Mosnier, M. Obersteiner, E. Schmid, and B. Elbersen. 2013. How effective are the sustainability criteria accompanying the European Union 2020 biofuel targets? *Global Change Biology Bioenergy* 5(3):306-314.

Georgescu, M., D. B. Lobell, and C. B. Field. 2009. Potential impact of U.S. biofuels on regional climate. *Geophysical Research Letters* 36(21):1-6.

Hertel, T. W., A. A. Golub, A. D. Jones, M. O'Hare, R. J. Plevin, and D. M. Kammen. 2010a. Effects of U.S. maize ethanol on global land use and greenhouse gas emissions: Estimating market-mediated responses. *BioScience* 60(3):223-231.

Hertel, T. W., W. E. Tyner, and D. K. Birur. 2010b. The global impacts of biofuel mandates. *Energy Journal* 31(1):75-100.

Hill, J., E. Nelson, D. Tilman, S. Polasky, and D. Tiffany. 2006. Environmental, economic, and energetic costs and benefits of biodiesel and ethanol biofuels. *Proceedings of the National Academy of Sciences of the United States of America* 103(30):11206-11210.

Hill, J., S. Polasky, E. Nelson, D. Tilman, H. Huo, L. Ludwig, J. Neumann, H. Zheng, and D. Bonta. 2009. Climate change and health costs of air emissions from biofuels and gasoline. *Proceedings of the National Academy of Sciences of the United States of America* 106(6):2077-2082.

IEA (International Energy Agency). 2012. *World energy outlook 2012*. Paris, France: IEA.

IMF (International Monetary Fund). 2013. *Energy subsidy reform: Lessons and implications*. Washington, DC: IMF.

Khanal, S., R. P. Anex, C. J. Anderson, D. E. Herzmann, and M. K. Jha. 2013. Implications of biofuel policy-driven land cover change for rainfall erosivity and soil erosion in the United States. *Global Change Biology Bioenergy* 5(6):713-722.

Koplow, D. 2009. State and federal subsidies to biofuels: Magnitude and options for redirection. *International Journal of Biotechnology* 11(1-2):92-126.

Landis, D. A., and B. P. Werling. 2010. Arthropods and biofuel production systems in North America. *Insect Science* 17(3):220-236.

Liaquat, A. M., M. A. Kalam, H. H. Masjuki, and M. H. Jayed. 2010. Potential emissions reduction in road transport sector using biofuel in developing countries. *Atmospheric Environment* (44)32:3869-3877.

MacKenzie, D., L. Bedsworth, and D. Friedman. 2005. *Fuel economy fraud: Closing the loopholes that increase U.S. oil dependence*. Cambridge, MA: Union of Concerned Scientists.

Malcolm, S., and M. Aillery. 2009. Growing crops for biofuels has spillover effects. *Amber Waves* 7(1):10-15.

Meehan, T. D., B. P. Werling, D. A. Landis, and C. Gratton. 2012. Pest-suppression potential of Midwestern landscapes under contrasting bioenergy scenarios. *PLoS ONE* 7(7):e41728.

The National Academies. 2012. *Disaster resilience: A national imperative*. Washington, DC: The National Academies Press. P. 1.

NRC (National Research Council). 2010. *Hidden costs of energy: Unpriced consequences of energy production and use*. Washington, DC: The National Academies Press.

NRC. 2011. *Renewable fuel standard: Potential economic and environmental effects of U.S. biofuel policy*. Washington, DC: The National Academies Press.

OECD (Organisation for Economic Co-operation and Development). 2012. *Inventory of estimated budgetary support and tax expenditures for fossil fuels 2013*. Paris, France: OECD Publishing.

Oladosu, G., and S. Msangi. 2013. Biofuel-food market interactions: A review of modeling approaches and findings. *Agriculture* 3(1):53-71.

ORNL and RFF (Oak Ridge National Laboratory and Resources for the Future). 1992-1998. *External costs and benefits of fuel cycles: Reports 1-8*. ORNL, Oak Ridge, TN, and RFF, Washington, DC: McGraw-Hill/Utility Data Institute.

Ottinger, R. L., D. R. Wooley, N. A. Robinson, D. R. Hodas, and S. E. Babb. 1990. *Environmental costs of electricity*. New York: Oceana Publications.

Palmer, K., A. Paul, and M. Woerman. 2012. *The variability of potential revenue from a tax on carbon*. Issue Brief 12-03. Washington, DC: Resources for the Future.

RFA (Renewable Fuels Association). 2014. *Statistics*. http://www.ethanolrfa.org/pages/statistics (accessed December 28, 2014).

Ridley, C. E., C. M. Clark, S. D. LeDuc, B. G. Bierwagen, B. B. Lin, A. Mehl, and D. A. Tobias. 2012. Biofuels: Network analysis of the literature reveals key environmental and economic unknowns. *Environmental Science and Technology* 46(3):1309-1315.

Robertson, B. A., P. J. Doran, L. R. Loomis, J. Robertson, and D. W. Schemske. 2011. Perennial biomass feedstocks enhance avian diversity. *Global Change Biology Bioenergy* 3(3):235-246.

Sarica, K., and W. E. Tyner. 2013. Alternative policy impacts on US GHG emissions and energy security: A hybrid modeling approach. *Energy Economics* 40:40-50.

Scavia, D., and Y. Liu. 2009. *2009 Gulf of Mexico hypoxia forecast and measurement.* http://sitemaker.umich.edu/scavia/files/2009_gulf_of_mexico_hypoxic_forecast_and_observation.pdf (accessed December 23, 2014).

Schiesari, L., and B. Grillitsch. 2011. Pesticides meet megadiversity in the expansion of biofuel crops. *Frontiers in Ecology and the Environment* 9(4):215-221.

Schnepf, R., and B. D. Yacobucci. 2013. *Renewable Fuel Standard (RFS): Overview and issues.* CRS Report for Congress. Washington, DC: Congressional Research Service.

Scovronick, N., and P. Wilkinson. 2014. Health impacts of liquid biofuel production and use: A review. *Global Environmental Change-Human and Policy Dimensions* 24:155-164.

Searchinger, T., R. Heimlich, R. A. Houghton, F. X. Dong, A. Elobeid, J. Fabiosa, S. Tokgoz, D. Hayes, and T. H. Yu. 2008. Use of US croplands for biofuels increases greenhouse gases through emissions from land-use change. *Science* 319(5867):1238-1240.

Smeets, E., A. Tabeau, S. van Berkum, J. Moorad, H. van Meil, and G. Woltjer. 2014. The impact of the rebound effect of the use of first generation biofuels in the EU on greenhouse gas emissions: A critical review. *Renewable & Sustainable Energy Reviews* 38:393-403.

Sprague, L. A., R. M. Hirsch, and B. T. Aulenbach. 2011. Nitrate in the Mississippi River and its tributaries, 1980 to 2008: Are we making progress? *Environmental Science and Technology* 45(17):7209-7216.

Stallings, C. C. 2009. *Distiller's grains for dairy cattle and potential environmental impact.* Virginia Cooperative Extension, Publication 404-135. http://pubs.ext.vt.edu/404/404-135/404-135.html (accessed December 23, 2014).

Taheripour, F., T. W. Hertel, W. E. Tyner, J. F. Beckman, and D. K. Birur. 2010. Biofuels and their by-products: Global economic and environmental implications. *Biomass & Bioenergy* 34(3):278-289.

Tyner, W. E. 2008. The U.S. ethanol and biofuels boom: Its origins, current status, and future prospects. *Bioscience* 58(7):646-653.

Tyner, W. E. 2013. Biofuels and food prices: Separating wheat from chaff. *Global Food Security* 2(2):126-130.

Wagstrom, K., and J. Hill. 2012. Air pollution impacts of biofuels. In *Socioeconomic and environmental impacts of biofuels: Evidence from developing nations*, edited by A. Gasparatos and P. Stromberg. New York: Cambridge University Press. Pp. 53-68.

Wise, T. A. 2012. *The cost to developing countries of U.S. corn ethanol expansion.* Working Paper No. 12-02. Medford, MA: Global Development and Environment Institute at Tufts University.

ANNEX 3: ATTAINING RECOMMENDED AMOUNTS OF FRUITS AND VEGETABLES IN THE AMERICAN DIET

Understanding the Consumption of Fruits and Vegetables Within the Context of a Complex System

The *Dietary Guidelines for Americans* encourage the U.S. population to consume more fruits and vegetables in order to maintain health and to prevent chronic disease. However, individual consumers make choices about what to eat within a broader context of what foods are available, affordable, and acceptable. This broader context is shaped by numerous actors and processes within the complex food system. Therefore, consideration of how the population could move toward increased consumption of fruits and vegetables is an ideal problem to be addressed with this framework.

The recommendation to consume more fruits and vegetables, although well intentioned, may not reach its goals if consideration is not given to the whole food supply chain and the associated environmental, social, and economic context in which consumers operate. This example explores the imbalance between dietary recommendations and consumption of fruits and vegetables and its implications for the food system, the environment, and society. An integrated assessment using the committee's framework can provide insights into points along the supply chain where interventions would be most efficacious.

The importance of fruit and vegetable intake to the prevention of chronic disease has been long established through a large body of literature and confirmed through a series of systematic reviews (USDA, 2014; WCRF/AICR, 2007). Consistent evidence suggests fruit and vegetable intakes by adults are inversely associated with risk of myocardial infarction and stroke, especially with intakes above five servings per day. Also, evidence indicates that consumption of many fruits and vegetables decreases the risk of several types of cancer. Although limited, further evidence suggests that fruit and vegetable consumption also protects against adiposity in children and adolescents. The health-promoting properties of fruits and vegetables could stem from their high nutrient density (e.g., the amount of nutrients relative to energy) compared to other foods; their being rich sources of fiber or phytochemicals, which may be beneficial; and even their effects on the gut flora.

Although fruits and vegetables may be protective for a range of chronic diseases, the consumption of raw products may increase risk for foodborne illness. Raw vegetables, fruits, and nuts were major sources of foodborne illness for the years 1998-2008, leading to nearly half of all cases and nearly a quarter of deaths with identified etiology of disease (Painter et al., 2013). Although the number of illnesses and deaths are small in comparison to the numbers associated with coronary heart disease, cancer, and other chronic disease, the sudden onset of foodborne illness can have an immediate impact on consumption patterns, especially following large outbreaks. For example, following a 2006 *E. coli* O157:H7 outbreak associated with fresh, ready-to-eat spinach grown in California, the Texas spinach industry lost at least 20 percent in sales for all types of spinach—fresh and processed (CNAS and TAMU, 2007).

For the past 30 years, the *Dietary Guidelines for Americans* (DGA) have encouraged the population to increase their intakes of fruits and vegetables (HHS and USDA, 2014). The guidelines are a statement of federal nutrition policy and form the standards against which all federal nutrition programs are gauged. Their guidance for increasing fruit and vegetable consumption have always been made within the context of concomitant recommendations regarding other aspects of the diet, notably increased whole grains and decreased added sugars, solid fats, and sodium, and, in more recent editions, food safety. The implication has been that fruits and vegetables should be used as substitutes for less nutrient-dense foods because simply adding fruits and vegetables to an already energy-rich diet would aggravate the problem of overweight and obesity. The point of the guidelines has always been that the overall composition of the diet is critical.

Identify the Problem

As described in the committee's framework, the first step of an assessment is to identify the problem. For this example, the problem is the imbalance between dietary recommendations and consumption of fruits and vegetables and its implications for the food system, the environment, and society.

Despite the continued federal guidance, fruit and vegetable intakes have remained well below recommendations over the past several decades (Krebs-Smith and Kantor, 2001; NCI, 2014). Recent estimates suggest that mean daily intakes for the whole population are slightly more than 1 cup of fruits and 1.5 cups of vegetables. As recommended intakes for the average 2,000 kcal diet are 2 cups and 2.5 cups, respectively, this suggests the average gap for each is approximately 1 cup per day. To conform to recommendations, the average person would need to nearly double fruit intake and increase vegetable intake by about 65 percent. Changes of this magnitude on individual consumption would reverberate throughout the entire food supply chain.

Define the Scope of the Problem

Once a problem has been identified, the next step in an assessment is to frame its scope. This is done by characterizing the boundaries, components, processes, actors, and linkages encompassed by the system under consideration. This is particularly important for this example because the issue of fruit and vegetable consumption sits squarely along the entire supply chain portion of the food system, from "farm to fork" (see Figure 7-A-2). The aggregate supply of available fruits and vegetables falls short of the total needed for the entire population to eat the recommended amount per day (Buzby et al., 2006); many processed foods entering retail distribution channels contain little if any fruits or vegetables; many places where foods are sold do not offer fruits or vegetables in any form; and food service outlets tend to offer relatively few. Consumers, for their part, often choose other foods over fruits and vegetables, for reasons of cost, convenience, or preference. Thus, the mismatch between recommendations and availability/consumption occurs across the entire food chain.

Like any complex system, the key aspects of the U.S. food system in relation to fruits and vegetables include numerous drivers, actors, processes, outcomes, stocks, and flows. Supply and demand are the major drivers, with diverse external forces, such as weather, agricultural and immigration policies, and labor also exerting influences. Farmers, farm workers, food manufacturers, retailers, restaurateurs and chefs, school food service directors,

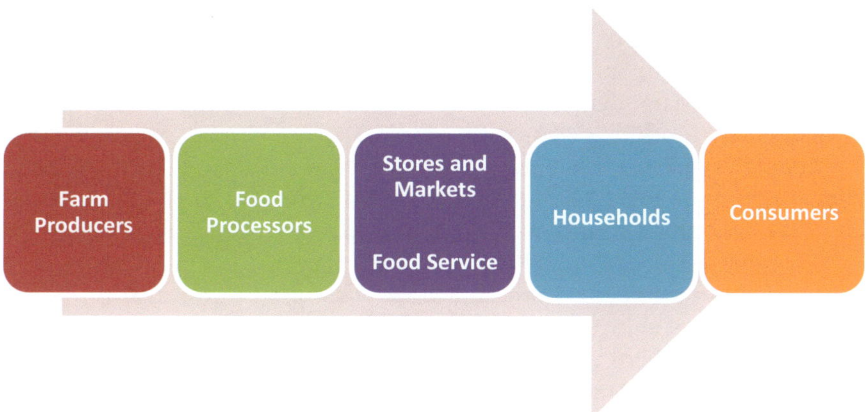

FIGURE 7-A-2 Fruits and vegetables supply chain and selected drivers.

and household food gatekeepers are all actors in this system, controlling the processes of planting, harvesting, transporting, processing, distribution, marketing, and preparation of fruits and vegetables. Figure 7-A-2 illustrates the main steps in the supply chain that can be influenced by various drivers.

Farm Level

Within the United States, fruit and vegetable production is a major business enterprise. Between 2000 and 2008, the sale of fruits and vegetables averaged about $35 billion annually (ERS, 2014a,b). Three-quarters of all fruit and vegetable production comes from irrigated land, which reflects a large capital investment and has implications for water ecology. Although less than 10 percent of all vegetable farms have sales exceeding $500,000, they account for about 90 percent of all vegetable sales. Most of the vegetable farms in this country are small, producing their yields on fewer than 15 acres.

Fruit and vegetable production comes from only 3 percent of U.S. cropland (UCS, 2013), but it accounts for about a third of all U.S. crop value (ERS, 2014a,b). Whether fruits and vegetables are destined for fresh markets or intended for future processing determines the varieties grown and the harvesting processes used. The Upper Midwest and some Pacific states are the largest producers of vegetables that go into processed foods, whereas Arizona, California, Florida, Georgia, and New York send more vegetables to markets as raw produce. California produces the largest share of fruit and vegetable crops among all of the states.

Market forces (supply and demand), productivity, and other external factors are key drivers in determining which crops are grown or imported. Oversupply at any point in time brings prices down, which decreases profitability. For this reason, the 2014 Farm Bill maintained a provision that prevents the planting of fruits and vegetables on acreage for which growers receive federal payments. Perishability of fruits and vegetables makes the timing of harvesting, distribution, and retail sales more important than for less perishable food products.

Regardless of the final use, fruit and vegetable production is labor intensive, and the produce industry in the United States pays higher wages than do many other countries (Calvin and Martin, 2010). This means the U.S. farming sector can attract the workers it needs. However, the work is seasonal and dependent on migrant labor. Changes in immigration policy could alter domestic production dramatically. As described below, for some crops, the cost of labor and land results in the movement of production out of the United States to other regions, especially for fruits and vegetables that are seasonal, frozen, canned, or dehydrated.

In addition to domestic output, international production is essential to the aggregate U.S. fruit and vegetable supply. Imports of fruits and vegetables have risen substantially in the past 25 years, leading to a growing trade deficit in this sector of the economy (Johnson, 2014). Whereas the value of imports approximately equaled that of exports in the early 1990s, a trade deficit for fruits and vegetables of more than $11 billion had developed by 2011, despite the fact that exports have continued to grow. A number of domestic and global market conditions have affected this situation, including differences among countries in production costs, tariffs, and import requirements, and the increased demand in the United States for off-season produce.

Food Processors Level

Product innovation can have a major influence on demand. The introduction of pre-packaged, pre-cut, and other value-added raw, ready-to-eat fruit and vegetable products has boosted consumption. Examples of this are small-cut carrots, broccoli florets, bagged salads, and sliced apples.

Contrary to popular belief, fruits and vegetables do not need to be consumed raw or prepared from "fresh" to be healthy. The term "fresh" is often used to describe any raw produce, whereas it implies a reference to the time since harvesting. Ironically, frozen and canned fruits and vegetables are often processed closer to the point of harvest and thus frequently have greater nutrient retention than do so-called fresh items purchased from a grocery store for later preparation in the home. Fresh fruit and vegetable use far exceeds that of canned and frozen forms in the United States.

Marketing

Between the farm and consumer levels of the food supply chain is the essential influence of marketing, including product development, promotion, placement, and pricing. Promotion is a critical factor, as the food industry spends $11 billion per year on advertising, and grocery stores earn more from companies paying for optimal locations within the store to display their products than they do from customers (IOM, 2006). An example of an industry effort to promote fruit and vegetable consumption is the "Let's Move Salad Bars to Schools" project, in which a coalition of private partners donates equipment required to display fresh salad components in a safe and hygienic manner to minimize food safety and regulatory compliance issues. To date, more than 2,600 schools have received donated salad bars for use in their school lunch program. However, the food and beverage industry also spent $149 million on marketing in schools in 2009, and advertising for sugar-sweetened beverages accounted for 90 percent of that (NPR, 2014). To the extent that industry efforts to promote less nutrient-dense foods and beverages are successful, consumers may be influenced to choose relatively fewer fruits and vegetables.

In addition to the marketing efforts conducted by individual food companies, the U.S. Department of Agriculture (USDA) coordinates federally legislated promotion programs for various commodities (AMS, 2014b). Known as "check-off" programs, they are requested, administered, and funded by the industries themselves. They are designed to increase domestic demand and increase foreign markets for the relevant commodities. However, only a small fraction of these funds are appropriated to the promotion of fruits and vegetables; most of the funds go to the promotion of meats and dairy (Wilde, 2014).

Food Markets

Most fruits and vegetables are consumed at home, having been purchased in grocery stores or other markets. Since 1980, the number of produce items available in the average grocery store has doubled, and the availability of convenience items such as short-cut carrots, pre-packaged salads, and supermarket salad bars has expanded (Krebs-Smith and Kantor, 2001). Consumers now have a wide choice of fruits such as grapes, stone fruit, and berries that previously were available only in summer months due to increases in off-season imports of fruits from the southern hemisphere. In addition, since 1994, the number of farmers' markets has increased severalfold in the United States to more than 8,000 in 2013 (AMS, 2014a).

Although supermarkets typically carry more than 400 produce items (Krebs-Smith and Kantor, 2001), it is important to note that, in many geographical areas, stores that sell food offer little, if any, fruits and vegetables. More than 40 percent of retail establishments in this country—including one in two hardware stores, and many auto repair shops, pharmacies, and furniture stores—sell food, and most of that is energy-dense and nutrient-deficient candy, snacks, and sugar-sweetened beverages (Cohen, 2014). This may be due to a number of factors, among them food safety concerns, regulatory requirements, profitability, turnover, ease of consumption, and other factors. These types of snacks are generally shelf-stable, single-serve items that have a low food safety risk profile.

When examined geographically, greater availability of such calorie-dense choices and restricted availability of fruits and vegetables seems to be of particular concern among lower-income and minority neighborhoods (Larson et al., 2009).

Fast-Food Outlets, Schools, and Other Food Service

Away-from-home food is a growing portion of all food ingested in this country. The overall number of restaurants has tripled in the past 40 years (Cohen, 2014), and if this trend continues, it could have a substantial impact on fruit and vegetable consumption because consumers are more likely to eat fruit and several healthful varieties of vegetables at home than away from home. Menu offerings from the country's top fast-food restaurant chains in 2010 were low in overall diet quality and particularly out of line with dietary recommendations for fruits and vegetables (Kirkpatrick et al., 2014).

Several recent efforts have been launched to improve the availability of fruits and vegetables in America's schools. USDA's Farm-to-School Initiative was designed to help farmers in all 50 states sell fresh fruits and vegetables directly to local schools participating in the National School Lunch Program (NSLP). The Healthy Hunger-Free Kids Act of 2010 led to more stringent school meal nutrition standards, which were instituted in the 2012-2013 school year and included increased quantities of fruits and vegetables. Through its food distribution programs, USDA purchases a variety of foods, including fruits and vegetables, to help supplement the diets of children participating in the NSLP and Child and Adult Care Food Program. A recent evaluation of the foods distributed through these programs revealed that the overall quality of the mix of foods was considerably healthier than typical U.S. diets, including a greater proportion of fruits and vegetables (Zimmerman et al., 2012).

The prominence of healthy food offerings at schools and other food service operations is important because of the power of "optimal defaults." This term refers to the provision of pre-selected, best interest options as the default, while still allowing free choice (Radnitz et al., 2013). It has long been known to be enormously influential in areas such as organ donation and retirement savings, and it has more recently been tried with success in schools by, for example, putting carrot sticks within easier reach than the French fries in the lunch line.

Consumers Level

Numerous economic, social, and behavioral factors affect consumers' fruit and vegetable choices, only some of which are under their control. Spending on foods for at-home consumption is out of line with dietary recommendations: The average U.S. household underspends on vegetables (except potatoes) and whole fruits as well as whole grains, low-fat dairy, nuts, poultry and fish; it overspends on refined grains, fruit juices, whole-fat dairy, red meats, beverages, sugar, and candies (Volpe and Okrent, 2012).

Prices of fruits and vegetables have risen faster than has the Consumer Price Index, but the latest data from USDA indicate that $2.50 was sufficient to meet an individual's daily recommendations for these foods in 2008.

Food prices are lower in suburban communities, where supermarkets are plentiful, and higher in central cities, where retail food stores tend to be smaller. Retail food prices are highest in the Northeast and West and lowest in the Midwest and South. The regional variation in food prices can be explained by differences in consumer demand, distribution, and operating costs, and the presence or absence of warehouse stores such as Costco and Walmart.

In addition to affordability, availability of fruits and vegetables where individuals live and work is an important factor that can affect decisions to consume healthful diets. Bodor et al. (2008) found that availability of vegetables within 100 m (300 ft) of a residence was positively associated with vegetable intake. Each additional meter of shelf space devoted to vegetables within the retail outlet was associated with one-third of a serving per day of increased intake.

Nutrition knowledge is positively associated with making healthful food choices, including more dark green and deep yellow vegetables and tomatoes and fewer fried potatoes (Guthrie, 2004). However, fewer than 2 percent of adults can correctly identify how much they should consume of all food groups. Use of food labels when buying food has declined since the mid-1990s. However, they do not indicate how many cups of fruits and vegetables are contained in a product.

Although the diets of nearly all Americans fare poorly when compared with recommendations (Krebs-Smith et al., 2010), some subgroups are doing worse than others. In an analysis comparing dietary intakes among income groups, adults in the high-income group generally had greater adherence to recommendations than did the low- and middle-income groups. Intakes of whole fruits, total vegetables, and some vegetable subgroups are especially concerning among lower-income groups and non-Hispanic blacks (Kirkpatrick et al., 2012). French fry consumption does not vary by income, but high-income consumers were found to eat more celery, garlic, cucumbers, peppers, mushrooms, and tomatoes than did other groups (Lin et al., 2004).

Obviously, the constraint of limited resources makes choosing a healthful diet that much less likely for low-income households. The minimal cost of a healthy diet, as estimated by USDA's Thrifty Food Plan (TFP), was $146 per week for a four-person household in 2013 (CNPP, 2014). According to the TFP, nearly half of that should go toward fruits and vegetables, but in 2008 they accounted for only 16 to 18 percent of at-home food dollars for both low- and high-income households. Furthermore, low-income households spend less on total food purchases than the cost of the TFP. Low-income women who work full time spend an average of only

46 minutes per day on meal preparation (Hamrick et al., 2011), and foods requiring minimal preparation are more expensive. Although a wide variety of fruits and vegetables are eligible for purchase through the Supplemental Nutrition Assistance Program (SNAP), the allowed products require preparation time, and ready-to-eat meals are not allowed for purchase. The extra time for preparation and perhaps unfamiliarity with preparation techniques can be a disincentive for increased fruit and vegetable consumption in this population. This illustrates the need to account for social considerations when attempting to change health outcomes.

Identify the Scenarios

To understand the effects of a new intervention, policy, or technology, an assessment compares the performance of the current system as described in the scope—the baseline—with one or more alternative scenarios that reflect the proposed change. For this example, an assessment team would compare the current supply and consumption of fruits and vegetables (baseline) with an alternative scenario in which supply and consumption are in accordance with recommendations. It implies a hypothetical change in the distribution of many commodities in the American diet, because fruits and vegetables would be expected to replace other foodstuffs that are currently consumed in excess. The step also would involve identifying what elements of the food system could affect that change, and what the ripple effects would be in health, environmental, and social spheres. There is some question whether a change of the magnitude required for intakes to match recommendations is realistic.

Conduct the Analysis

In this step of an assessment, data, metrics, and analysis tools are used to examine the likely health, environmental, social, and economic effects associated with the alternative scenario. Before beginning an analysis, it is always a good idea to determine what types of assessments have been done previously related to the problem or question.

Previous Analyses

Previous assessments have been relatively few in number but may be useful in providing data that could be used as inputs for future simulations or other complex analyses. These analyses focused on three key questions.

What changes might be necessary to alter the inducements and barriers to fruit and vegetable consumption throughout the food system? The perception that fruits and vegetables are expensive relative to other foods has raised the question of whether increasing incomes might overcome the potential barrier of price. Frazao et al. (2007) examined how individuals might change their spending on different categories of food if provided with additional income, and how this might vary across income levels. They used the Bureau of Labor Statistics' Consumer Expenditure Survey data on household food purchases and considered all forms of fruits and vegetables—fresh as well as canned, frozen, dried, and juice. Low-income households were found to spend 26 cents of every food dollar on food away from home; the remainder was spent on groceries, of which only 12 cents was spent on fruits and vegetables. As incomes rose, more money was spent on food in absolute terms, but the percentage of income spent on food declined. Furthermore, the greater spending on food with rising incomes was more likely to be on food away from home or non-staple foods, such as snack foods, sweets, fats and oils, and beverages. The authors concluded that additional income or untargeted food assistance was unlikely to improve fruit and vegetable consumption.

Another study examined the effect of targeted price incentives, which may have a different effect on consumer behavior than would increased income. The Healthy Incentives Pilot (HIP) was a relatively small-scale program (HIP, 2014) designed to determine whether point-of-sale incentives within SNAP would encourage the purchase of healthy foods. The treatment group received 30 cents back on their benefits card for every dollar spent on targeted fruits and vegetables, and their subsequent intakes of fruits and vegetables were compared to those of a control group. The treatment group consumed 25 percent more fruits and vegetables than did the control group, with more of the observed difference being due to vegetables (60 percent) than fruits (40 percent). Nearly all participants in the Healthy Incentives Pilot indicated they would like to continue in the program, and HIP households more frequently had fruits and vegetables available at home than did households in the control group.

The societal trend in consuming ever more food away from home also has been examined as a barrier to fruit and vegetable intakes. Todd et al. (2010) compared meals consumed away from home to those at home in terms of their influence on food group intakes among adults. They found that meals consumed away from home contained fewer servings of whole fruit and dark green and orange vegetables per 1,000 kcal, but that these effects varied by meal. The density of fruit in snacks eaten away from home was 9 percent less than those eaten at home, whereas breakfast, lunch, and dinner were 18, 22, and 16 percent less, respectively. Differences were more extreme for whole fruits. Differences in dark green and orange vegetables were greater at dinner (31 percent less) than at lunch (11 percent less).

What changes would be needed throughout the food supply chain in order for fruit and vegetable intakes of the U.S. population to conform to, or move in the direction of, guidance? The most recent assessment to have examined the divide between fruit and vegetable intakes and their recommendations was an examination of the 2007-2010 National Health and Nutrition Examination Survey (NHANES) (NCI, 2014) data, which reported on the distribution of intakes and the prevalence of intakes below the recommendation. That analysis indicated 25 percent of the population consumed less than half a cup of fruit per day, and 75 percent of the population had intakes below the minimum recommendation for their sex–age group. Considering vegetables, the usual intake at the 75th percentile for the entire population was two cups per day; 87 percent of the population had a usual intake below the minimum recommendation for their sex–age group, with percentages running even higher for adolescents and young adults. In short, nearly the entire U.S. population consumes a diet with fewer vegetables than recommended and a large majority underconsume fruits relative to recommendations.

A number of studies have examined the extent of change necessary for different levels of the food supply chain to realize concordance with fruit and vegetable recommendations. Kantor (1998) developed the Loss Adjusted Food Availability Data to examine the nation's aggregate supply of food in relation to dietary guidelines. In an early analysis of those data, Young and Kantor (1999) found that if Americans were to follow dietary recommendations, changes would be needed in the type and quantity of food produced and where and how it is produced. Furthermore, adjustments would be needed in "agricultural production, trade, non-food uses and prices" as well as the "crop acreage devoted to food and feed." Buzby et al. (2006) replicated that analysis in 2006 and reached similar conclusions. However, although these studies suggest that changes in production and trade of fruits and vegetables would be needed if the U.S. population were to follow dietary guidelines, they did not imply that such changes would be sufficient to induce the public to eat more fruits and vegetables. Understanding the impediments to eating more fruits and vegetables and determining how to overcome them would also be needed.

McNamara et al. (1999) took these analyses a step further by examining the gap between the current food supply and the estimated future demand for food commodities, based on a hypothetical population-wide adoption of the DGA and Census projections. The projected population growth over 20 years meant that supplies of commodities that people are advised to eat more of needed to increase dramatically. Substantial increases in supplies of fruit and most subgroups of vegetables were found to be needed to close the gap between then-current and future intakes. The magnitude of the gap between intakes and the projections suggested "the need for continued increases in agricultural productivity, higher resource use, and greater levels of international trade." Others have examined marketing and retail influences on the extent to which the food supply conforms to dietary guidelines, and they have concluded that lower prices for some commodities may be needed (Kinsey and Bowland, 1999).

What would be the expected environmental, social, and acute and chronic health effects of changes in fruit and vegetable consumption? In a landmark study, Doll and Peto (1981) estimated the number of avoidable cancer deaths in the United States if diets were to conform to dietary recommendations. The changes they considered included not just the addition of fruits and vegetables, but rather the substitution of fruits, vegetables, and whole grains for meat, refined grains, and sugars in the diet. Their estimate that about one-third of cancer deaths could be prevented with dietary changes was a revelation. Willett (1995) reexamined this issue and determined the original estimate was still appropriate, although he estimated that the confidence interval around the estimate could be narrowed. The World Cancer Research Fund and the American Institute for Cancer Research issued a comprehensive review of food, physical activity, and the prevention of cancer in 2007 (WCRF/AICR, 2007). Although that report did not provide an estimate of prevented cancers across all types, it found "probable" associations between many fruits and vegetables and the prevention of cancers of the mouth, pharynx, larynx, esophagus, and stomach.

Several studies have examined the environmental effects of widespread shifts away from a meat-centric diet toward a more plant-based diet. Peters et al. (2007) found that diets higher in meat generally increased land requirements, but this varied by the amount of fat in the diet, so that high-fat vegetarian diets had a greater environmental footprint than did lower-fat diets with a small amount of meat. Land-use requirements for different types of diets vary not only in quantity but in quality as well. Meat-centric diets rely on greater amounts of land that can be used for pasture or hay, whereas plant-based diets require relatively more land that is only suitable for cultivated crops. Individual food rankings regarding environmental impact can shift dramatically, depending on whether emissions generated as a result of production is measured per kilogram or per 1,000 calories (EWG, 2011; Haspel, 2014).

New Analyses

Each of these previous analyses has focused on relatively narrow sections of the food supply chain and thus provides only limited insights. A more holistic assessment would likely result in a more comprehensive understanding of the nature of the problem, the viability of various solutions, and the trade-offs to be expected if change could be enacted.

One type of analysis suggested from the committee's framework is agent-based modeling (ABM), which could be used to identify the inducements and barriers to fruit and vegetable consumption throughout the food system, and how consumption might respond to shifts. The individual-level focus of ABM and its ability to capture heterogeneity (e.g., in socioeconomic status [SES] or body mass index), spatial effects (e.g., food availability and advertising), and adaptation (e.g., formation of preferences or habits) would help to address important features of this question. An ABM might take as inputs starting distributions of consumption and SES, spatial configurations, and exposure conditions, and it might yield as outputs key metrics such as means and distributions of fruit and vegetable intakes across the population (and across subgroups).

Another type of analysis well suited for questions raised in this example is system dynamics modeling, which could be used to assess the magnitude and timing of changes that might be needed in order for fruit and vegetable intakes of the U.S. population to attain (or move in the direction of) guidelines. By capturing a broad set of factors in the system, along with dynamic processes like feedback and delay, a system dynamics model might provide system-level insights. Such a model might allow mapping of varying magnitudes of shifts in input assumptions (e.g., about production or advertising) into corresponding expected shifts in key outcome metrics like per-capita quantities of fruits and vegetables in the U.S. food supply.

A third type of an analysis—life cycle assessment—could be used to examine what the health, environmental, and social effects of such a change might be. The important feature of life cycle assessment is that it assesses impacts across the full spectrum of a product's life cycle. In the case of fruits and vegetables, and other foods that would replace them in the diet, the life cycle coincides with the food supply chain. Starting with the seeds and other farm inputs, and ending with consumption and waste, the life cycles of various food commodities are associated with numerous health, environmental, social, and economic effects. Some of these, such as improved health outcomes as a result of dietary changes, can take many years to be realized (and measured). Key effects expected to emerge in this case would depend on the extent of the increase in fruit and vegetable intakes and the concomitant changes, if any, in the intakes of other food commodities. Analyses of this type would probably look for changes in:

- The health of the population (nutritional status, chronic disease incidence); incidence of foodborne illnesses; and health of farm workers and food producers (potentially greater risk of injury or exposure to harmful chemicals).

- Environmental effects (unless dominant farming practices changed, there would be greater use of fertilizers, pesticides, and other chemicals to produce the fruits and vegetables).
- Social and economic effects (fruit and vegetable production requires a supply of seasonal workers, so employment would be affected, and immigration policies could dramatically affect availability of workers). If fruits and vegetables replace other calories in the diet, sales of other foods would go down, which may have economic effects on other commodity markets. Also, there may be synergistic effects among the areas above.

REFERENCES

AMS (Agriculture Marketing Service). 2014a. *National count of farmers market directory listing graph: 1994-2013.* http://www.ams.usda.gov/AMSv1.0/ams.fetchTemplateData.do?template=TemplateS&leftNav=WholesaleandFarmersMarkets&page=WFMFarmersMarketGrowth&description=Farmers%20Market%20Growth (accessed March 21, 2014).

AMS. 2014b. *Research and promotion programs.* http://www.ams.usda.gov/AMSv1.0/lsmarketingprograms (accessed March 21, 2014).

Bodor, J. N., D. Rose, T. A. Farley, C. Swalm, and S. K. Scott. 2008. Neighbourhood fruit and vegetable availability and consumption: the role of small food stores in an urban environment. *Public Health Nutrition* 11(4):413-420.

Buzby, J. C., H. F. Wells, and G. Vocke. 2006. *Possible implications for U.S. agriculture from adoption of select dietary guidelines.* Agricultural Economic Report No. 31. Washington, DC: U.S. Department of Agriculture, Economic Research Service.

Calvin, L., and P. Martin. 2010. Labor-intensive US fruit and vegetable industry competes in a global market. *Amber Waves.* Washington, DC: U.S. Department of Agriculture, Economic Research Service.

CNAS and TAMU (Center for North American Studies and Texas A&M University). 2007. An initial assessment of the economic impacts of E. coli on the Texas spinach industry. *CNAS Issue Brief.* http://cnas.tamu.edu/Spinach%20E%20Coli%20Impacts%20Final.pdf (accessed December 30, 2014).

CNPP (Center for Nutrition Policy and Promotion). 2014. *USDA food plans: Cost of food report for December 2013.* http://www.cnpp.usda.gov/USDAFoodPlansCostofFood/reports (accessed December 30, 2014).

Cohen, D. A. 2014. *A big fat crisis: The hidden forces behind the obesity epidemic—and how we can end it.* New York: Nation Books.

Doll, R., and R. Peto. 1981. The causes of cancer: Quantitative estimates of avoidable risks of cancer in the United States today. *Journal of the National Cancer Institute* 66(6):1191-1308.

ERS (Economic Research Service). 2014a. *Fruits and tree nuts: Overview.* http://www.ers.usda.gov/topics/crops/fruit-tree-nuts.aspx (accessed March 21, 2014).

ERS. 2014b. *Vegetables and pulses: Overview.* http://www.ers.usda.gov/topics/crops/vegetables-pulses.aspx (accessed March 21, 2014).

EWG (Environmental Working Group). 2011. *Meat eater's guide to climate change and health.* http://www.ewg.org/meateatersguide/ (accessed December 30, 2014).

Frazao, E., M. Andrews, D. Smallwood, and M. Prell. 2007. *Can food stamps do more to improve food choices? An economic perspective—food spending patterns of low-income households: Will increasing purchasing power result in healthier food choices?* Economic Information Bulletin No. EIB-29-4. Washington, DC: U.S. Department of Agriculture, Economic Research Service.

Guthrie, J. 2004. *Understanding fruit and vegetable choices: Economic and behavioral influences.* Agriculture Information Bulletin No. 792-1. Washington, DC: U.S. Department of Agriculture, Economic Research Service.

Hamrick, K. S., M. Andrews, J. Guthrie, D. Hopkins, and K. McClelland. 2011. *How much time do Americans spend on food?* Washington, DC: U.S. Department of Agriculture, Economic Research Service.

Haspel, T. 2014. Vegetarian or omnivore: The environmental implications of diet. *The Washington Post,* March 10. http://www.washingtonpost.com/lifestyle/food/vegetarian-or-omnivore-the-environmental-implications-of-diet/2014/03/10/648fdbe8-a495-11e3-a5fa-55f0c77bf39c_story.html (accessed December 30, 2014).

HHS and USDA (U.S. Department of Health and Human Services and U.S. Department of Agriculture). 2014. *Dietary guidelines for Americans. Previous guidelines and reports.* http://www.health.gov/dietaryguidelines/pubs.asp (accessed November 21, 2014).

HIP (Healthy Incentives Pilot). 2014. Healthy Incentives Pilot. http://www.fns.usda.gov/hip/healthy-incentives-pilot (accessed December 30, 2014).

IOM (Institute of Medicine). 2006. *Food marketing to children and youth: Threat or opportunity?* Washington, DC: The National Academies Press.

Johnson, R. 2014. *The U.S. trade situation for fruit and vegetable products.* Congressional Research Service Report. http://www.fas.org/sgp/crs/misc/RL34468.pdf (accessed December 30, 2014).

Kantor, L. S. 1998. *A dietary assessment of the U.S. food supply: Comparing per capita food consumption with Food Guide Pyramid serving recommendations.* Washington, DC: U.S. Department of Agriculture, Economic Research Service.

Kinsey, J., and B. Bowland. 1999. How can the US food system deliver food products consistent with the Dietary Guidelines? Food marketing and retailing: An economist's view. *Food Policy* 24(2-3):237-253.

Kirkpatrick, S. I., K. W. Dodd, J. Reedy, and S. M. Krebs-Smith. 2012. Income and race/ethnicity are associated with adherence to food-based dietary guidance among US adults and children. *Journal of the Academy of Nutrition and Dietetics* 112(5):624-635.

Kirkpatrick, S. I., J. Reedy, L. L. Kahle, J. L. Harris, P. Ohri-Vachaspati, and S. M. Krebs-Smith. 2014. Fast-food menu offerings vary in dietary quality, but are consistently poor. *Public Health Nutrition* 17(4):924-931.

Krebs-Smith, S. M., and L. S. Kantor. 2001. Choose a variety of fruits and vegetables daily: Understanding the complexities. *Journal of Nutrition* 131(2S-1):487S-501S.

Krebs-Smith, S. M., P. M. Guenther, A. F. Subar, S. I. Kirkpatrick, and K. W. Dodd. 2010. Americans do not meet federal dietary recommendations. *Journal of Nutrition* 140(10):1832-1838.

Larson, N. I., M. T. Story, and M. C. Nelson. 2009. Neighborhood environments: Disparities in access to healthy foods in the U.S. *American Journal of Preventive Medicine* 36(1):74-81.

Lin, B.-H., J. Reed, and G. Lucier. 2004. *U.S. fruit and vegetable consumption: Who, what, where, and how much.* Agriculture Information Bulletin No. 792-2. Washington, DC: U.S. Department of Agriculture, Economic Research Service.

McNamara, P. E., C. K. Ranney, L. S. Kantor, and S. M. Krebs-Smith. 1999. The gap between food intakes and the Pyramid recommendations: Measurement and food system ramifications. *Food Policy* 24(2-3):117-133.

NCI (National Cancer Institute). 2014. *Usual dietary intakes: Food intakes, US population, 2007-10.* http://appliedresearch.cancer.gov/diet/usualintakes/pop (accessed December 30, 2014).

NPR (National Public Radio). 2014. *New rules would curb how kids are sold junk food at school.* http://www.npr.org/blogs/thesalt/2014/02/25/282507974/new-rules-would-curb-how-kids-are-sold-junk-food-at-school (accessed May 9, 2014).

Painter, J. A., R. M. Hoekstra, T. Ayers, R. V. Tauxe, C. R. Braden, F. J. Angulo, and P. M. Griffin. 2013. Attribution of foodborne illnesses, hospitalizations, and deaths to food commodities by using outbreak data, United States, 1998-2008. *Emerging Infectious Diseases* 19(3):407-415.

Peters, C. J., J. L. Wilkins, and G. W. Fick. 2007. Testing a complete-diet model for estimating the land resource requirements of food consumption and agricultural carrying capacity: The New York state example. *Renewable Agriculture and Food Systems* 22(2):145-153.

Radnitz, C., K. L. Loeb, J. DiMatteo, K. L. Keller, N. Zucker, and M. B. Schwartz. 2013. Optimal defaults in the prevention of pediatric obesity: From platform to practice. *Journal of Food and Nutritional Disorders* 2(5):1-8.

Todd, J. E., L. Mancino, and B.-H. Lin. 2010. *The impact of food away from home on adult diet quality.* Washington, DC: U.S. Department of Agriculture, Economic Research Service.

UCS (Union of Concerned Scientists). 2013. *The healthy farmland diet.* Cambridge, MA: Union of Concerned Scientists. http://www.ucsusa.org/food_and_agriculture/solutions/expand-healthy-food-access/the-healthy-farmland-diet.html (accessed December 30, 2014).

USDA (U.S. Department of Agriculture). 2014. *Nutrition Evidence Library.* http://www.nel.gov (accessed March 21, 2014).

Volpe, R., and A. Okrent. 2012. *Assessing the healthfulness of consumers' grocery purchases.* No. EIB-102. Washington, DC: U.S. Department of Agriculture, Economic Research Service.

WCRF and AICR (World Cancer Research Fund and American Institute for Cancer Research). 2007. *Food, nutrition, physical activity, and the prevention of cancer: A global perspective.* Washington, DC: AICR.

Wilde, P. 2014. *U.S. Food Policy Blog.* http://usfoodpolicy.blogspot.com/2014/02/usda-reports-on-pizza-consumption-and.html (accessed October 28, 2014).

Willett, W. C. 1995. Diet, nutrition, and avoidable cancer. *Environmental Health Perspectives* 103(Suppl 8):165-170.

Young, C. E., and L. S. Kantor. 1999. *Moving toward the food guide pyramid: Implications for US agriculture.* Agricultural Economic Report No. 779. Washington, DC: U.S. Department of Agriculture, Economic Research Service.

Zimmerman, T. P., S. Dixit-Joshi, B. Sun, D. Douglass, J. Hu, F. Glantz, and E. Eaker. 2012. *Nutrient and MyPyramid analysis of USDA foods in the NSLP, CACFP, CSFP, TEFAP, and FDPIR.* Alexandria, VA: Food and Nutrition Service, Office of Research and Analysis.

ANNEX 4: NITROGEN IN AGROECOSYSTEMS

Nitrogen Dynamics and Management in Agroecosystems

Nitrogen (N) is essential for agricultural productivity, but in its more reactive forms, it can pose significant threats to humans and the environment. Quantifying the abundance of nitrogen in different chemical forms and understanding its pathways through soil, air, water, plants, and animals under different management scenarios are essential to minimize threats to human health and environmental quality. Nonetheless, studying multiple forms of nitrogen in the environment presents many challenges and calls for the use of a systems analysis framework.

This example illustrates several principles contained within the committee's framework. First, it shows that the use and management of nitrogen in agroecosystems have effects that can be manifest in health, environmental, social, and economic domains. Second, it indicates that N-related farming practices can affect numerous different populations and components of managed and natural ecosystems, including members of the general public, farmers and farm workers, fish and shellfish, and wildland plant communities. Third, it makes clear that these effects can be manifest in geographical areas both near and far from sites of agricultural production and N use. Fourth, it illustrates how various drivers, especially government policies, can have significant impacts on N-related farming practices and subsequent health, environmental, social, and economic effects. Finally, the example illustrates the value of both empirical measurements and modeling analyses in assessing contrasting systems for using and managing N for food production. Although the example is presented from the perspective of the U.S. food system, the conceptual model included within it could apply to other systems in other countries as well.

The example points to research gaps. Although multiple analyses of N dynamics in agroecosystems have been conducted already, most have focused on N fluxes and transformations in a limited set of farm production systems. Recognizing that such data are difficult to obtain and costly, data collection over the long term is nonetheless critical to understanding N dynamics as they are affected by year-to-year variations in weather and by heterogeneity in soil conditions. Data collection is also needed on health, environmental, social, and economic effects and costs of N emissions over time and at regional and national scales.

Nitrogen (N) is the most limiting element for plant growth in many ecosystems, despite being the most plentiful element in the earth's atmosphere. In its most abundant form, gaseous dinitrogen (N_2), N is unavailable to most organisms. However, following transformation to other forms, especially nitrate (NO_3^-) and ammonium (NH_4^+), N becomes highly reactive in the biosphere and can be highly mobile in water and air.

Nitrogen is a key component of proteins in both plants and animals, including the enzymes responsible for photosynthesis and other critical biological reactions, and the muscles used for movement and other body functions. Consequently, most crops, especially cereals, require sizable supplies of N to yield well, and livestock and poultry need a diet rich in N to produce large quantities of milk, eggs, and meat.

Agriculture now uses more reactive N than does any other economic sector in the United States (EPA, 2011). However, it is also the sector responsible for the greatest losses of reactive N to the environment (EPA, 2011), where N has multiple unintended consequences, including threats to human health, degradation of air and water quality, and stress on terrestrial and aquatic organisms (Ribaudo et al., 2011; UNEP, 2007; Vitousek et al., 2009). Because reactive N strongly affects crop production and farm profitability, as well as human health and environmental quality, managing N efficiently and in an environmentally harmonious manner is a critically important component of agricultural sustainability (Foley et al., 2011; Robertson and Vitousek, 2009).

Identify the Problem

Assessments are typically triggered by a broad problem or concern. The first step in an assessment, identifying the problem, is often based on consultation with stakeholders and reviews of relevant literature. The problem identified for this assessment is the multiple unintended consequences of certain N management applications in agriculture. Its purpose is to compare management practices for N application in terms of the stocks and flows of nitrogen. The ideal management practice would result in high crop yields while minimizing N emissions that are harmful for the environment and, indirectly, human health and economic development.

Define the Scope of the Problem

Once a problem has been identified, the next step in an assessment is to frame its scope. This is done by characterizing the boundaries, components, processes, actors, and linkages encompassed by the system under consideration. For this example, we briefly describe the boundaries of the N system

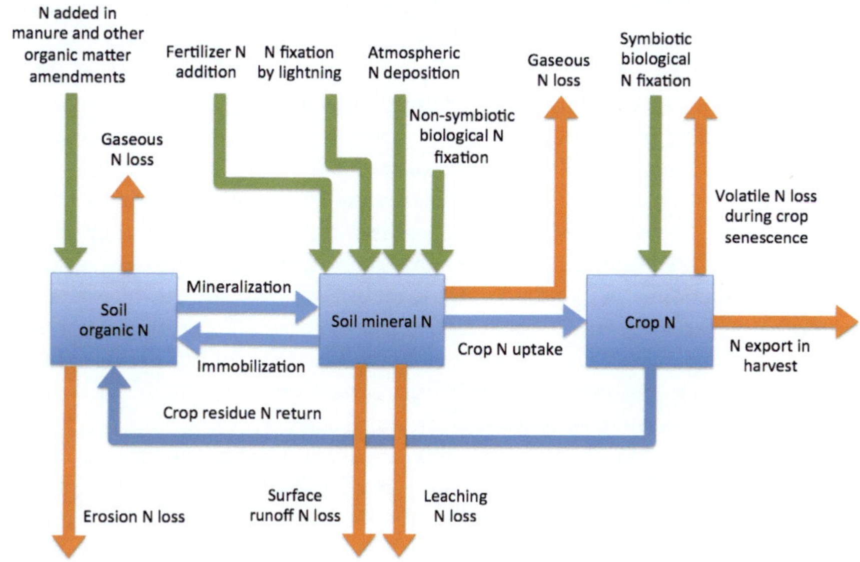

FIGURE 7-A-3 Major N stocks (boxes) and flows (arrows) for a cropping system. Nitrogen stocks and flows are not drawn to scale.

in terms of characterizing the N pathways under different environmental conditions and farming practices. We also describe what we know about the potential health, environmental, social, and economic effects over time and space. In addition, this step identifies various policies as drivers of the system.

Nitrogen Dynamics in Agroecosystems

Nitrogen can exist in multiple forms whose concentrations and movements are strongly influenced by environmental conditions and farming practices. Consequently, understanding the fate of N in agroecosystems is challenging. Models developed from the study of dynamic systems constitute one set of tools for assessing different options for configuring agroecosystems for improved N management. A simple model depicting relevant stocks and flows of N in agroecosystems used for crop production is shown in Figure 7-A-3.

Mineral N fertilizers produced through the Haber-Bosch process constitute the single greatest source of reactive N introduced into the United States, with about 11 teragrams (Tg[1]) of fertilizer N being used in U.S.

[1] A teragram is the equivalent of 1 billion kilograms.

agriculture each year (EPA, 2011). Mineral forms of N fertilizer are energetically expensive to synthesize (57 MJ fossil energy/kg N) and sensitive to increases in the price of natural gas used in their production (ERS, 2008; Shapouri et al., 2010). Thus, the fact that typically only 40 to 60 percent of applied N fertilizer is absorbed by crop plants (Dinnes et al., 2002; Drinkwater and Snapp, 2007; Robertson and Vitousek, 2009) implies large agronomic, economic, and energetic inefficiencies, as well as a large potential for excess N to move downstream and downwind from crop fields. The exact fate of N fertilizer is heavily dependent on farm management decisions influencing N cycle processes, including crop selection, irrigation management, and the rate, formulation, placement, and timing of fertilizer applications. The fate of fertilizer N also can be highly dependent on weather conditions, especially precipitation patterns.

In addition to the application of mineral fertilizers, N may enter crop fields by several other pathways. Biological fixation of atmospheric N_2 by microbes associated with the roots of leguminous crops like soybean and alfalfa (symbiotic fixation) adds about 8 Tg N per year to U.S. agroecosystems (EPA, 2011). About 6.8 Tg of N is present in manure produced each year in the United States, but of that quantity, only 0.5 to 1.3 Tg N is applied to cropland and 3.7 Tg N is deposited on pastures and rangelands (EPA, 2011; MacDonald et al., 2009), indicating that a substantial proportion of manure N is not recycled effectively. Moreover, manure application rates vary greatly among fields, with most fields receiving none and some receiving high rates (MacDonald et al., 2009). Consequently, excessive concentrations of nutrients, especially phosphorus and N, can occur in the vicinity of concentrated animal feeding operations and can lead to water pollution (Jackson et al., 2000). Additional pathways by which reactive N is introduced into agroecosystems include lightning, fixation by non-symbiotic microbes living in soil, and atmospheric deposition. The former two processes are responsible for adding only small quantities of N; the latter input can be locally important (Galloway et al., 2004).

Large amounts of N are present within soil organic matter, accruing from residues of plants and soil microbes and applications of manure and other organic matter amendments. Nitrogen comprises about 5 percent of soil organic matter by weight, and for soils with appreciable amounts of organic matter, such as many of those found in the U.S. Corn Belt, the surface 30 cm contains thousands of kilograms of N, most of which is contained in organic forms. Decomposition of soil organic matter by microbes transforms organic forms of N ($R\text{-}NH_2$) into mineral forms (ammonium [NH_4] and nitrate [NO_3]) that are available to plants but also are subject to loss through leaching and runoff as water moves through and over the soil, and through denitrification as microbes transform nitrate to nitrogen oxide (N_2O), N_2, and other N gases. Mineral forms of N in the soil also can be consumed by microbes and immobilized in organic forms. The processes involved in mineralization and immobilization transformations are dependent on temperature and moisture conditions and the relative amounts of carbon, nitrogen, and oxygen present in decomposing materials and the associated soil, all of which can be quite variable in space and over time. Mineralization and immobilization processes, as mentioned previously, also are influenced by farm management decisions.

Losses of N through leaching, runoff, and denitrification are critical components of agroecosystem N dynamics, farm profitability, and environmental quality (EPA, 2011; Robertson and Vitousek, 2009). Nitrogen also can be lost from agroecosystems as gaseous ammonia emitted from fertilizer and manure applied to the soil, or from senescing crops (EPA, 2011; Smil, 1999). Erosion of topsoil and the organic forms of N it contains constitutes another pathway for N loss from agroecosystems (Smil, 1999). In situations where large amounts of crop residue are harvested from fields, soil organic matter stocks may become depleted and the lack of protective soil cover may result in increased amounts of N lost through erosion and runoff (Blanco-Canqui, 2010). Overall, the magnitudes of various N losses from agroecosystems are highly variable in space and time, and they are strongly influenced by weather conditions and management practices.

Human Health and Environmental Concerns

Reactive N released from agroecosystems is responsible for a number of adverse public health and environmental effects. Four of the most salient effects for the United States are noted here.

Drinking water contamination Nitrate coming from farmland is an important contaminant of drinking water in many agricultural regions (EPA, 2011). It constitutes a potential health threat due to its ability to (1) induce methemoglobinemia, a condition in which the oxygen-carrying capacity of blood is inhibited; (2) promote endogenous formation of *N*-nitroso compounds, which are carcinogens and teratogens; and (3) inhibit iodine uptake, thereby inducing hypertrophic changes in the thyroid (Ward, 2009). These health concerns are not restricted to members of the farm population. Nitrate contamination of surface water is common in the Corn Belt and is a recurrent challenge to cities such as Des Moines, Iowa, which draws drinking water from the Raccoon and Des Moines Rivers, both of which drain intensively farmed areas. After repeatedly violating the U.S. Environmental Protection Agency's (EPA's) drinking water standard of 10 mg L^{-1} for nitrate-nitrogen, and challenged by increasing levels of nitrate in its source water, the Des Moines Water Works constructed the largest ion exchange nitrate removal facility in the world in 1991 (Hatfield et al.,

2009). The need for this facility, which provides service to 500,000 people, has not abated, as record high levels of nitrate were encountered in Des Moines' drinking water sources in 2013. Nitrate also poses a significant threat to groundwater used for drinking water. A recent report focusing on the Tulare Lake Basin and Salinas Valley of California, which together contain 40 percent of the state's irrigated cropland and more than 50 percent of its dairy cattle, found that nitrate poses a significant threat to the health of rural communities dependent on well water, with nearly 1 in 10 people in the two regions now at risk (Harter et al., 2012). The report identified agricultural fertilizers and animal wastes as the largest sources of nitrate in groundwater in the areas investigated; it also noted that 40 out of the 51 community public water systems in the study area that had excessive nitrate levels are in "severely disadvantaged communities" with high poverty rates. These populations are especially susceptible to nitrate pollution because they generally cannot afford drinking water treatment or capital-intensive alternative water supplies.

Eutrophication and hypoxia Reactive N in water draining from agricultural regions can be responsible for eutrophication of freshwater bodies and hypoxia in coastal waters (Galloway et al., 2003). High levels of N in water stimulate harmful algal blooms, leading to suppression of desired aquatic vegetation, and when the algae die, their subsequent decomposition by bacteria leads to large reductions in dissolved oxygen concentrations, with concomitant reductions in populations of shellfish, game fish, and commercial fish.

Eutrophication and hypoxia effects are often spatially separated from their causes. For example, an estimated 71 percent of the N entering the northern Gulf of Mexico, the largest hypoxic zone in the United States and the second largest hypoxic zone worldwide, comes from croplands, rangelands, and pastures upstream in the Mississippi River Basin, with 17 percent of the total N load coming from Illinois, 11 percent from Iowa, and 10 percent from Indiana (Alexander et al., 2008). Thus, because of the mobility of reactive N, agricultural practices and land uses in one region can affect water quality, recreational activities, and economic sectors like fisheries hundreds of miles downstream.

Greenhouse gas loading Agricultural practices, principally fertilizer use, are responsible for about 74 percent of U.S. emissions of nitrous oxide (N_2O), a greenhouse gas with a global warming potential 300-fold greater than that of carbon dioxide (EPA, 2013). Although the agricultural sector is responsible for only 6.3 percent of total U.S. greenhouse gas emissions (EPA, 2013), it is notable that agricultural emissions can offset efforts to use agricultural systems to mitigate climate change by sequestering carbon dioxide or providing alternative energy sources (Robertson and Vitousek, 2009). Nitrous oxide emissions from agriculture also are notable as illustrations of how practices taking place locally on farmlands can have global-scale effects.

Ecological and human health effects of ammonia and other NH_x-N emissions In 2002, the United States emitted 3.1 Tg of N into the atmosphere as ammonia and other NH_x-N compounds, with agricultural practices, principally manure and fertilizer management, estimated to be responsible for 84 percent of that total (EPA, 2011). Most of these emissions are deposited within 1,000 km downwind as ammonia or ammonium in rainwater and aerosols (Robertson and Vitousek, 2009). Ammonia emissions can lead to the formation of fine inorganic particulate matter ($PM_{2.5}$) as ammonium-sulfate-nitrate salts, which are a factor for premature human mortality (Paulot and Jacob, 2014).

Deposition of reactive N from the atmosphere can acidify soils and waters and alter plant and soil community composition in grasslands and forests, leading to reductions in overall biological diversity and increases in the abundance of certain weedy species (EPA, 2011; Robertson and Vitousek, 2009). Like the movement of reactive N in water from agricultural regions to coastal ecosystems, the aerial movement and deposition of NH_x-N compounds illustrates that agriculture's impact on the environment can extend into other ecosystems that may be located considerable distances from farmlands.

Using models of ammonia sources and transport and $PM_{2.5}$ formation and deposition, Paulot and Jacob (2014) calculated the quantities of atmospheric ammonia and $PM_{2.5}$ that are related to U.S. food exports and the associated impacts of these pollutants on human health. They concluded that over the study period of 2000 to 2009, 5,100 people died annually due to these emissions, incurring a cost of $36 billion. This value greatly exceeded the net value of the exported food ($23.5 billion per year). The investigators noted that these human health and economic costs indicated "extensive negative externalities," and that taking into account other environmental impacts of agriculture, such as eutrophication, loss of biodiversity, and greenhouse gas emissions, would further diminish the value of agricultural production and exports.

Policy and Educational Considerations

Environmental quality and human health concerns related to the use of N for crop production have important policy dimensions. In an analysis of 29 watersheds covering 28 percent of the United States, Broussard et al. (2012) noted that increases in federal farm program payments were significantly correlated with greater dominance of cropland by corn and soybean, more expansive fertilizer applications, and higher riverine nitrate concentrations. They suggested that federal farm policies, expressed through farm payments, are a potent policy instrument that affects land-use decisions, cropping patterns, and water quality. Based on focus group interviews with farmers and residents of the Wells Creek and Chippewa River watersheds in Minnesota, Boody et al. (2005) noted that recent federal programs have encouraged the production of a narrow set of commodity crops while discouraging diversified agriculture and conservation efforts that better protect environmental quality. Similarly, Nassauer (2010, p. 190) observed that "for more than 50 years, production subsidies have vastly exceeded conservation spending—by almost ten times today—and this ratio has been clearly understood by farmers making production decisions." Consequently, fewer opportunities exist for reducing N emissions to air and water from arable croplands through the increased use of conservation buffer strips and grasslands, reconstructed wetlands, and diversified cropping systems that include hay and other non-commodity crops.

Federal energy policies that have promoted ethanol production from corn grain have been linked to reactive N emissions. Donner and Kucharik (2008) used process-based models to simulate hydrological and nutrient fluxes in the Mississippi River Basin under different corn production scenarios. They found that the increase in corn cultivation required to meet the federal goal of producing 15 to 36 billion gallons of renewable fuels by the year 2022 would increase average annual discharge of dissolved inorganic N into the Gulf of Mexico by 10 to 34 percent.

A recent report from the EPA-specified federal policy options (EPA, 2011) for reducing emissions of reactive N from U.S. agroecosystems to better protect environmental quality and human health. Existing government policies and programs for reactive-N reduction included the Conservation Reserve Program, the Wetland Reserve Program, and the Environmental Quality Incentives Program. Market-based instruments for pollution control identified by the report included tradable water quality credits, auction-based contracting, individual transferable quotas, risk indemnification to protect farmers adopting new practices from uncertainty, and conservation easements. Biophysical and technical approaches identified by the report included decreasing the amount of N fertilizer needed through changes in human diet (principally a reduction in animal protein consumption); removing croplands susceptible to reactive N loss from crop production; increasing fertilizer use efficiency through changes in crop management practices and improved fertilizer technology; engineering and restoring wetlands to decrease nitrate loading of aquatic systems; and developing new technologies to minimize ammonia emissions from manure.

At the other end of the spectrum from federal policies that influence

N use and reactive N emissions are local and statewide efforts to change practices through education. Successful implementation of management practices, such as improved irrigation strategies, diversified crop rotations, conservation buffer strips, and improved crop N use efficiency, requires a focus on policy incentives and research as well as substantial investments in education for end-users. This can be done through established networks of science and communication and by engaging a broad spectrum of the general public and members of the agricultural community through the development of local and regional watershed groups (Dzurella et al., 2012; Morton and Brown, 2011; MPCA, 2014).

Identify the Scenarios

To understand the effects of a new intervention, policy, or technology, an assessment compares the performance of the current system as described in the scope—the baseline—with one or more alternative scenarios that reflect the proposed change. For this example, an assessment team would identify the alternative systems for N management. We illustrate this step through a literature review about prior comparisons under different circumstances.

The conceptual model shown in Figure 7-A-3 shows stocks and flows of N for a crop-soil system and illustrates that improving crop N uptake, promoting recycling within the system, and regulating flows out of the system affect N use efficiency by crops and N emissions to water and air.

Use of this conceptual model fosters comparisons of alternative configurations of farming systems and promotes the use of multiple criteria when evaluating the performance of different systems. For example, in a field experiment conducted in Michigan, McSwiney and Robertson (2005) found that corn yield increased with additions of mineral N fertilizer up to a rate of about 100 kg N ha^{-1} ($hectares^{-1}$), but that additional fertilizer failed to increase yield. In contrast, emissions of the greenhouse gas N_2O from the soil were low at fertilizer rates up to 100 kg N ha^{-1}, but they more than doubled as fertilizer rates exceeded that threshold. Nonlinear, exponentially increasing rates of nitrogen oxide emissions in response to increases in N fertilizer rates also were observed by Hoben et al. (2011) on five commercially farmed fields used for corn production in Michigan. At the two N fertilizer rates above those recommended for maximum economic return (135 kg N ha^{-1}), average nitrogen oxide fluxes were 43 and 115 percent higher than were fluxes at the recommended rate. Other studies have found that nitrate leaching increases with increasing rates of N fertilization (Drinkwater and Snapp, 2007). Thus, in terms of the model shown in Figure 7-A-3, carefully managing the rate of fertilizer N addition to meet but not exceed crop demand could optimize the amount of soil mineral N and crop N uptake, while minimizing N loss to the atmosphere through denitrification and N loss to water through leaching and runoff.

Crops differ in their effects on nitrate emissions to ground and surface waters, due to crop-specific rates of N fertilizer application, biological N fixation, N uptake, and N return in residue (Robertson and Vitousek, 2009). In the Mississippi River Basin, nitrate-N concentrations in streams and rivers are directly proportional to the amount of land within watersheds planted with corn and soybean (Broussard and Turner, 2009; Schilling and Libra, 2000), largely because those crops are small in size or not actively growing during periods of the year when substantial quantities of dissolved N are moving from fields in runoff and leachate (Hatfield et al., 2009; Randall et al., 1997). Consequently, as noted previously, nitrate contamination of surface and groundwaters within the Corn Belt that supply drinking water is a major concern, as is the flow of nitrate-laden river water into the Gulf of Mexico, where it contributes to hypoxia.

In contrast to corn and soybeans, which are relatively ineffective at preventing N emissions to water, small grains, such as oat, and perennial grasses and legumes used for forage production are more effective in preventing N from entering drainage and surface waters, due to their greater use of water-carrying dissolved N during spring and autumn and, in the case of forage crops, a longer period of growth and N uptake throughout the year (Hatfield et al., 2009; Randall et al., 1997). Cover crops, which take up N during periods of the year when cash and feed crops like corn and soybean are not present in fields, can strongly reduce N losses to water by reducing soil mineral N stocks (Kaspar et al., 2007; Syswerda et al., 2012; Tonitto et al., 2006). Diversified crop rotation systems that use small grain, forage, and cover crops in addition to corn and soybeans can reduce N emissions to water by increasing inputs of N through biological fixation, increasing the size of soil organic N stocks, reducing requirements for mineral fertilizer, and maximizing crop uptake of soil mineral N (Blesh and Drinkwater, 2013; Drinkwater et al., 1998; Gardner and Drinkwater, 2009; Oquist et al., 2007).

Unlike the Corn Belt, where most crop production occurs under rainfed conditions, most production in California is irrigated, especially in intensively cropped regions. Because the movement of reactive N is related to soil moisture conditions and water fluxes, water management and N management are linked closely. Dzurella et al. (2012) recommended that reductions of nitrate in California groundwater aquifers should be pursued by optimizing application rates and timing of water, fertilizer, and manure applications to better match crop need. In addition, they recommended that adjustments and improvements be made to crop rotation strategies and storage and handling of fertilizers and manure, and that manure N be accounted for by reducing mineral fertilizer N applications accordingly.

Alternative configurations of cropping systems and N sources may be particularly useful in addressing emissions of reactive N from California cropping systems. For example, Wyland et al. (1996) investigated the effects of winter cover crops (phacelia and rye) in broccoli-based cropping systems in the Salinas Valley and found that the cover crops reduced nitrate leaching by 65 to 70 percent relative to a winter fallow treatment. The effect was attributed to the cover crops' ability to capture N and water that would otherwise have been lost from the soil profile. In a long-term field experiment conducted in California's Sacramento Valley, soil N storage was greater and N losses were smaller for cropping systems that relied largely or exclusively on N inputs from leguminous cover crops and manure and that minimized or eliminated the use of mineral N fertilizer (Poudel et al., 2001). Using the same experiment site, Kramer et al. (2002) measured N uptake by corn from mineral fertilizer, residues of a vetch cover crop, and poultry manure and found that as compared to relying exclusively on mineral fertilizer, combinations of organic sources of N with low rates of fertilizer were sufficient to produce high yields while better matching N supply with crop demand in the latter part of the growing season. The investigators concluded that combining organic N sources with mineral fertilizer "holds promise for reducing the use of inorganic fertilizers and possible N losses from agroecosystems" (Kramer et al., 2002, p. 242).

The fate of N in cropping systems managed with different forms of N inputs and different cropping practices can be depicted in two contrasting conceptual models. Figure 7-A-4 shows possible N dynamics in a system that mostly relies on mineral fertilizers and that does not use cover crops or perennial crops to increase N uptake and retention. Losses of N to air and water could be substantial in such systems, with concomitant costs to farmers, due to low use efficiency for purchased N fertilizer, and to society, due to degradation of water resources and impairment of human health.

Figure 7-A-5 depicts possible N dynamics in an alternative cropping system that relies less on mineral N fertilizer and places greater emphasis on biological N fixation, manure and organic matter amendments, cover crops, and perennial crops. Losses of N to air and water in this alternative system could be much smaller than in the fertilizer-dependent system, with concomitant reductions in environmental and health costs to society. Farmers, however, might incur greater costs through the use of manure and other soil amendments rather than mineral fertilizer and through the production of non-cash crops.

With adequate confidence in the accuracy and precision of plot- and field-level measurements, system-level comparisons of N dynamics can be extended to landscape and watershed scales using biogeochemical process models that are spatially referenced for site-specific soil, climate, and management conditions. For example, De Gryze et al. (2009) employed data

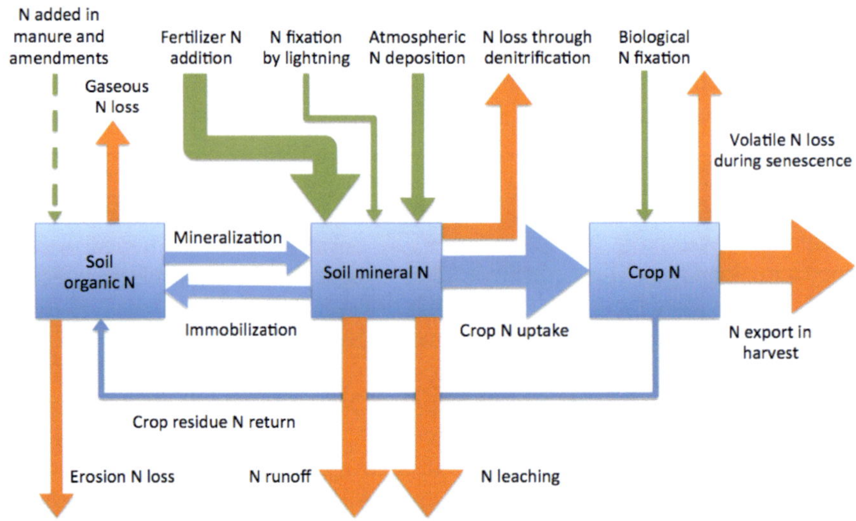

FIGURE 7-A-4 Hypothetical N stocks and flows for a cropping system using mainly mineral N inputs. Boxes representing N stocks and arrows representing N flows are not drawn to scale.

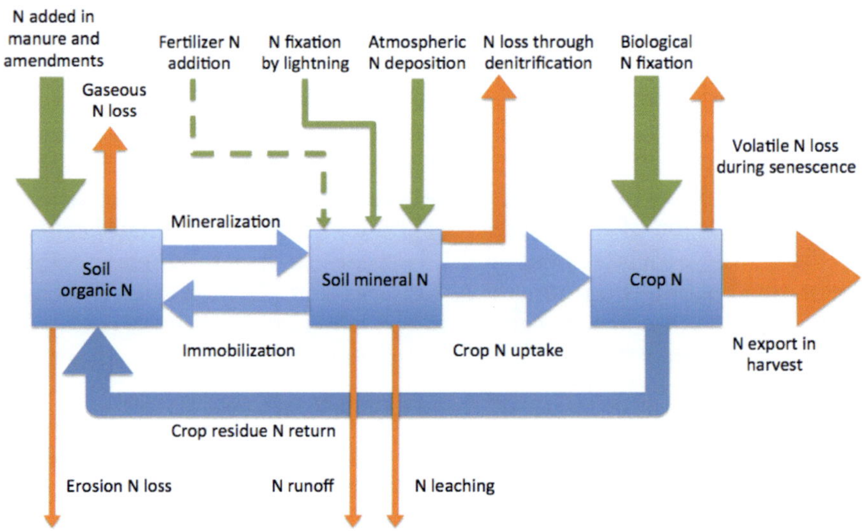

FIGURE 7-A-5 Hypothetical N stocks and flows for a cropping with low reliance on mineral N fertilizer, but with emphasis on biological N fixation, manure and organic matter amendments, cover crops, and perennial crops. Boxes representing N stocks and arrows representing N flows are not drawn to scale.

from four long-term field experiment sites and the CENTURY/DAYCENT model to examine nitrous oxide emissions from regions of the Sacramento and San Joaquin Valleys used for the production of the seven most abundant crops in both valleys: rice, alfalfa, cotton, tomatoes, winter wheat, corn, and safflower. When manure was used instead of mineral fertilizer or when 25 percent less mineral fertilizer was used, predicted nitrous oxide emissions were reduced by 0.5 to 1.2 Mg CO_2 equivalent ha^{-1} yr^{-1}. The investigators noted that manure releases N to the soil system slowly, resulting in better synchrony between nutrient supply and crop demand, and that reducing use of inorganic fertilizer decreases the amount of mineral N in the soil available for loss through denitrification. Though the modeling results indicated greater reliance on manure, and fertilizer rate adjustments would result in only modest reductions in nitrous oxide emissions, the modeling process illustrated how region-wide impacts of alternative crop and soil management systems on reactive N emissions might be assessed.

Biophysical process models that describe N dynamics can be extended from the field level to landscape and watershed levels for assessment of the water quality impacts of alternative patterns of land use. For example, Boody et al. (2005) used the ADAPT (Agricultural Drainage and Pesticide Transport) model to evaluate N emissions to streams under four different scenarios for land use in two agriculturally dominated watersheds in Minnesota: Wells Creek (16,264 ha), and Chippewa River (17,994 ha). The scenarios included (1) a continuation of current patterns of land use, mostly corn, soybean, and sugar beet production; (2) the use of "Best Management Practices," including conservation tillage practices, 30-meter wide buffer strips along stream banks, and application of fertilizer rates to match but not exceed crop demands; (3) increased landscape and cropping system diversity through wetland restoration, greater use of long rotations that included small grains and perennial forage crops with corn, soybean, and sugar beet, and increased use of pastures; and (4) an extension of the third scenario that further increased vegetative cover by shifting more arable cropland to grasslands, increasing the width of riparian buffers to 90 meters, and planting cover crops wherever row crops were produced. In addition to changes in water quality, changes in farm production inputs and net farm income were assessed using economic databases.

Under scenarios 3 and 4 in both watersheds, N fertilizer use fell 62 to 90 percent, N exported from land to streams decreased 51 to 74 percent, and government payments for commodity price support declined 44 to 70 percent, while net farm income rose 12 to 105 percent over the current baseline. Boody et al. (2005) concluded that environmental and economic benefits could be attained through changes in agricultural land management without increasing public costs. Landscape and cropping system diversification also resulted in large predicted reductions in stream N concentrations in simulations conducted for two watersheds in Iowa by Santelmann et al. (2004) using the SWAT (Soil and Water Assessment Tool) model.

Conduct the Analysis

In this step of an assessment, data, metrics, and analysis tools are used to examine the likely health, environmental, social, and economic effects associated with the alternative scenarios. For this example, we consider the data, metrics, and tools that would be used to compare the N management scenarios described above.

Empirical datasets with which to account for the full complement of N dynamics in different agricultural production systems are difficult to obtain (Vitousek et al., 2009). Although it can be relatively easy to monitor N inputs in the form of mineral fertilizers and manure, and N outputs in the form of harvested crop materials and marketed animal products, accurate measurements of biological N fixation, gaseous losses through denitrification, aqueous losses due to leaching, and N transformations between organic and mineral forms can be technically challenging, subject to considerable temporal and spatial variation, and expensive (Galloway et al., 2004). Consequently, despite the centrality of N dynamics for agricultural production, most experimental and observational studies have focused on a limited subset of N fluxes and transformations.

Building complete N budgets for contrasting management systems will require longer-term commitments and greater investment than are typical for the majority of more narrowly focused agricultural research projects. The Long-Term Ecological Research site operated by Michigan State University (Robertson et al., 2014; Syswerda and Robertson, 2014; Syswerda et al., 2012) is one of the few large-scale, long-term, multidisciplinary cropping system experiments conducted within the United States in which a large number of N stocks and flows have been studied with sufficient detail to provide insight into system-level characteristics. If N dynamics in all of the major agricultural production systems of the United States are to be understood, long-term investment in a distributed network of agroecosystem research sites is critically important, due to the need to (1) observe soil conditions for multiple years to detect slow impacts of farm management practices, (2) accommodate interannual variability in weather and pest conditions, and (3) effectively address the wide range of geographic conditions in which farming takes place. As noted by Robertson et al. (2008), this approach is largely lacking from the U.S. agricultural research portfolio.

The earlier scoping and scenario sections should make it clear that additional measurements and assessments, beyond yields, N fluxes, and N use efficiency, are necessary to understand the full impacts of N use and management in agroecosystems. These include quantification of the off-site health, environmental, and economic effects and costs of N emissions. Given the long distances that reactive forms of N can move downstream and downwind and the long lag times that may occur before effects are observed (Galloway et al., 2003), such measurements and assessments must be conducted at spatial scales much greater than individual fields, must be conducted for multiple years, and must include a much wider spectrum of plants, animals, microbes, and human populations than those encountered on farms. Socioeconomic investigations also must be integrated with biophysical research to (1) understand the signals and types of information that most affect farmers' decisions concerning N use and management; (2) determine the economic impacts of using alternative N management and cropping systems at farm, regional, and national scales; and (3) identify changes in policy that might affect the N-related impacts of agroecosystem management (Robertson and Vitousek, 2009; Robertson et al., 2008).

The use and management of N in agroecosystems is not restricted to the United States alone; it is an issue of worldwide concern (UNEP, 2007; Vitousek et al., 2009). Thus, improvements in analytical methods and approaches may be gained from investigations conducted internationally.

REFERENCES

Alexander, R. B., R. A. Smith, G. E. Schwarz, E. W. Boyer, J. V. Nolan, and J. W. Brakebill. 2008. Differences in phosphorus and nitrogen delivery to the Gulf of Mexico from the Mississippi River Basin. *Environmental Science and Technology* 42:822-830.

Blanco-Canqui, H. 2010. Energy crops and their implications on soil and environment. *Agronomy Journal* 102:403-419.

Blesh, J., and L. E. Drinkwater. 2013. The impact of nitrogen source and crop rotation on nitrogen mass balances in the Mississippi River Basin. *Ecological Applications* 23:1017-1035.

Boody, G., B. Vondracek, D. A. Andow, M. Krinke, J. Westra, J. Zimmerman, and P. Welle. 2005. Multifunctional agriculture in the United States. *Bioscience* 55:27-38.

Broussard, W., and R. E. Turner. 2009. A century of changing land-use and water-quality relationships in the continental U.S. *Frontiers in Ecology and the Environment* 7:302-307.

Broussard, W. P., R. E. Turner, and J. V. Westra. 2012. Do federal farm policies influence surface water quality? *Agriculture, Ecosystems and Environment* 158:103-109.

De Gryze, S., M. V. Albarracin, R. Catala-Luque, R. E. Howitt, and J. Six. 2009. Modeling shows that alternative soil management can decrease greenhouse gases. *California Agriculture* 63(2):84-90.

Dinnes, D. L., D. L. Karlen, D. B. Jaynes, T. C. Kaspar, J. L. Hatfield, T. S. Colvin, and C. A. Cambardella. 2002. Nitrogen management strategies to reduce nitrate leaching in tile-drained Midwestern soils. *Agronomy Journal* 94:153-171.

Donner, S. D., and C. J. Kucharik. 2008. Corn-based ethanol production compromises goal of reducing nitrogen export by the Mississippi River. *Proceedings of the National Academy of Sciences of the United States of America* 105:4513-4518.

Drinkwater, L. E., and S. S. Snapp. 2007. Nutrients in agroecosystems: Rethinking the management paradigm. *Advances in Agronomy* 92:63-186.

Drinkwater, L. E., P. Wagoner, and M. Sarrantonio. 1998. Legume-based cropping systems have reduced carbon and nitrogen losses. *Nature* 396:262-265.

Dzurella, K. N., J. Medellin-Azuara, V. B. Jensen, A. M. King, N. De La Mora, A. Fryjoff-Hung, T. S. Rosenstock, T. Harter, R. Howitt, A. D. Hollander, J. Darby, K. Jessoe, J. R. Lund, and G. S. Pettygrove. 2012. Nitrogen source reduction to protect groundwater quality. Technical Report 3. In *Addressing nitrate in California's drinking water with a focus on Tulare Lake Basin and Salinas Valley groundwater.* Center for Watershed Sciences, University of California, Davis. http://groundwaternitrate.ucdavis.edu (accessed December 23, 2014).

EPA (U.S. Environmental Protection Agency). 2011. *Reactive nitrogen in the United States—an analysis of inputs, flows, consequences, and management options.* EPA-SAB-11-013. Washington, DC: Environmental Protection Agency. http://yosemite.epa.gov/sab/sabproduct.nsf/WebBOARD/INCSupplemental?OpenDocument (accessed December 23, 2014).

EPA. 2013. *Inventory of U.S. greenhouse gas emissions and sinks: 1990-2011.* EPA 430-R-13-001, Washington, DC: EPA. http://www.epa.gov/climatechange/Downloads/ghgemissions/US-GHG-Inventory-2013-Main-Text.pdf (accessed December 23, 2014).

ERS (Economic Research Service). 2008. *Agricultural projections to 2017.* Washington, DC: U.S. Department of Agriculture, Economic Research Service. http://www.ers.usda.gov/publications/oce-usda-agricultural-projections/oce-2008-1.aspx (accessed December 23, 2014).

Foley, J. A., N. Ramankutty, K. A. Brauman, E. S. Cassidy, J. S. Gerber, M. Johnston, N. D. Mueller, C. O'Connell, D. K. Ray, P. C. West, C. Balzer, E. M. Bennett, S. R. Carpenter, J. Hill, C. Monfreda, S. Polasky, J. Rockstrom, J. Sheehan, S. Siebert, D. Tilman, and D. P. M. Zaks. 2011. Solutions for a cultivated planet. *Nature* 478(7369):337-342.

Galloway, J. N., J. D. Aber, J. W. Erisman, S. P. Seitzinger, R. W. Howarth, E. B. Cowling, and B. J. Cosby. 2003. The nitrogen cascade. *BioScience* 53:341-356.

Galloway, J. N., F. J. Dentener, D. G. Capone, E. W. Boyer, R. W. Howarth, S. P. Seitzinger, G. P. Asner, C. C. Cleveland, P. A. Green, E. A. Holland, D. M. Karl, A. F. Michaels, J. H. Porter, A. R. Townsend, and C. J. Vorosmarty. 2004. Nitrogen cycles: Past, present, and future. *Biogeochemistry* 70:153-226.

Gardner, J. B., and L. E. Drinkwater. 2009. The fate of nitrogen in grain cropping systems: A meta-analysis of N-15 field experiments. *Ecological Applications* 19:2167-2184.

Harter, T., J. R. Lund, J. Darby, G. E. Fogg, R. Howitt, K. Jessoe, G. S. Pettygrove, J. F. Quinn, J. H. Viers, D. B. Boyle, H. E. Canada, N. De La Mora, K. N. Dzurella, A. Fryjoff-Hung, A. D. Hollander, K. L. Honeycutt, M. W. Jenkins, V. B. Jensen, A. M. King, G. Kourakos, D. Liptzin, E. M. Lopez, M. M. Mayzelle, A. McNally, J. Medellin-Azuara, and T. S. Rosenstock. 2012. *Addressing nitrate in California's drinking water with a focus on Tulare Lake Basin and Salinas Valley groundwater.* Center for Watershed Sciences, University of California, Davis. http://groundwaternitrate.ucdavis.edu (accessed December 23, 2014).

Hatfield, J. L., L. D. McMullen, and C. S. Jones. 2009. Nitrate–nitrogen patterns in the Raccoon River Basin related to agricultural practices. *Journal of Soil and Water Conservation* 64:190-199.

Hoben, J. P., R. J. Gehl, N. Millar, P. R. Grace, and G. P. Robertson. 2011. Nonlinear nitrous oxide (N_2O) response to nitrogen fertilizer in on-farm corn crops of the US Midwest. *Global Change Biology* 17:1140-1152.

Jackson, L. L., D. R. Keeney, and E. M. Gilbert. 2000. Swine manure management plans in north-central Iowa: Nutrient loading and policy implications. *Journal of Soil and Water Conservation* 55:205-212.

Kaspar, T. C., D. B. Jaynes, T. B. Parkin, and T. B. Moorman. 2007. Rye cover crop and gamagrass strip effects on NO_3 concentration and load in tile drainage. *Journal of Environmental Quality* 36:1503-1511.

Kramer, A. W., T. A. Doane, W. R. Horwath, and C. van Kessel. 2002. Combining fertilizer and organic inputs to synchronize N supply in alternative cropping systems in California. *Agriculture, Ecosystems and Environment* 91:233-243.

MacDonald, J., M. Ribaudo, M. Livingston, J. Beckman, and W. Y. Huang. 2009. *Manure use for fertilizer and for energy.* Administrative Publication No. AP-037. Washington, DC: U.S. Department of Agriculture, Economic Research Service.

McSwiney, C. P., and G. P. Robertson. 2005. Nonlinear response of N_2O flux to incremental fertilizer addition in a continuous maize (*Zea mays* L.) cropping system. *Global Change Biology* 11:1712-1719.

Morton, L. W., and S. S. Brown (eds.). 2011. *Pathways for getting to better water quality: The citizen effect.* New York: Springer.

MPCA (Minnesota Pollution Control Agency). 2014. *The Minnesota nutrient reduction strategy.* St. Paul, MN. http://www.pca.state.mn.us/index.php/view-document.html?gid=20213 (accessed December 23, 2014).

Nassauer, J. I. 2010. Rural landscape change as a product of U.S. federal policy. In *Globalisation and agricultural landscapes: Change patterns and policy trends in developed countries*, edited by J. Primdahl and S. Swaffield. Cambridge, UK: Cambridge University Press. Pp. 185-200.

Oquist, K. A., J. S. Strock, and D. J. Mulla. 2007. Influence of alternative and conventional farming practices on subsurface drainage and water quality. *Journal of Environmental Quality* 36:1194-1204.

Paulot, F., and D. J. Jacob. 2014. Hidden cost of U.S. agricultural exports: Particulate matter from ammonia emissions. *Environmental Science and Technology* 48:903-908.

Poudel, D. D., W. R. Horwath, J. P. Mitchell, and S. R. Temple. 2001. Impacts of cropping systems on soil nitrogen storage and loss. *Agricultural Systems* 68:253-268.

Randall, G. W., D. R. Huggins, M. P. Russelle, D. J. Fuchs, W. W. Nelson, and J. L. Anderson. 1997. Nitrate losses through subsurface tile drainage in conservation reserve program, alfalfa, and row crop systems. *Journal of Environmental Quality* 26:1240-1247.

Ribaudo, M., J. Delgado, L. Hansen, M. Livingston, R. Mosheim, and J. Williamson. 2011. *Nitrogen in agricultural systems—implications for conservation policy.* Economic Research Service Report No. 127. Washington, DC: U.S. Department of Agriculture, Economic Research Service.

Robertson, G. P., and P. M. Vitousek. 2009. Nitrogen in agriculture: Balancing the cost of an essential resource. *Annual Review of Environment and Resources* 34:97-125.

Robertson, G. P., V. G. Allen, G. Boody, E. R. Boose, N. G. Creamer, L. E. Drinkwater, J. R. Gosz, L. Lynch, J. L. Havlin, L. E. Jackson, S. T. A. Pickett, L. Pitelka, A. Randall, A. S. Reed, T. R. Seastedt, R. B. Waide, and D. H. Wall. 2008. Long-term agricultural research: A research, education, and extension imperative. *BioScience* 58:640-645.

Robertson, G. P., K. L. Gross, S. K. Hamilton, D. A. Landis, T. M. Schmidt, S. S. Snapp, and S. M. Swinton. 2014. Farming for ecosystem services: An ecological approach to production agriculture. *Bioscience* 64(5):404-415.

Santelmann, M. V., D. White, K. Freemark, J. I. Nassauer, J. M. Eilers, K. B. Vache, B. J. Danielson, R. C. Corry, M. E. Clark, S. Polasky, R. M. Cruse, J. Sifneos, H. Rustigian, C. Coiner, J. Wu, and D. Debinski. 2004. Assessing alternative futures for agriculture in Iowa, U.S.A. *Landscape Ecology* 19:357-374.

Schilling, K. E., and R. D. Libra. 2000. The relationship of nitrate concentration in streams to row crop land use in Iowa. *Journal of Environmental Quality* 29:1846-1851.

Shapouri, H., P. W. Gallagher, W. Nefstead, R. Schwartz, R. Noe, and R. Conway. 2010. *2008 Energy balance for the corn–ethanol industry.* Agricultural Economic Report 846. Office of the Chief Economist. Washington, DC: U.S. Department of Agriculture.

Smil, V. 1999. Nitrogen in crop production: An account of global flows. *Global Biogeochemical Cycles* 13:647-662.

Syswerda, S. P., and G. P. Robertson. 2014. Ecosystem services along a management gradient in Michigan (USA) cropping systems. *Agriculture, Ecosystems and Environment* 189:28-35.

Syswerda, S. P., B. Basso, S. K. Hamilton, J. B. Tausig, and G. P. Robertson. 2012. Long-term nitrate loss along an agricultural intensity gradient in the Upper Midwest USA. *Agriculture, Ecosystems and Environment* 149:10-19.

Tonitto, C., M. B. David, and L. E. Drinkwater. 2006. Replacing bare fallows with cover crops in fertilizer-intensive cropping systems: A meta-analysis of crop yield and N dynamics. *Agriculture, Ecosystems and Environment* 112:58-72.

UNEP (United Nations Environment Programme). 2007. *Reactive nitrogen in the environment—too much or too little of a good thing.* Paris, France: UNEP. http://www.whrc.org/resources/publications/pdf/UNEPetal.2007.pdf (accessed December 23, 2014).

Vitousek, P., R. Naylor, T. Crews, M. B. David, L. E. Drinkwater, E. Holland, P. J. Johnes, J. Katzenberger, L. A. Martinelli, P. A. Matson, G. Nziguheba, D. Ojima, C. A. Palm, G. P. Robertson, P. A. Sanchez, A. R. Townsend, and F. S. Zhang. 2009. Nutrient imbalances in agricultural development. *Science* 324:1519-1520.

Ward, M. H. 2009. Too much of a good thing? Nitrate from nitrogen fertilizers and cancer. *Reviews on Environmental Health* 24:357-363.

Wyland, L. J., L. E. Jackson, W. E. Chaney, K. Klonsky, S. T. Koike, and B. Kemple. 1996. Winter cover crops in a vegetable cropping system: Impacts on nitrate leaching, soil water, crop yield, pests and management costs. *Agriculture, Ecosystems and Environment* 59:1-17.

ANNEX 5: COMPARING HEN HOUSING PRACTICES AND THEIR EFFECTS ON VARIOUS DOMAINS

A Systems Approach to Exploring the Effects of Hen Housing

In contrast to the previous examples, in this annex the case study is based on an actual assessment, in which data on various dimensions of effects are being collected and analyzed for various hen housing alternatives. Interestingly, the planning, data collection, and analysis that occurred for this project closely parallel the principles and steps of this committee's framework.

This unique project allows simultaneous assessment of the magnitude of effects across all of the domains of effects of egg production on a commercial scale. This effort could not be assessed by conducting independent studies alone.

The project also is unique in bringing together a large group of stakeholders to share information and participate in evaluation and decision-making processes. The example shows the importance of involving a multidisciplinary team of researchers and other stakeholders from the beginning of the planning stages throughout the analysis step.

This project, however, does not address some dimensions of the committee's proposed framework, specifically distribution and resilience. These dimensions encompass economic effects that the policy intervention could have on farms of differing sizes. In addition, the project does not attempt to understand public attitudes toward farm animal welfare and the role that those attitudes played in consumer purchasing behavior or how an increase in the cost of eggs would affect consumer behavior. Significant knowledge gaps exist in this area.

The study illustrates the need to carefully choose alternative interventions for comparison. It shows that an intervention that might positively affect hen welfare, for example, also affects human health, the environment, and the economy of the sector.

The primary limitation of the project is that it is being conducted on a single farm, with one genetic strain of hens. This may constrain applicability to other U.S. regions and management practices, although the project will provide an overall framework and methodology for assessment that can be used across contexts. It should be noted that the goal of the project is to identify

continued

synergies and trade-offs, not to attempt to provide a formal integration of the data into an index that will "rank" the different housing systems. Each member stakeholder in the coalition can use the information obtained to make its own purchasing and supply decisions, based on its own organization's values with respect to sustainability.

Eggs are a primary source of animal protein worldwide. As early as in the 1950s, commercial egg producers began to adopt conventional cages to house laying hens. Before this intensification of egg production, hens were kept in small to medium-sized flocks in barns or in free-range systems. Although the latter allowed the hens to perform a wide range of natural behaviors, they also exposed them to diseases and predation. In addition, food safety concerns arose because hens could lay eggs outside their nesting areas (potentially allowing for contact with manure), and these eggs were soiled and dirtier than nest-laid eggs and potentially contaminated with manure-borne pathogens. Cage housing greatly reduced food safety issues because the birds' excreta fell through the cage floor and was removed by belt systems from the barn, thus preventing both birds and eggs from contacting manure. In general, cage flooring is sloped to allow eggs to roll out onto an egg collection belt. This prompt collection ensures improved cleanliness and freshness of the egg product. In general, cages facilitated the expansion and integration of the laying industry by allowing larger flock sizes and more automation of feeding, watering, and egg collection, which reduced the cost of eggs. Today, the vast majority of U.S. eggs (>95 percent) are from hens raised in conventional cage barns.

Starting in the 1960s, conventional cage housing began to be criticized, particularly in the European Union (EU), because it restricted the behavior of the hens and did not allow for the resources hens needed to perch, nest, or forage. In 1976, the Council of Europe published a convention stating that farm animals should be given "space appropriate to their physiological and ethological [behavioral] needs." The European Union established minimum space standards for laying hens, and cages were entirely banned in 1999. In 2008, California voters passed a referendum named Proposition 2 (i.e., the Prevention of Farm Animal Cruelty Act) that, although ambiguously worded, effectively outlawed conventional cages for laying hens. Legislation that either outlawed or restricted the use of conventional cages was passed in Michigan, Ohio, Oregon, and Washington during the following 2 years.

After its ban on conventional cages for egg-laying hens, the European Union undertook considerable efforts to develop alternatives to conventional cage housing. The two alternative types of housing systems now acceptable under EU regulations are non-cage (also known as cage-free) systems, and furnished cages (also known in the United States as enriched colony systems). Non-cage systems include large buildings (i.e., aviaries) that provide indoor housing for tens or hundreds of thousands of hens that are allowed to move freely. The hens are provided with perches and nest boxes that largely allow for automated egg collection. A portion of the floor of the house contains bedding (e.g., wood shavings), which facilitates the pecking, scratching, and dustbathing behaviors of the hens. On the downside, this space also allows manure to accumulate over long time periods.

Several types of furnished cages exist, and in general they provide more space to birds than do conventional cages. Furnished cages, which each house a group of 20 to 60 hens, offer perches, a nest box, and an area on to which loose material is delivered to facilitate pecking, scratching, and dustbathing. As with conventional cages, the cage floor is made entirely of wire and is sloped so that the eggs roll out onto an automatic egg collection belt[1] and the manure falls onto manure collection belts that remove waste from the building.

Identify the Problem

The first step of an assessment is to identify the problem. This is typically done based on consultation with stakeholders and reviews of relevant literature. The problem identified for this assessment is that changes in hen housing potentially have far-reaching economic consequences and may also have unintended consequences in the areas of environmental quality, human and animal health, and worker safety. The objective of the current study has been to learn about interconnections and trade-offs in various alternative poultry housing configurations. Results of the current study may be used to inform public policy related to practices and management of egg-laying hens in the United States.

Define the Scope of the Problem and Identify the Scenarios

Once a problem has been identified, the next steps of an assessment are to frame its scope and to identify alternative scenarios. Framing the scope is done by characterizing the boundaries, components, processes, actors, and linkages encompassed by the system under consideration. Identifying alternative scenarios compares the performance of the current system—the baseline—with one or more alternative scenarios. This is done to understand the potential effects of a new policy or intervention under consideration.

---

[1] Videos showing the features of different systems can be found at http://www2.sustainableeggcoalition.org/resources (accessed January 20, 2015).

For this example, these two steps have been combined, and the scope of the problem and alternative scenarios are described by summarizing selected studies that have compared the effects of various hen housing systems.

Effects of Bans on Conventional Cage Systems

When the hen housing laws in the United States were passed, it became apparent that moving to alternative production systems would affect sustainability domains other than just hen health and welfare, including egg safety and quality, environmental quality, food affordability, worker health and safety, and public values and attitudes. In 2008, the American Egg Board[2] funded Michigan State University and the University of California, Davis, to review existing knowledge in these sustainability areas and to identify gaps. A series of papers resulted that identified effects and knowledge gaps as discussed below. Significant knowledge gaps exist in understanding the public attitudes and values toward farm animal welfare. This area will be the subject of future studies and it is not listed below.

Hen health and welfare This area has been more intensively studied than any of the other sustainability areas (Lay et al., 2011). Conventional cages restrict hen behavior the most, whereas non-cage systems provide more space for movement and provide behavioral resources, with furnished cages being intermediate. However, non-cage systems are known to be more associated with hen health problems than are cage systems. These problems include higher risks of infection with diseases and parasites and higher rates of bone breakage due to hens' contact with manure and vectors. Incidences of cannibalism and pecking also are more abundant in non-cage versus cage systems. These factors are important drivers of mortality, which is often higher in non-cage than in cage systems.

Egg safety and quality Although a number of European studies have characterized egg quality in different hen housing systems, results have been contradictory with respect to attributes, such as egg size, shell strength, shell quality and integrity, egg interior quality, and egg nutritional quality (Holt et al., 2011). The major egg safety factor is *Salmonella* enteriditis contamination. When eggs are laid on top of manure or soil (which is often the case in cage-free systems), they become soiled with manure, and fecal

[2] The American Egg Board is the promotion, education, and research organization for the U.S. egg industry. It is composed of 18 members who are egg producers appointed by the Secretary of Agriculture to administer the program on behalf of all egg producers in the 48 contiguous states. The Board was authorized by the Egg Research and Consumer Information Act passed by the 93rd Congress and its activities are conducted under the oversight of the U.S. Department of Agriculture.

pathogens on the shell can enter the egg through the egg pores. However, little conclusive research has been conducted on the effects of various housing systems on *Salmonella*.

Environmental quality Environmental impacts of laying hen production systems include air quality (particulate matter and ammonia), water quality (run-off), manure management (due to effects on ammonia production), and resource usage (feed, energy, land) (Xin et al., 2011). In general, particulate matter is lower in cage versus non-cage systems because the barns contain no manure that can be aerosolized. Manure is a primary contributor to higher ammonia concentrations in cage-free houses because it is generally not removed until the end of the laying cycle. Hens are stocked at lower density in furnished cages than in conventional cages, and at even lower density in non-cage systems. These lower densities are associated with greater land use and more feed consumption, thus contributing to reduced resource usage efficiency and a higher carbon footprint. Knowledge gaps included comparisons of environmental effects and footprints among the different hen housing systems in the United States, lack of process-based models for air emissions, lack of knowledge about the effectiveness of mitigation strategies, and limited understanding of interactions among environmental effects, worker safety, and hen health and welfare.

Food affordability Studies from Europe have shown that the cost of producing eggs was higher in non-cage versus cage systems, with costs of production in furnished cage systems intermediate. Data from California producers indicated that the shift from conventional cages to indoor non-cage systems would cause farm-level cost increases of about 40 percent per dozen eggs, but no U.S. data were available for furnished cages (Sumner et al., 2011). Gaps in knowledge include those related to costs of production in alternative production systems in the United States, impacts on smaller producers of having to make significant capital investments to adopt new housing systems, and the effects of increased egg prices on retailer and consumer behavior.

Worker health and safety Little information is available on worker health and safety issues associated with alternative production systems. Although it can be assumed that factors which affect hen health and comfort (e.g., dust, ammonia) also potentially affect workers, a lack of empirical information exists about the impacts of either environmental factors or ergonomic challenges.

Conduct the Analysis

The review conducted in this project to define the scope of the problem and identify alternative scenarios provided justification for the data collection, metrics, and analysis proposed by the stakeholder team assembled to assess this problem. The goal of their analysis was to outline trade-offs and ramifications of potential hen housing decisions.

This analysis provides an excellent example of a series of challenges within a major food production area. Decisions about the weight or importance of every major effect depend on reconciling competing value judgments. For example, is behavioral freedom more or less important than hen health as a consideration when deciding which housing system is more sustainable? To what extent do the magnitudes of each effect and the potential costs of mitigation affect decision making about hen welfare? Competing value judgments again come into play when weighing the importance of one area of sustainability against another when the information is conflicting. Various integration methods have been employed to address these challenges, including deliberative approaches, informal decision making, and quantitative analyses. The latter are appealing because they result in the assignment of numerical outcomes to the various sustainability attributes. However, because no empirically or logically "correct" way exists to assign such numbers, ultimately they also depend on value judgments. Participatory decision-making strategies that involve a broad array of stakeholders are a promising method for value integration, and a group of stakeholders was convened to begin this process for sustainable egg production.

Stakeholder Participation

The data gaps and approaches identified above were influential in informing the next stage in the process of evaluating the sustainability of egg production, which was the formation of the Coalition for a Sustainable Egg Supply (CSES), described by Swanson et al. (in press). CSES is a multi-stakeholder group collaborating on a study of housing alternatives for egg-laying hens in the United States. It has more than 30 members, including research institutions, trade organizations, scientific societies, nongovernmental organizations, egg suppliers, food manufacturers, and restaurant/retail/food service companies. Leadership for the project is provided by McDonald's, Cargill, Michigan State University, the University of California, Davis, and the American Humane Association, with the American Veterinary Medical Association, the U.S. Department of Agriculture's Agricultural Research Service, and the Environmental Defense Fund serving as advisors. Retailers have assumed a central role in discussions about animal welfare and the sustainability of the food supply in general because they have been increasingly subject to public activity (e.g., shareholders' resolutions, advertising campaigns) designed to influence their purchasing practices. CSES is facilitated by the Center for Food Integrity (CFI), a not-for-profit organization dedicated to building consumer trust and confidence in the food system. CFI members represent each segment of the food chain.

Metrics and Data Collection

The goal of CSES is to collect data to understand the magnitude of effects and the trade-offs in terms of hen welfare, worker health and safety, food affordability, environmental impacts, and egg safety and quality in different hen housing systems under U.S. conditions. The data are being collected over two full hen flock cycles from a commercial farm in the Midwest that contains three types of housing facilities: conventional cage, cage-free aviary, and furnished cage systems.

The following effects/outcomes are being compared among the alternative hen housing systems:

- *Hen health and welfare:* Hen behavior and resource/space use, physiological indicators of stress, comprehensive physical condition, and health outcomes measured using a standardized evaluation system plus clinical observation and testing, bone quality, and bone-breaking strength (i.e., force required to break a bone).
- *Egg safety and quality:* Interior and exterior egg quality; egg shelf life; microbial contamination levels of eggs, egg-processing areas, and housing areas; immunological responses of hens to the *Salmonella* vaccine.
- *Environmental quality:* Indoor air quality and thermal conditions, gaseous and particulate emissions from houses and manure storage areas, efficiency of resource (feed, water, energy), nitrogen mass balance, life cycle analysis.
- *Food affordability:* Production costs (feed, land and buildings, labor, hen disease and health costs, pullet costs) and revenue (marketable output flows).
- *Worker health and safety:* Personnel exposure to gaseous and particulate matter, respiratory health, ergonomic stressors, musculoskeletal disorders.

The CSES provided more than $6.5 million for this research to be conducted, with additional significant costs incurred to construct or renovate the commercial houses to enable the project to be operated. In addition, CFI is conducting parallel research using focus groups to understand consumer attitudes toward hen housing systems and the sustainability of egg production, as well as to determine how those attitudes may be influenced when consumers are provided with the information obtained from the CSES research project.

REFERENCES

Holt, P. S., R. H. Davies, J. Dewulf, R. K. Gast, J. K. Huwe, D. R. Jones, D. Waltman, and K. R. Willian. 2011. The impact of different housing systems on egg safety and quality. *Poultry Science* 90(1):251-262.

Lay, D. C., Jr., R. M. Fulton, P. Y. Hester, D. M. Karcher, J. B. Kjaer, J. A. Mench, B. A. Mullens, R. C. Newberry, C. J. Nicol, N. P. O'Sullivan, and R. E. Porter. 2011. Hen welfare in different housing systems. *Poultry Science* 90(1):278-294.

Sumner, D. A., H. Gow, D. Hayes, W. Matthews, B. Norwood, J. T. Rosen-Molina, and W. Thurman. 2011. Economic and market issues on the sustainability of egg production in the United States: Analysis of alternative production systems. *Poultry Science* 90(1):241-250.

Swanson, J. C., J. A. Mench, and D. Karcher. In press. The coalition for sustainable egg supply project: An introduction. *Poultry Science.*

Xin, H., R. S. Gates, A. R. Green, F. M. Mitloehner, P. A. Moore, Jr., and C. M. Wathes. 2011. Environmental impacts and sustainability of egg production systems. *Poultry Science* 90(1):263-277.

8

Epilogue

The committee was charged with developing a framework for assessing the health, environmental, social, and economic effects associated with the way food is grown, processed, distributed, marketed, sold, and consumed, as well as regulated, within the U.S. component of the global food system. To address this responsibility effectively, the committee believed it necessary to develop an understanding of the current food system and its evolution over time. The committee sought to describe some of the salient effects of the food system on human health and well-being and on the environment. The food system has evolved and will continue to evolve as a result of the natural resource endowment and changing government policies, societal norms, market forces, and scientific discoveries. Although it is difficult to predict the shape and characteristics of the U.S. food system in the future, the framework developed by the committee is intended both to facilitate retrospective and prospective analyses of the system and to foster improved decision making on how it might be better organized, altered, and maintained.

CONCLUDING THOUGHTS

Examples abound in which decisions about the food system have resulted in consequences in multiple domains well beyond their immediate objective. Researchers are still analyzing the causes and the effects even after policies have been implemented. While collecting information and illustrating the application of the framework to the various examples selected,[1] the committee reached the following conclusions:

1. *Comprehensive studies of food systems that use all principles of the committee's framework are rare in published literature. For example, the committee could not find a single example where all four domains (health, environment, social, and economic effects) and the four key dimensions (quantity, quality, distribution, and resilience) were considered. More importantly, most studies lack clear statements of boundaries and assumptions about the affected domains, their interactions, or dynamic feedbacks.*
2. *Studies that consider the entire food supply chain and address multiple domains (and dimensions) of effects of an intervention and its drivers can identify outcomes and trade-offs that are not visible in more narrowly focused assessments.*
3. *Policies or actions that aim for an outcome in one domain of the food system (e.g., health) can have consequences not only in the same domain but also in other ones (e.g., environmental, social, and economic domains). These consequences may be positive or negative, intended or unintended. They can be substantial and are often not proportional to the change incurred. That is, what might appear as a small intervention may have disproportionately large consequences in various domains across time and space.*
4. *The data and methodologies used to study the food system have been collected and developed both by public and by private initiatives, depending on the questions they help to address (e.g., public health or climate change questions versus questions related to the environmental effects of a specific company). Methodologies include not only those to describe and assess the effects of the system but also those that serve to synthesize and interpret the results. Publicly collected data and publicly supported models have been and continue to be critically important in assessing and comparing the effects of the food system in various domains and dimensions. The lack of access to data collected by industry can be a major challenge for public research aimed at understanding the drivers and effects of the food system.*

[1] The committee selected the following examples: (1) the use of antibiotics in animal feeding (see Box 7-7); (2) recommendations for fish consumption and health (see Annex 1); (3) policies mandating biofuel production (see Annex 2); (4) recommendations to increase fruit and vegetable consumption (see Annex 3); (5) nitrogen application to obtain maximum crop yields (see Annex 4); and (6) policies on animal welfare dealing with commercial egg production (see Annex 5).

5. *Stakeholders are important audiences of any assessment exercise, but they also can play an important role throughout the process by contributing to, identifying, or scoping the problem or potential effects that may not have been apparent to the researchers. They also can be important sources of data when public sources are not readily available. Effectively engaging stakeholders has challenges, such as avoiding conflicts of interest, ensuring equitable engagement, and addressing potential lack of trust by the public. Therefore, this type of participatory process requires careful planning about whom to involve, when to involve them, and how much involvement is appropriate.*
6. *Even though major improvements in the U.S. food system have resulted in the past from the introduction of new technologies, needed future improvements in the system may not be achievable solely through technological innovation. Achieving them may require more comprehensive approaches that incorporate non-technological factors to reach long-term solutions. Systemic approaches that take full account of social, economic, ecological, and evolutionary factors and processes will be required to meet challenges to the U.S. food system in the 21st century. Such challenges include antibiotic and pesticide resistance; chemical contamination of air and water; soil erosion and degradation; water deficits; diet-related chronic disease, obesity, domestic and global hunger, and malnutrition; and food safety.*
7. *To discover the best solutions to these problems, it is important not only to identify the effects of the current system but also to understand the drivers (e.g., human behavior, markets, policy) and how they interact with each other and with the observable system effects. Such understanding can help decision makers to identify the best opportunities to intervene and to anticipate the potential consequences of any intervention.*

These conclusions support the development of an analytical, systems approach framework that can be used to broaden insights into the consequences of food and agriculturally related activities and policies, assisting decision makers in becoming aware of trade-offs and potential unintended consequences. When considering alternative configurations[2] (e.g., policies

---

[2] Configurations are elements within the food system, such as policy interventions, technologies, market conditions, or organizational structure of different segments of the food system, that can be modified to achieve a particular goal or to explore how potential drivers (e.g., growth in demand for foods with particular traits) might impact the distribution of health, environmental, social, and economic effects.

or practices) that affect the food system, the framework provided by the committee should be used to examine policies or proposed changes in the food system that may have wide implications. Applying the framework also will help to identify uncertainties and identify and prioritize research needs.

The committee recognizes that in some cases, limited resources might preclude a comprehensive analysis of the food system. Also, discrete questions may not require a full systemic analysis. In such instances, not all steps or methods will apply equally, depending on the scope and topic chosen by a researcher. Regardless of the scope of the analysis, assessors still need to recognize boundaries and implications and to take into account the various interrelationships of the food system.

The use of such an analytical framework relies on good data, metrics, and methodologies. Organized and systematic collection of data on a national and international basis, in addition to local, regional, and state levels, is vital to improving the ability to answer critical questions on U.S. food system impacts. The U.S. government maintains major datasets that are useful for assessing the health, environmental, social, and economic effects of the food system. These include the U.S. Department of Agriculture's (USDA's) Food Availability Data, Loss-Adjusted Food Availability Data, and Nutrient Availability Data databases, which are critical as a proxy for the food consumption and food losses in the United States for more than 200 commodities. Another critical database is the Centers for Disease Control and Prevention's National Health and Nutrition Examination Survey, which estimates the health and nutritional status of the U.S. population. In the environmental domain, the National Agricultural Statistics Service's Agricultural Chemical Use Program collects data on pesticide use in farms, which is important to estimate the risks to farmers and the environment. The USDA National Agriculture Statistics Service data series (e.g., the Farm Labor Survey; the Census of Agriculture; and the Agricultural Resource Management Survey) are also important. Many other databases also are crucial for conducting assessments; a list of selected databases can be found in Table B-3, Appendix B. The design, collection, and analysis of data should be reviewed periodically so that it matches the needs of researchers and decision makers as new questions arise. Many specific needs also could be identified in the social and economic domains, but some general areas of concern are the overall lack of segregated datasets (e.g., data by sociodemographic factors at regional or local levels) and of validated metrics for some variables, such as the well-being of individuals or groups.

The committee recommends that Congress and federal agencies continue funding and supporting the collection (and improvement) of federally supported datasets that can be used for food system assessment studies along with giving consideration to creating new data collection programs as priorities arise. Likewise, continued support for developing and advancing methods and models is necessary for a more comprehensive understanding of U.S. food system effects across all domains. The National Institutes of Health's Office of Behavioral and Social Sciences Research has supported systems science research to advance health promotion and public health efforts, but more could be done to advance multidisciplinary studies among the agricultural, economic, environmental, social science, and health research communities. The government, academic, and private sectors have recognized the need to share data. The committee supports federal efforts to share data and encourages further development of improved methods for more efficiently sharing data across disciplines and agencies and with the private sector. The committee urges that government–industry collaboration mechanisms be developed to make industry-collected information more readily available for use in research and policy analysis.

The committee also notes the need to build human capacity in the field of systems science research. As this report has pointed out, a fuller understanding of the implications of changes to the food system could be gained by more integrated analyses, yet much research in these domains remains narrowly focused and linear in its design. Training scientists in academia, the private sector, and government agencies in all aspects of complex systems approaches—including systems research design, data collection and analytical methodologies, and the use of models—would remove some of the barriers impeding progress. Continued support for research on and demonstration of systems analysis methodologies will be important to ensure that innovation in this field continues. It is particularly important that government institutions such as USDA, the U.S. Food and Drug Administration, the U.S. Environmental Protection Agency, the U.S. Department of Labor, and other relevant federal agencies have the human and analytical capacity to undertake assessments using the principles of the framework as they consider policies that have domestic and global consequences.

The committee intends the report to stimulate broad thinking about the consequences of food system policies and actions beyond a single dimension. The recognition that the U.S. food system represents a complex adaptive system set within local, national, and global biophysical and social/institutional contexts should bring new methodologies to the study of the potential consequences of new policies, technologies, and configurations. Such analyses may provide better guidance to decision makers. The description of the food system and its effects has intentionally been presented from a U.S. perspective, and it omits important interactions and effects for the rest of the world. However, its application is aimed not only at those attempting to understand the U.S. food system and its consequences but also at others outside the United States who are conducting similar research and making similar decisions about their food systems.

Appendix A

Open Session Agendas

The committee held data-gathering sessions that were open to the public in Washington, DC, on July 16, 2013, September 16-17, 2013, and December 16, 2013. The open session agendas for the public meetings and a workshop are presented below.

COMMITTEE ON A FRAMEWORK FOR ASSESSING THE HEALTH, ENVIRONMENTAL, AND SOCIAL EFFECTS OF THE FOOD SYSTEM

Tuesday, July 16, 2013

The Keck Center, National Academy of Sciences
500 Fifth Street, NW, Room 110
Washington, DC

Open Session

1:00 p.m. **Welcome and Introductions**
Malden Nesheim, *Committee Chair*

1:05 p.m. **Sponsor Perspectives on the Study**
Dana Bourland and Barbara Picower, The JPB Foundation

1:30 p.m. **Exploring the True Cost of Food**
Helen Jensen, Iowa State University

2:00 p.m.	**Overview of the U.S. Food System** August "Gus" Schumacher, Wholesome Wave Foundation
2:30 p.m.	**Q&A**
3:00 p.m.	**Break**
3:15 p.m.	**Overview of the Health Effects of the Food System** Robert Lawrence, Johns Hopkins University
3:45 p.m.	**Overview of the Environmental Effects of the Food System** David Tilman, University of Minnesota
4:15 p.m.	**Overview of the Social Effects of the Food System** Cornelia Flora, Iowa State University
4:45 p.m.	**Q&A**
5:15 p.m.	**Public Comments**
5:35 p.m.	**Closing Remarks**
5:45 p.m.	**Adjourn Open Session**

MAPPING THE FOOD SYSTEM AND ITS EFFECTS: A WORKSHOP

September 16-17, 2013

The Keck Center, National Academy of Sciences
500 Fifth Street, NW, Room 100
Washington, DC

Workshop Goals

1. Describe the components of the food system and their relationships.
2. Explore a broad range of key environmental, socioeconomic, and health effects.
3. Describe current efforts to identify indicators and develop frameworks that take into consideration environmental, socioeconomic, and health effects of the food system.

Monday, September 16, 2013

12:30 p.m.	**Registration**
1:30 p.m.	**Welcome and Introductory Remarks** Malden Nesheim, *Committee Chair*

Session 1 – Defining the U.S. Food System

1:40 p.m.	**Introduction** Moderator: Kate Clancy, *Committee Member*
1:45 p.m.	**The U.S. Food System from the Perspective of Fruit and Vegetable Producers** Tom Stenzel, United Fresh Produce Association
2:15 p.m.	**The U.S. Food System from a Manufacturer's Perspective** Joan Menke Schaenzer, ConAgra Foods
2:45 p.m.	**Break**
3:00 p.m.	**Broad Overview of the U.S. Food System** Catherine Woteki, U.S. Department of Agriculture
3:30 p.m.	**The U.S. Role in a Global Food System** K. Scott Portnoy, Cargill Inc.
3:50 p.m.	**Discussion with Session 1 Speakers**

Session 2 – Environmental Effects of the Food System

4:15 p.m.	**Introduction** Moderator: Scott Swinton, *Committee Member*
4:20 p.m.	**Global Challenges to Food Security and the Environment** Jonathan Foley, University of Minnesota
4:40 p.m.	**Methods to Measure and Value Ecosystem Services and Trade-offs** Jim Boyd, Resources for the Future

5:00 p.m.	**Economic Determinants of Agricultural Land Use in the Long Run** Tom Hertel, Purdue University
5:20 p.m.	**Modeling the Bio-Geochemistry of Nutrient Flow into Ground and Surface Waters and Air from Various Agro-Ecosystems** R. Cesar Izaurralde, Pacific Northwest National Laboratory and University of Maryland
5:40 p.m.	**Discussion with Session 2 Speakers**
6:15 p.m.	**Adjourn**

Tuesday, September 17, 2013

8:00 a.m.	**Registration**
8:30 a.m.	**Welcome and Recap of Day 1** Malden Nesheim, *Committee Chair*

Session 3 – Socioeconomic Effects of the Food System

8:40 a.m.	**Introduction** Moderator: Robbin Johnson, *Committee Member*
8:45 a.m.	**Agriculture, Trade, and Rural Development** Robert Thompson, Johns Hopkins University
9:05 a.m.	**Market Responses to Sustainability in U.S. Agricultural and Food Policies and Practices** Bruce Babcock, Iowa State University
9:25 a.m.	**Discussion with Session 3 Speakers**
9:45 a.m.	**Break**

Session 4 – Health Effects of the Food System

10:00 a.m.	**Introduction** Moderator: Keshia Pollack, *Committee Member*

10:05 a.m.	**Consumer Preferences and Marketing as Drivers of the Food Supply** David Just, Cornell University
10:25 a.m.	**Food Access: Prices and the Retail Environment** Parke Wilde, Tufts University
10:45 a.m.	**Assessing Food System Effects on Chronic Diseases and Related Health Inequities** Shiriki Kumanyika, University of Pennsylvania
11:05 a.m.	**Assessing and Managing Health Risks from Chemical Constituents and Contaminants of Food** Joseph Rodricks, ENVIRON
11:25 a.m.	**Networks of Exchanging Antibiotic Resistance in Human-Associated and Environmental Bacteria** Gautam Dantas, Washington University
11:45 a.m.	**Discussion with Session 4 Speakers**
12:30 p.m.	**Lunch**

Session 5 – Use of Frameworks and Sustainability Indicators

1:30 p.m.	**Introduction** Moderator: Ross Hammond, *Committee Member*
1:35 p.m.	**Use of a Corporate Framework for Social and Environmental Responsibility** Robert Langert, McDonald's
1:55 p.m.	**Use of a Corporate Framework for Social and Environmental Responsibility in Contracted Food Service** Helene York, Bon Appetit Management Co.
2:15 p.m.	**Use of Standards and Indicators to Monitor Food Systems Sustainability** Molly Anderson, College of the Atlantic

2:35 p.m.	**Life Cycle Assessment as a Conceptual and Analytical Framework for Linking Food Production and Consumption** Martin Heller, University of Michigan
2:55 p.m.	**Use of Cost–Benefit Analysis at FDA** Amber Jessup, U.S. Department of Health and Human Services
3:15 p.m.	**Use of Cost–Benefit Analysis at EPA** Charles Griffiths, Environmental Protection Agency
3:35 p.m.	**Break**
3:50 p.m.	**Discussion with Session 5 Speakers**
4:40 p.m.	**Public Comments**
5:00 p.m.	**Closing Remarks** Malden Nesheim, *Committee Chair*
5:15 p.m.	**Adjourn**

December 16, 2013

The Keck Center, National Academy of Sciences
500 Fifth Street, NW, Room 201
Washington, DC

Open Session

12:00 p.m.	**Food System Workers, United States** Lorann Stallones, Colorado State University
12:45 p.m.	**Immigration, Farm Workers, and the Food System** Philip Martin, University of California, Davis
1:30 p.m.	**Adjourn**

Appendix B

Selected Metrics, Methodologies, Data, and Models

This appendix includes four tables—one each on metrics, methodologies, data sources, and models—that provide samples of existing resources for assessing food system effects. All of the tables have entries pertaining to health, environmental, social, and economic effects. They are meant to help researchers and assessors understand the availability of resources as they engage in complex system assessments.

The metrics table (see Table B-1) is designed to highlight measures commonly used to gauge key constructs that might be considered in doing an assessment. Each metric includes the purpose, the targeted group of persons or things that can be assessed with the measure, and basic information about how the measure is derived. Some of these metrics are indexes that provide an indication of several components simultaneously (e.g., the Healthy Eating Index). Other indicators are direct measurements of a variable.

The methodologies table (see Table B-2) provides key study designs, methodologies, and general models that can be used in complex system analyses or otherwise used to examine the effects of the food system.

The data sources table (see Table B-3) provides a list of some commonly used datasets that can be used in assessments of food system effects. Some of these are government funded, while others are proprietary; some are free, while others charge a fee. But all are publicly available. For each data source, the table includes the purpose of the resource, the target population of persons or things about which inferences can be drawn using the data, and sources of further information. Some data sources can be used to assess effects in various domains or to describe the food system itself. For example, food availability data can be considered an economic outcome of the food system or can be used to describe the nutritional quality of the food supply and to infer the health status of the population. To avoid duplication, only one entry was included in cases where a data source has more than one purpose across various domains of effects.

Finally, the models table (see Table B-4) includes examples of specific models that have been used to simulate effects of the food system. There is not a direct correspondence between the model entries in Table B-2 (methodologies) and Table B-4 (models), however. The models described in Table B-2 are broad, while those in Table B-4 are for specific realizations of a subset of methodologies.

The tables are meant to be illustrative, not comprehensive, and to show a selection of the most common metrics, methodologies, data sources, and models used. Furthermore, it is expected that research related to health, environmental, social, and economic effects as well as to the food system itself will continue to expand, leading to the evolution of these resources and the development of new ones.

APPENDIX B TABLES FOLLOW

TABLE B-1 Selected Metrics for Assessing Health, Environmental, Social, and Economic Effects of Food System

Metric	Purpose	Target Population	How Measured	For Further Information
HEALTH EFFECTS				
Body mass index	Indicator of appropriateness of weight for height; used to define and screen for overweight and obesity	General population	$\frac{\text{Mass (kg)}}{\text{Height (m)}^2}$	http://www.cdc.gov/healthyweight/assessing/bmi http://nccor.org/projects/catalogue/index.php http://nccor.org/projects/measures/index.php
Prevalence of disease	Indicator of the number of affected persons at a given time	General population	Number of cases of disease in the population at a given time; Number of persons in the population at same time	Gordis, L. 1996. *Epidemiology*. Philadelphia, PA: W.B. Saunders.
Incidence of disease	Indicator of the number of new cases of a disease that occur during a given period of time	General population	Number of new cases of disease in the population during a given period of time; Number of persons at risk of developing the disease during same time	Gordis, L. 1996. *Epidemiology*. Philadelphia, PA: W.B. Saunders.
Mortality rate	Indicator of proportion of population dying from particular cause or all causes	General population	Total number of deaths from particular cause (or all causes); Number of persons in the population at mid-year	Gordis, L. 1996. *Epidemiology*. Philadelphia, PA: W.B. Saunders.

Cholesterol	The total concentration of cholesterol present in blood, including low-density lipoprotein, high-density lipoprotein, and very-low-density lipoprotein; sometimes used as a screening test for heart disease	General population	Total amount of cholesterol (mg)/dL of blood	http://wwwn.cdc.gov/nchs/nhanes/2011-2012/TCHOL_G.htm
Blood mercury	An indicator of mercury exposure from all sources	General population, especially women of childbearing age	Total amount of mercury (elemental, inorganic, and organic) (ng)/mL of blood	http://www.cdc.gov/nchs/nhanes/nhanes2007-2008/pbcd_e.htm
Healthy Eating Index	Measure of diet quality that assesses conformance to federal dietary guidance	Individuals Foods available in markets or outlets Menus National food supply	Weighted score based on amounts of fruits; whole fruits; vegetables; greens and beans; whole grains; dairy; protein foods; seafood and plant proteins; refined grains; sodium; and empty calories per 1,000 kcal, and the amount of poly- plus mono-unsaturated fatty acids per amount of saturated fatty acids	http://www.cnpp.usda.gov/HealthyEatingIndex.htm http://www.cnpp.usda.gov/Publications/HEI/HEI-2010/CNPPFactSheetNo2.pdf

continued

TABLE B-1 Continued

Metric	Purpose	Target Population	How Measured	For Further Information
FoodNet	Measure national trends in outbreaks from year to year based on FoodNet database (see Table B-3)	General population	Estimate of the burden of illness for the most common or the most severe foodborne illness etiological agents, based on FoodNet outbreak database corrected for various factors, including rate of visiting the hospital when individuals suffer from diarrheal disease, how often specimens are collected in an attempt to identify the etiological agent involved, and specific tests that are run on samples provided	http://www.cdc.gov/foodborneburden/trends-in-foodborne-illness.htm
ENVIRONMENTAL EFFECTS				
Nitrate Groundwater Pollution Hazard Index		Farmers	The index works with an overlay of soil, crop, and irrigation information; based on the three components, an overall potential hazard number is assigned and management practices are suggested where necessary	http://ciwr.ucanr.edu/Tools/Nitrogen_Hazard_Index

Air Quality Index (AQI)	Index for reporting daily air quality	Local conditions for a variety of target populations	AQI is calculated using five major air pollutants regulated by the Clean Air Act: ground-level ozone, particle pollution (also known as particulate matter), carbon monoxide, sulfur dioxide, and nitrogen dioxide	http://www.airnow.gov/index.cfm?action=topics.about_airnow
Erodibility Index	Provides information on the potential of the soil to erode based on physical and chemical properties of the soil and climatic conditions	Farmers Resource managers	Combines the effects of slope and soil type, rainfall intensity, and land use	http://www.nrcs.usda.gov/wps/portal/nrcs/detail/national/technical/?cid=stelprdb1041925
SOCIAL AND ECONOMIC EFFECTS				
Income, Wealth, Equity				
Gross sectoral output and factor productivity	Assess the productivity of the use of different factors (labor, capital, land, etc.) in producing food	Aggregate farm sector	Index values are assigned to the various inputs and outputs associated with farm production; indexes allow comparisons across disparate types of inputs and commodities and across time	http://www.ers.usda.gov/data-products/agricultural-productivity-in-the-us.aspx

continued

TABLE B-1 Continued

Metric	Purpose	Target Population	How Measured	For Further Information
Sector profitability	Assess the economic performance of key industrial actors in food supply chain	Major food industry firms	Estimated profit margins for top U.S. companies	http://pages.stern.nyu.edu/~adamodar/New_Home_Page/datafile/margin.html http://money.cnn.com/magazines/fortune/fortune500/2009/performers/industries/profits
Industry structure (concentration)	Track changes in the concentration of production and ownership in different food supply chain sectors	Farm producers, food processors, manufacturers, distributors, and retailers	Four-Firm Index Gini Coefficient	http://www.ers.usda.gov/topics/farm-economy/farm-structure-and-organization/research-on-farm-structure-and-organization.aspx http://www.foodcircles.missouri.edu/consol.htm
Average net farm income	Document trends in the income and wealth position of farm operator households	Farm operator households	Indicators of average income and wealth position, distribution of farm households by income class	http://www.ers.usda.gov/data-products/farm-income-and-wealth-statistics.aspx http://www.ers.usda.gov/topics/farm-economy/farm-household-well-being.aspx http://ers.usda.gov/data-products/arms-farm-financial-and-crop-production-practices.aspx

Employment in food system industries	Determine levels and conditions of employment across different segments of food supply chain	Food supply chain sector	Indicators of employment level by sector	http://www.bls.gov/bls/employment.htm http://www.bls.gov/cps
Worker compensation; average and median household income; poverty rate in worker households	Track changes in wages and poverty among workers in different segments of food supply chain	Workers in food supply chain sectors	Mean wages, weeks of employment, and household poverty rates for workers in different sectors	http://www.bls.gov/bls/blswage.htm http://www.bls.gov/cps/earnings.htm#occind http://www.bls.gov/opub/ted/2003/jun/wk5/art04.htm http://www.bls.gov/cps
Quality of Life				
Farm operator managerial control (contracting, debt: asset ratio)	Track trends in economic relationships that affect independence of farm operators	Farm operator households	Levels of debt, presence of formal production, or marketing contracts	http://www.ers.usda.gov/topics/farm-economy/farm-sector-income-finances/assets,-debt,-and-wealth.aspx http://www.ers.usda.gov/topics/farm-economy/farm-structure-and-organization.aspx

continued

TABLE B-1 Continued

Metric	Purpose	Target Population	How Measured	For Further Information
Working conditions (hours, safety, stability, housing, access to benefits, opportunity for career mobility)	Examine quality of working conditions, pay and benefits for workers in different segments of food supply chain	Workers in different food supply chain sectors	Mean wages, hours of work, access to benefits, duration of employment	http://www.doleta.gov/agworker/naws.cfm http://www.ers.usda.gov/topics/farm-economy/farm-labor.aspx http://foodchainworkers.org/wp-content/uploads/2012/06/Hands-That-Feed-Us-Report.pdf http://www.bls.gov/bls/blswage.htm http://www.bls.gov/ncs/ebs/home.htm http://www.bls.gov/cps/lfcharacteristics.htm#tenure
Economic power (citizenship status of workers, unionization)	Examine social status and organization of workers in different food system industries	Food system industry sectors	Levels of unionization and citizenship status of workers by sector	http://www.bls.gov/cps/lfcharacteristics.htm#union http://www.bls.gov/cps/demographics.htm#foreignborn

Gender and racial equality	Examine differences in social and economic effects among genders and races	General population	Data are stratified by gender or race in order to identify differences	See discipline of topic-specific readings. For example, for health disparities see http://www.nlm.nih.gov/hsrinfo/disparities.html http://www.cdc.gov/chronicdisease/healthequity/index.htm
Worker Health and Safety				
Occupational injury rates (fatal and nonfatal)	Measure magnitude of workplace safety risks	Private-sector employers and employees	Provides injury and illness counts and rates by employer and employee characteristics	http://www.bls.gov/iif http://www.cdc.gov/niosh/injury
Food Availability				
Food Costs and Expenditures				
Food costs (prices and elasticities)		General population	Measures of the Consumer Price Index (CPI) as an indicator of changes in retail food prices, food expenditures, the food dollar series, which measures annual expenditures by U.S. consumers; and price spreads, which compare the prices paid by consumers for food with the prices received by farmers for their corresponding commodities	http://www.ers.usda.gov/topics/food-markets-prices/food-prices,-expenditures-costs.aspx#.VACGK2MXNkg http://www.fapri.iastate.edu/tools/elasticity.aspx http://www.ers.usda.gov/data-products/commodity-and-food-elasticities.aspx#.VACPUWMXNkg

continued

TABLE B-1 Continued

Metric	Purpose	Target Population	How Measured	For Further Information
Percentage of income spent on food (overall, by income, job, or health status)		General population		http://www.ers.usda.gov/data-products/food-expenditures.aspx#.VACPk2MXNkg
Percentage of food expenditures by food category, place of consumption		General population		http://www.ers.usda.gov/data-products/food-expenditures.aspx#.VACPk2MXNkg
				http://www.bls.gov/cex/2012/combined/quintile.pdf
Food Security				
Household and individual food security and insecurity		General population		http://www.ers.usda.gov/topics/food-nutrition-assistance/food-security-in-the-us/definitions-of-food-security.aspx#.VACQB2MXNkg
Participation in different nutrition programs (Supplemental Nutrition Assistance Programs [SNAP] and others)		General population		http://www.ers.usda.gov/topics/food-nutrition-assistance/supplemental-nutrition-assistance-program-%28snap%29.aspx#.VACQUWMXNkh

Food Access		
Density of full-service grocery stores; fast food operations	General population	http://www.ers.usda.gov/data-products/food-environment-atlas/about-the-atlas.aspx#.VACTF2MXNkg
		http://www.ers.usda.gov/data-products/food-access-research-atlas/.aspx
SNAP redemption at supermarkets	General population	http://www.ers.usda.gov/topics/food-nutrition-assistance/food-nutrition-assistance-research.aspx#.VACQ2mMXNkg
		Castner, L., and J. Henke. 2011. *Benefit redemption patterns in the Supplemental Nutrition Assistance Program*. Alexandria, VA: U.S. Department of Agriculture, Food and Nutrition Service, Office of Research and Analysis.

continued

TABLE B-1 Continued

Metric	Purpose	Target Population	How Measured	For Further Information
Availability of farmers' markets				http://www.ers.usda.gov/data-products/food-environment-atlas/about-the-atlas.aspx#.VACTF2MXNkg
Food Quality				
Changes in types of foods advertised				http://www.nielsen.com/content/corporate/us/en.html
				http://kff.org/other/food-for-thought-television-food-advertising-to
Changes in the number of healthful food offerings in food venues				
Sales of organic and other sustainably produced foods				http://www.ers.usda.gov/publications/eib-economic-information-bulletin/eib58.aspx#.U63LyqhGyTY
				https://www.ota.com/bookstore/14.html
				http://www.nationalsustainablesales.com/research-library

Sales of locally produced foods		http://www.usda.gov/wps/portal/usda/knowyourfarmer?navid=KNOWYOURFARMER
Time spent on food preparation		http://www.bls.gov/tus/atusfaqs.htm#1
Daily energy intake from home-prepared foods	General population	http://www.ers.usda.gov/topics/food-choices-health/food-consumption-demand/food-away-from-home.aspx#.VADUsWMXNkg
		http://www.ers.usda.gov/data-products/food-expenditures.aspx#.VADWFGMXNkg
Percentage of people who cook	General population	http://www.bls.gov/tus/atusfaqs.htm#1

TABLE B-2 Selected Methodologies for Assessing Health, Environmental, Social, and Economic Effects of Food System

Name	Description	Application (scientific paper where method has been used)	For Further Information
HEALTH EFFECTS			
Clinical trials	Study design that involves examining narrowly defined questions in the biomedical or behavioral fields, using an experimental design, with as much control over bias as possible	Appel, L. J., T. J. Moore, E. Obarzanek, W. M. Vollmer, L. P. Svetkey, F. M. Sacks, G. A. Bray, T. M. Vogt, J. A. Cutler, M. M. Windhauser, P. H. Lin, and N. Karanja. 1997. A clinical trial of the effects of dietary patterns on blood pressure. Dash collaborative research group. *New England Journal of Medicine* 336(16):1117-1124.	Gordis, L. 1996. *Epidemiology*. Philadelphia, PA: W.B. Saunders.
Cohort studies	Study design in which exposures of interest are assessed at baseline in a group (cohort) of people, and health outcomes occurring over time are then related to baseline exposures	Oh, K., F. B. Hu, J. E. Manson, M. J. Stampfer, and W. C. Willett. 2005. Dietary fat intake and risk of coronary heart disease in women: 20 years of follow-up of the Nurses' Health Study. *American Journal of Epidemiology* 161(7):672-679.	Gordis, L. 1996. *Epidemiology*. Philadelphia, PA: W.B. Saunders.
Case-control studies	Study design that involves comparing two groups of people, those with the disease or condition under study (cases) and a very similar group of people who do	Dahm, C. C., R. H. Keogh, E. A. Spencer, D. C. Greenwood, T. J. Key, I. S. Fentiman, M. J. Shipley, E. J. Brunner, J. E. Cade, V. J. Burley, G. Mishra, A. M. Stephen,	Gordis, L. 1996. *Epidemiology*. Philadelphia, PA: W.B. Saunders.

	not have the disease or condition (controls)	D. Kuh, I. R. White, R. Luben, M. A. Lentjes, K. T. Khaw, and S. A. Rodwell Bingham. 2010. Dietary fiber and colorectal cancer risk: A nested case-control study using food diaries. *Journal of the National Cancer Institute* 102(9):614-626.	
Microbial risk assessment for food and water	Standardized methodology for evaluating how likely it is that human health will be impacted by pathogenic microorganisms in foods and water	Akingbade, D., N. Bauer, S. Dennis, D. Gallagher, K. Hoelzer, J. Kause, R. Pouillot, M. Silverman, and J. Tang. 2013. *Draft interagency risk assessment—*Listeria monocytogenes *in retail delicatessens technical report.* Washington, DC: U.S. Department of Agriculture Food Safety and Inspection Service.	http://www.who.int/foodsafety/micro/jemra/en http://www.cdc.gov/foodsafety/microbial-risk-assessment.html
Chemical risk assessment for food and water	Standardized methodology for evaluating how likely it is that human health will be impacted by chemical additives and contaminants in foods	Food and Agriculture Organization. 2014. *Residue evaluation of certain veterinary drugs*. FAO JECFA Monographs 15. Rome, Italy: FAO.	http://www.who.int/foodsafety/chem/en

continued

TABLE B-2 Continued

Name	Description	Application (scientific paper where method has been used)	For Further Information
Health Impact Assessment	Systematic process that uses an array of data sources and analytic methods and considers input from stakeholders to determine the potential effects of a proposed policy, plan, program, or project on the health of a population and the distribution of those effects within the population; provides recommendations on monitoring and managing those effects	Health Impact Project. 2013. *Health impact assessment of proposed changes to the Supplemental Nutrition Assistance Program*. Washington, DC: The Pew Charitable Trusts and Robert Wood Johnson Foundation.	http://www.healthimpactproject.org
ENVIRONMENTAL EFFECTS			
Ecological Risk Assessment	Standardized process for evaluating how likely it is that the environment may be impacted as a result of exposure to environmental stressors such as chemicals, land change, disease, invasive species, and climate change	Solomon, K. R., J. P. Giesy, T. W. LaPoint, J. M. Giddings, and R. P. Richards. 2013. Ecological risk assessment of atrazine in North American surface waters. *Environmental Toxicology and Chemistry* 32(1):10-11.	http://www.epa.gov/risk
Environmental Assessment/ Environmental Impact Statement	A detailed analysis that serves to ensure that the policies and goals defined in the National Environmental Policy Act (NEPA) of 1969 (see 40 CFR Part 6) are addressed; NEPA requires federal	http://www.healthimpactproject.org/hia/us/red-dog-mine-extension-aqqaluk-project-final-supplemental-environmental-impact-statement	http://www.epa.ie/monitoringassessment/assessment/eia/#.Uz1ItFc9DK0

	agencies and others using federal funds or assets to assess the environmental impacts of major federal projects or decisions such as issuing permits, spending federal money, or affecting federal lands		
Life cycle assessment	Methodology to assess environmental impacts associated with a product's life from raw material to consumption, including waste disposal or recycling	Heller, M. C., and G. A. Keoleian. 2011. Life cycle energy and greenhouse gas analysis of a large-scale vertically integrated organic dairy in the united states. *Environmental Science and Technology* 45(5):1903-1910.	http://www.eiolca.net/Method/LCA_Primer.html Hendrickson, C. T., L. B. Lave, and H. S. Matthews. 2006. *Environmental life cycle assessment of goods and services: An input–output approach.* Washington, DC: Resources for the Future Press.
Rapid Bioassessment Protocols for Use in Streams and Wadeable Rivers	Practical technical reference for conducting cost-effective biological assessments of lotic systems	Jack, J., R. H. Kelley, and D. Stiles. 2006. Using stream bioassessment protocols to monitor impacts of a confined swine operation. *Journal of the American Water Resources Association* 42(3):747-753.	http://water.epa.gov/scitech/monitoring/rsl/bioassessment

continued

TABLE B-2 Continued

Name	Description	Application (scientific paper where method has been used)	For Further Information
SOCIAL AND ECONOMIC EFFECTS			
Social Impact Assessment	Processes of analyzing, monitoring, and managing the intended and unintended social consequences, both positive and negative, of planned interventions and any social change processes invoked by those interventions; primarily used outside of the United States	Mahmoudi, H., O. Renn, F. Vanclay, V. Hoffmann, and E. Karami. 2013. A framework for combining social impact assessment and risk assessment. *Environmental Impact Assessment Review* 43:1-8.	http://www.nmfs.noaa.gov/sfa/reg_svcs/social_impact_assess.htm
Benefit–cost analysis	Method to calculate a monetary measure of the aggregate change in individual well-being resulting from a project or a policy decision	Roberts, T., J. C. Buzby, and M. Ollinger. 1996. Using benefit and cost information to evaluate a food safety regulation: HACCP for meat and poultry. *American Journal of Agricultural Economics* 78(5):1297-1301.	http://evans.uw.edu/centers-projects/bcac/benefit-cost-analysis-center Boardman, A.E., D.H. Greenberg, A.R. Vining, and D.L. Weimer. 2011. *Cost-benefit analysis: Concepts and practice*, 4th ed. Upper Saddle River, NJ: Prentice-Hall.
Cost-effectiveness analysis	Methodology to compare the relative costs and outcomes (effects) from a project or a policy decision; cost-effectiveness analysis is distinct from benefit–cost analysis, which assigns a monetary value to the measure of effect	Sacks, G., J. L. Veerman, M. Moodie, and B. Swinburn. 2011. "Traffic-light" nutrition labelling and "junk-food" tax: A modelled comparison of cost-effectiveness for obesity prevention. *International Journal of Obesity* 35(7):1001-1009.	Drummond, M. F., M. J. Sculpher, G. W. Torrance, B. J. O'Brien, and G. L. Stoddart. 2005. *Methods for the economic evaluation of health care programmes*. Oxford, UK: Oxford University Press.

			Gold, M. R., J. E. Siegel, L. B. Russell, and M. C. Weinstein. 1996. *Cost-effectiveness in health and medicine.* New York: Oxford University Press.
Computable General Equilibrium	Method for measuring economic welfare changes due to market price and quantity feedbacks in response to changes in policy, technology, or another exogenous variable (e.g., climate)	Hertel, T. W., A. A. Golub, A. D. Jones, M. O'Hare, R. J. Plevin, and D. M. Kammen. 2010. Effects of US maize ethanol on global land use and greenhouse gas emissions: Estimating market-mediated responses. *BioScience* 60(3):223-231.	http://www.iadb.org/en/topics/trade/understanding-a-computable-general-equilibrium-model,1283.html
Total Factor Productivity Analysis	Index of the economic factors that contribute to growth in productivity (e.g., of agriculture)	Ball, V. E., C. A. K. Lovell, H. Luu, and R. Nehring. 2004. Incorporating environmental impacts in the measurement of agricultural productivity growth. *Journal of Agricultural and Resource Economics* 29(3):436-460.	http://www.ers.usda.gov/data-products/agricultural-productivity-in-the-us/findings,-documentation,-and-methods.aspx#.U1qm5aIeCdc
Non-market valuation	Method for placing monetary values on changes in levels of goods and services that lack markets, including health and environmental effects	Champ, P. A., K. J. Boyle, and T. C. Brown. 2003. *A primer on nonmarket valuation*. Dordrecht, The Netherlands: Kluwer Academic Publishers.	

continued

TABLE B-2 Continued

Name	Description	Application (scientific paper where method has been used)	For Further Information
Agent-based modeling	Methods for simulating the actions and interactions of individuals, organizations, and groups to assess their affects on the whole system	See Table B-4 on selected models.	http://www2.econ.iastate.edu/tesfatsi/abmread.htm Epstein, J. M. 2006. *Generative social science.* Princeton, NJ: Princeton University Press.
Systems dynamics modeling	Methods for simulating key dynamic stocks and flows, and key feedback cycles in operation within a system, to provide quantitative estimates of the potential system response to changes	Sterman, J. M. 2006. Learning from evidence in a complex world. *American Journal of Public Health* 96(3):505-514.	Sterman, J. M. 2000. *Business dynamics: Systems thinking for a complex world.* Boston, MA: Irwin/McGraw-Hill.
Food demand analysis/time series	To study the food demand response to prices, total expenditures, and other economic factors	Huang, K. S., and R. C. Haidacher. 1983. Estimation of a composite food demand system for the United States. *Journal of Business & Economic Statistics* 1(4):285-291.	

Food demand analysis/ cross-sectional analysis	Food consumption by individual household units is regressed on prices, income, and household characteristics to determine how demand varies by household characteristics; it allows for the incorporation of behavior and household environmental characteristics in the analysis	Okrent, A., and J. M. Alston. 2012. *The demand for disaggregated food-away-from-home and food-at-home products in the United States*. Economic Research Report No. ERR-139. Washington, DC: U.S. Department of Agriculture, Economic Research Service.

NOTE: Additional resources:
National Collaborative on Childhood Obesity's Catalogue of Surveillance Systems: http://nccor.org/projects/catalogue/index.php (accessed May 21, 2015).
National Collaborative on Childhood Obesity's Measures Registry: http://nccor.org/projects/measures/index.php (accessed May 21, 2015).

TABLE B-3 Selected Data Sources for Assessing Health, Environmental, Social, and Economic Effects of Food System

	Purpose	Target Population	Key Assessments	For Further Information
HEALTH EFFECTS				
National Health and Nutrition Examination Survey	Collect data about the health, nutritional status, and health behaviors of individuals in the United States	Civilian, non-institutionalized individuals in the United States; all ages	• Complete physical exam, including measured height and weight • Self-reported dietary intake • Demographics	http://www.cdc.gov/nchs/nhanes.htm
Behavioral Risk Factor Surveillance System	Collect state-specific data about preventive health practices and risk behaviors linked to chronic disease, injuries, and preventable infectious disease for adults in the United States	Adults living in households in all 50 states, the District of Columbia, Puerto Rico, the U.S. Virgin Islands, and Guam	• Demographics • Food security • Fruit and vegetable consumption • Quality of life	http://www.cdc.gov/BRFSS
Health and Diet Survey	Collect data about awareness, attitudes, and practices related to health and diet issues among consumers in the United States	Civilian, non-institutionalized adults age 18 and older in 50 states and the District of Columbia	• Demographics • Awareness of relationship between diet and specific diseases • Degree to which respondent makes household grocery purchasing decisions	http://www.fda.gov/Food/FoodScienceResearch/ConsumerBehaviorResearch/default.htm

			• Use of food labels • Knowledge of diet issues	
National Vital Statistics System	Collect data about births and deaths for individuals in the United States	Individuals in all 50 states, New York City, the District of Columbia, Puerto Rico, the U.S. Virgin Islands, Guam, American Samoa, and the Northern Mariana Islands	• Date of birth • Age at death • Race/ethnicity/sex • Cause of death	http://www.cdc.gov/nchs/nvss.htm
Food Patterns Equivalents Database	Convert foods and beverages to U.S. Department of Agriculture (USDA) Food Patterns components in order to characterize many kinds of foods and beverages reported in surveys and other types of studies into components that are relevant to dietary analysis and guidance	Foods reported on the 24-hour recalls in What We Eat in America portion of the National Health and Nutrition Examination Survey	• Total fruit (cup equivalents) • Total vegetables (cup equivalents) • Whole grains (oz equivalents) • Total protein foods (oz equivalents) • Dairy (cup equivalents) • Added sugars (teaspoons) • Solid fats (gram equivalents)	http://www.ars.usda.gov/Services/docs.htm?docid=23871

continued

TABLE B-3 Continued

	Purpose	Target Population	Key Assessments	For Further Information
Foodborne Diseases Active Surveillance Network	Outbreak data from active surveillance in 10 sentinel sites across the United States	10 sentinel sites (Connecticut, Georgia, Maryland, Minnesota, New Mexico, Oregon, Tennessee, and certain counties in California, Colorado, and New York), FDA and USDA-FSIS (Food Safety and Inspection Service); the information collected is used to estimate the burden of illness caused by the specific agent; breaks down estimates by age category and regions	Tracks foodborne illness from the most common agents: *Campylobacter*, *Listeria*, *Salmonella*, Shiga toxin-producing *Escherichia coli*, *Shigella*, *Vibrio* and *Yersinia*, and the parasites *Cryptosporidium* and *Cyclospora*	http://www.cdc.gov/foodnet/data/trends/index.html
Foodborne Outbreak Online Database	Provide access to national information on reported foodborne illness outbreak data	Outbreaks reported by state, local, and territorial public health departments through a Web-based program, the National Outbreak Reporting System	• Etiology; location of consumption; total ill, hospitalized, and deaths; food vehicle and contaminated vehicle where available • Insight into the types of foods involved in outbreaks • Some information on factors contributing to illness	http://wwwn.cdc.gov/foodborneoutbreaks

Estimates of Foodborne Illness Attribution	Estimate the most common food sources for specific foodborne illnesses	General population	• Etiology, illnesses and deaths • Breakdown by specific food categories	http://www.cdc.gov/foodborneburden/attribution/index.html
Risk and Safety Assessments for Food	Site contains formal microbial and chemical risk assessments conducted for foods	General population		http://www.fda.gov/Food/FoodScienceResearch/RiskSafetyAssessment/default.htm
National Antimicrobial Resistance Monitoring System	Monitor changes in susceptibility of select bacteria to antimicrobial agents of human and veterinary importance	Foodborne isolates collected from humans, animals, and retail meats	Antimicrobial resistance	http://www.cdc.gov/narms
Pesticide Data Program	Collect pesticide residue data	Meat, poultry, and egg products	Pesticide residues	http://www.ams.usda.gov/AMSv1.0/PDP
Total Diet Study	Ongoing market-based study to collect data on levels of contaminants and nutrients in foods	280 core foods in retail stores	Contaminants in foods (e.g., acrylamide and perchlorate)	http://www.fda.gov/food/foodscienceresearch/totaldietstudy/default.htm
Registration and chemical-specific information	Information about pesticides	Pesticides	Toxicity, use patterns, and registration status	http://www.epa.gov/pesticides/food/risks.htm

continued

TABLE B-3 Continued

	Purpose	Target Population	Key Assessments	For Further Information
ENVIRONMENTAL EFFECTS				
National Water Information System	Collect the occurrence, quantity, quality, distribution, and movement of surface and groundwater; analyzes the chemical, physical, and biological properties of water, sediment, and tissue samples from across the United States	Water-resources data collected at approximately 1.5 million sites in all 50 U.S. states, the District of Columbia, Puerto Rico, the U.S. Virgin Islands, Guam, American Samoa, and the Commonwealth of the Northern Mariana Islands	• Water flow and levels in streams and lakes • Water level in wells • Chemical and physical data for streams, lakes, wells, and other sites • Water use • Current and historical water-quality data and summary statistics	http://waterdata.usgs.gov/nwis http://water.usgs.gov/owq/data.html
Air Quality System	Repository of ambient air quality data	Data collected by Environmental Protection Agency and state, local, and tribal air pollution control agencies in the United States from more than 10,000 monitors, 5,000 of which are currently active	• Data include lead, ozone, particulate matter and fine particulate matter, sulfur dioxide, oxides of nitrogen (NO, NO_2, NO_x, NO_y), volatile organic compounds	http://www.epa.gov/ttn/airs/airsaqs

ECOTOX Database	Provide single-chemical toxicity information for aquatic life, terrestrial plants, and wildlife	Toxicity data derived predominately from the peer-reviewed literature, for aquatic life, terrestrial plants, and terrestrial wildlife	• Lethal, sublethal, and residue effects of chemicals on aquatic species, including plants and animals as well as freshwater and saltwater species • Toxicity information for use in characterizing, diagnosing, and predicting effects associated with chemical stressors and to support the development of ecocriteria and thresholds for natural resource use	http://cfpub.epa.gov/ecotox
Farm Financial and Crop Production Practices	Collect information on the financial condition, production practices, and resource use of America's farm businesses and rural households	National survey of agricultural producers that provides observations of field-level farm practices, the economics of the farm businesses, and the characteristics of farm operators	Data on nutrient use, pesticide use, conservation practices, pest management practices, irrigation technology and water use, etc., for select crops and U.S. states	http://www.ers.usda.gov/data-products/arms-farm-financial-and-crop-production-practices

continued

TABLE B-3 Continued

	Purpose	Target Population	Key Assessments	For Further Information
Geospatial Data Gateway	Provide a gateway to available geospatial environmental and natural resources data	Provides geospatial data produced or financed by USDA Service Center Agencies to any user; data outside these parameters is only available to USDA personnel	• Precipitation • Temperature • Elevation • Land-use cover • Hydrologic units • Soils • Topography	http://datagateway.nrcs.usda.gov
CropScape	Collect data about crop-specific and non-agricultural land cover in the United States	Farms within the contiguous continental United States	• Crop acreage • Crop type • Latitude/longitude, county, district, state	http://nassgeodata.gmu.edu/CropScape
Annual Agricultural Statistics	Collect data about the production, economics, and demographics of agriculture and its environment in the United States	Agricultural statistics in 50 U.S. states and the District of Columbia	• Acreage, yield, stock in storage, and volume production • Commodity sales volume and price • Commodity use • Commodity-based products production • Chemical usage • Prices paid by producers • Prices received by producers • Farm production expenditures	http://www.nass.usda.gov/Surveys/index.asp

Pesticide Data Program	Collect data about pesticide residues in food commodities and drinking water in the United States	More than 105 different commodities, including fresh and processed fruits and vegetables, meat and poultry, grains, specialty products, bottled water, municipal drinking water, and private and school/childcare facility well water	• Pesticide and compound class • Collection facility type • Commodity • Commodity type and origin • Residue level • State, Census region	http://www.ams.usda.gov/AMSv1.0/pdp
Quantis World Food life cycle assessments (LCAs) database	Provide reliable and up-to-date data for more accurate food and beverage LCAs, decisions, and communication. (Private, proprietary data.)	Reliable, transparent, and up-to-date database for environmental assessments, including more than 200 datasets within 10 categories	• Compliant with ecoinvent's quality guidelines • Compatible and coherent with existing software and databases, e.g., SimaPro, GaBi, Quantis	http://www.quantis-intl.com/wfldb

continued

TABLE B-3 Continued

	Purpose	Target Population	Key Assessments	For Further Information
SOCIAL AND ECONOMIC EFFECTS				
Consumer Expenditure Survey	Collect data about buying habits (e.g., food expenditures), income, and other characteristics of households in the United States	Households and families (referred to as "consumer units")	• Expenditures on specific types of foods purchased for home consumption and consumed away from home • Demographics • Geocodes • Inventory of durable goods in home (e.g., toys/games, electronic entertainment equipment, cooking equipment, exercise equipment)	http://www.bls.gov/cex
Center for Nutrition Policy and Promotion Food Prices Database	Collect data about estimated cost of specific food items consumed in the United States	Food items that were purchased by individuals and families in the 48 contiguous states and the District of Columbia	• Average national prices for individual foods • Census region	http://www.cnpp.usda.gov/usdafoodplanscostoffood.htm
Agricultural and food economic data	Data about U.S. and foreign agricultural prices, costs, inputs, production levels, incomes, and environmental effects	U.S. agriculture and food	• Crops • Farm economy • Farm practices and management • Food and nutrition assistance	http://www.ers.usda.gov/data-products.aspx http://www.nass.usda.gov/Surveys/index.asp

			• Food choices and health • Food markets and prices • Food safety • International markets and trade • Natural resources and environment • Rural economy	
Census of Agriculture	Collect data about production, sales, agricultural practices, and sales practices for farms, ranches, and the people who operate them in the United States and its territories	Farms, ranches, and their operators in all 50 states and territories, including American Samoa, Puerto Rico, Commonwealth of the Northern Mariana Islands, Guam, and the U.S. Virgin Islands	• Demographics such as age, race/ethnicity, and sex of farm operators; farm income • Farm locations (state and county) • Farm production • Farm production practices • Farm sizes • Gross annual sales of specific farm • Market value of farm products sold • Marketing practices • Number of organic farms by state • Types and amounts of specific commodities produced by farms	http://www.agcensus.usda.gov

continued

TABLE B-3 Continued

	Purpose	Target Population	Key Assessments	For Further Information
InfoUSA	Collect data about types of businesses in a community in the United States	Businesses and consumers in the United States and Canada	• Address, latitude and longitude, neighborhood, zip code • Business type and name • Housing type • Home value	http://www.infousa.com
National Survey of America's Families	Collect data on demographic, economic, housing, and other factors relevant to the well-being of children and adults younger than age 65 residing in households in the United States	Noninstitutionalized, civilian population younger than age 65 in the United States; the survey focuses on individuals residing in households with incomes below 200 percent of the federal poverty threshold	• Detailed information about income and income sources for low-income families with children • Food security • Detailed information about various types of food assistance	http://www.urban.org/center/anf/nsaf.cfm
Food Environment Atlas	Assemble statistics on food environment indicators to stimulate research on the determinants of food choices and diet quality, and to provide a spatial overview of a community's ability to access healthy food and its success in doing so	Counties in the United States	• Community's access to and acquisition of healthy, affordable food • Community's success in maintaining healthy diets • Demographics • Natural amenities	http://www.ers.usda.gov/data-products/food-environment-atlas/about-the-atlas.aspx

Household Food Security Survey Module	Assess food security within a household over the past 30 days or past 12 months	Households	18 items on food situation within the household, ranging in severity from worry about running out of food to adults and children going a whole day without food because of lack of financial resources; three-stage design with screeners	http://www.ers.usda.gov/topics/food-nutrition-assistance/food-security-in-the-us/survey-tools.aspx#household
Food Availability (per capita) Data System	Collect estimated data regarding foods, nutrients, and calories available for consumption for each individual in the United States	Commodity foods and nutrients available for consumption in the United States	• Food balance calculations • Food availability data, adjusted for loss and spoilage • Food availability data linked to nutrient composition data	http://www.ers.usda.gov/data-products/food-availability-(per-capita)-data-system.aspx

continued

TABLE B-3 Continued

	Purpose	Target Population	Key Assessments	For Further Information
Quarterly Food-at-Home Price Database	Provide estimates of average market-level prices for more than 50 food groups in the United States	U.S. households in the 48 contiguous states	• Average quarterly prices (dollars per 100 grams of food) for several categories of fruits and vegetables; grains and dairy products; meats, beans, nuts, and eggs; and fats/oils, beverages, and prepared foods • Geocode linkage: county, Census region, Census division	http://www.ers.usda.gov/data-products/quarterly-food-at-home-price-database.aspx
Food consumption and nutrient intake	Food consumption and nutrient intake by food source and demographic characteristics	U.S. households in the 48 contiguous states	• Average daily intake by food groups • Density (the amount of food for each 1,000 calories contained in an American diet) • Average daily intakes of fats, sodium, and cholesterol, but underconsume calcium, fiber, and iron • Mean nutrient intakes are reported by food source and by nutrient density	http://www.ers.usda.gov/data-products/food-consumption-and-nutrient-intakes.aspx

Gladson Nutrition Database	Collect data about ingredient content and nutrition labels for packaged food and beverage products sold in the United States	Food products sold in the United States	• Product ingredients • Product nutrition labeling information • Product package dimensions • Product package images • Serving size information (household unit and gram weight)	http://www.gladson.com/SERVICES/NutritionDatabase/tabid/89/Default.aspx
MenuStat	Collect nutrition data about menu items in the largest restaurant chains in the United States	Menu items from the largest chain restaurants in the United States	• Restaurant name • Year • Serving size • Calories and nutrients • Menu type (e.g., breakfast, kids)	http://menustat.org/about
Datamonitor Product Launch Analytics	Collect data about newly launched consumer packaged goods in retail markets around the world	Newly launched consumer packaged goods from around the world	• Product name, brand, and varieties • UPC code • Nutrition facts information • Product claim • Ingredients • Package format, material, and size	http://www.productscan.com

continued

TABLE B-3 Continued

	Purpose	Target Population	Key Assessments	For Further Information
Absolute difference in health disparities	Measure of absolute difference in health outcome among groups	Individuals and subgroups in a population	Health parameter measured in group A/ Health parameter measured in group B	http://seer.cancer.gov/publications/disparities2
Relative difference in health disparities	Measure of relative difference in health outcome among groups	Individuals and subgroups in a population	Health parameter measured in group A/ Health parameter measured in group B	http://seer.cancer.gov/publications/disparities2
Census of Fatal Occupational Injuries	Produce comprehensive, accurate, and timely annual counts of occupational injury fatalities	All fatal work injuries in the United States	Uses multiple data sources including death certificates, workers' compensation reports, and federal and state agency administrative reports to collect information on each workplace fatality	http://www.bls.gov/iif/oshcfoi1.htm
Survey of Occupational Injuries and Illnesses	Describe the magnitude of work-related injury and illnesses that are recordable, i.e., require at least 1 day away from work to recuperate	Data on nonfatal workplace injuries and illnesses from an annual survey of roughly 250,000 private employers, state governments, and local governments	Includes information about the case circumstances and worker characteristics for occupational injury and illnesses that involve lost work time, medical treatment other than first aid, restriction of work or motion, loss of consciousness, or	http://www.bls.gov/iif/oshcase1.htm

			transfer to another job; employers keep counts of injuries separate from illnesses	
Occupational Injury Surveillance of Production Agriculture Survey	Track nonfatal injuries occurring to adults working in agriculture	National surveillance system conducted in 2001, 2004, and 2009	Designed to produce national and regional estimates of the number of adults age 20 years and older working on farms and the number of occupational injuries that these workers incur	http://www.cdc.gov/niosh/topics/aginjury/OISPA/default.html
County Sprawl Index	A measure of urban sprawl, a pattern of land use epitomized by low-density development around urban areas	Counties in the United States	This updated sprawl index for 2000 and 2010 incorporates four dimensions of sprawl derived from 17 variables—density, land-use mix, population or employment concentrations ("centering"), and street characteristics; principal components analysis was used to extract factors from each of these dimensions and these were combined into a single index	http://gis.cancer.gov/tools/urban-sprawl

TABLE B-4 Selected Models for Assessing Health, Environmental, Social, and Economic Effects of Food System

Name	Description	Application (scientific paper where method has been used)	For More Information
HEALTH EFFECTS			
PMP (Pathogen Modeling Program)	Predict growth or inactivation of selected foodborne pathogens under different conditions, including temperature, water activity, pH, and other parameters	Numerous references available on the website provided in this table	http://pmp.errc.ars.usda.gov/PMPOnline.aspx
ENVIRONMENTAL EFFECTS			
RUSLE2 (Revised Universal Soil Loss Equation)	Predict rill and interrill erosion in response to runoff; based on climate, soil, topography, and management practices	Schipanski, M. E., M. Barbercheck, M. R. Douglas, D. M. Finney, K. Haider, J. P. Kaye, A. R. Kemanian, D. A. Mortensen, M. R. Ryan, J. Tooker, and C. White. 2014. A framework for evaluating ecosystem services provided by cover crops in agroecosystems. *Agricultural Systems* 125:12-22.	http://www.nrcs.usda.gov/wps/portal/nrcs/main/national/technical/tools/rusle2 http://www.ars.usda.gov/Research/docs.htm?docid=24403
WEPS (Wind Erosion Prediction System)	Predict wind erosion	Van Donk, S. J., and E. L. Skidmore. 2003. Measurement and simulation of wind erosion, roughness degradation and residue decomposition on an agricultural field. *Earth Surface Processes and Landforms* 28(11):1243-1258.	http://www.nrcs.usda.gov/wps/portal/nrcs/main/national/technical/tools/weps

GLEAMS (Groundwater Loading Effects on Agricultural Management Systems)	Evaluate the effects of agricultural practices on the movement of chemicals within and through the plant root zone	Bosch, D. J., M. L. Wolfe, and K. E. Knowlton. 2006. Reducing phosphorus runoff from dairy farms. *Journal of Environmental Quality* 35(3):918-927.	http://www.tifton.uga.edu/sewrl/Gleams/gleams_y2k_update.htm
WATSUIT (Water Suitability Determination Model)	Steady-state computer model to predict soil water salinity and sodicity under a particular irrigation water of given composition and leaching fraction	Visconti, F., J. M. de Paz, J. L. Rubio, and J. Sanchez. 2012. Comparison of four steady-state models of increasing complexity for assessing the leaching requirement in agricultural salt-threatened soils. *Spanish Journal of Agricultural Research* 10(1):222-237.	http://www.xuan-wu.com/2012-03-10-Watsuit
HYDRUS-1D	Microsoft Windows–based modeling environment for analysis of water flow and solute transport in variably saturated porous media	Shouse, P. J., J. E. Ayars, and J. Simunek. 2011. Simulating root water uptake from a shallow saline groundwater resource. *Agricultural Water Management* 98(5):784-790.	http://www.ars.usda.gov/Services/docs.htm?docid=8921
ENVIRO-GRO	Simulate subsurface variably saturated water flow, solute transport, root water uptake, nitrogen uptake, and relative yield for agricultural applications	Letey, J., and P. Vaughan. 2013. Soil type, crop and irrigation technique affect nitrogen leaching to groundwater. *California Agriculture* 67(4):231-241.	http://ciwr.ucanr.edu/Tools/ENVIRO-GRO

continued

TABLE B-4 Continued

Name	Description	Application (scientific paper where method has been used)	For More Information
EPIC (Environmental Policy Integrated Climate)	Simulate growth of approximately 80 crops using weather data. It predicts effects of management decisions on soil, water, nutrient, and pesticide movements, and their combined impact on soil loss, water quality, and crop yields for areas with homogeneous soils and management	Williams, J. R., C. A. Jones, J. R. Kiniry, and D. A. Spanel. 1989. The epic crop growth-model. *Transactions of the ASAE* 32(2):497-511. Gassman, P. W., J. R. Williams, V. W. Benson, R. C. Izaurralde, L. M. Hauck, C. A. Jones, J. R. Atwood, J. R. Kiniry, and J. D. Flowers. 2005. *Historical development and applications of the EPIC and APEX models.* Working paper 05-WP 397. Ames, IA: Center for Agriculture and Rural Development, Iowa State University.	http://epicapex.tamu.edu/epic
CENTURY and DAYCENT models	CENTURY is a general model of plant–soil nutrient cycling that is being used to simulate carbon and nutrient dynamics for different types of ecosystems, including grasslands, agricultural lands, forests, and savannas; DAYCENT is the daily time-step version	Parton, W. J., D. S. Schimel, C. V. Cole, and D. S. Ojima. 1987. Analysis of factors controlling soil organic-matter levels in Great-Plains grasslands. *Soil Science Society of America Journal* 51(5):1173-1179.	http://www.nrel.colostate.edu/projects/daycent https://www.nrel.colostate.edu/projects/century5

SWAT (Soil and Water Assessment Tool)	Small watershed to river basin-scale model to simulate soil erosion prevention and control, non-point source pollution control, and regional management in watersheds	Gassman, P. W., M. R. Reyes, C. H. Green, and J. G. Arnold. 2007. The soil and water assessment tool: Historical development, applications, and future research directions. *Transactions of the ASABE* 50(4):1211-1250.	http://swat.tamu.edu
GREET (Greenhouse Gases, Regulated Emissions, and Energy Use in Transportation Model)	Life cycle model of greenhouse gas emissions in the transportation sector developed to fully evaluate energy and emission impacts of advanced vehicle technologies and new transportation fuels, the fuel cycle from wells to wheels, and the vehicle cycle through material recovery and vehicle disposal need to be considered	Wang, M., J. Han, J. B. Dunn, H. Cai, and A. Elgowainy. 2012. Well-to-wheels energy use and greenhouse gas emissions of ethanol from corn, sugarcane and cellulosic biomass for US use. *Environmental Research Letters* 7(4):1-13.	https://greet.es.anl.gov https://greet.es.anl.gov/greet/documentation.html
EIO-LCA (Economic Input-Output Life Cycle Assessment)	Estimates the materials and energy resources required for, and the environmental emissions resulting from, activities in our economy	Hendrickson, C. T., L. B. Lave, and H. S. Matthews. 2006. *Environmental life cycle assessment of goods and service: An input–output approach*. Washington, DC: Resources for the Future Press.	http://www.eiolca.net

continued

TABLE B-4 Continued

Name	Description	Application (scientific paper where method has been used)	For More Information
SOCIAL AND ECONOMIC EFFECTS			
Global Trade Analysis Project (GTAP)	Multiregion, multisector, computable general equilibrium model, with perfect competition and constant returns to scale. The GTAP-E model estimates greenhouse gas effects related to international trade. The focus is on market and environmental effects of economic growth, policy changes, and changes in resource availability	Hertel, T. W., W. E. Tyner, and D. K. Birur. 2010. The global impacts of biofuel mandates. *Energy Journal* 31(1):75-100.	https://www.gtap.agecon.purdue.edu/about/getting_started.asp https://www.gtap.agecon.purdue.edu/products/gtap_book.asp
IMPACT Model	Computable general equilibrium model designed to examine alternative futures for global food supply, demand, trade, prices, and food security, along with bioenergy, climate change, water, changing diet/food preferences, and other themes	Rosegrant, M. W., M. Agcaoili-Sombilla, and N. D. Perez. 1995. *Global Food Projections to 2020: Implications for Investment*. 2020 Discussion Paper No. 5. Washington, DC: International Food Policy Research Institute.	http://www.ifpri.org/book-751/ourwork/program/impact-model http://www.ifpri.org/sites/default/files/publications/impactwater2012.pdf
FASOM-GHG (Forestry and Agricultural Sector Optimization Model with Greenhouse Gases Model)	Dynamic partial-equilibrium sectoral model used to simulate potential future impacts of policies on land use, GHG fluxes, and commodity markets within the agricultural and forestry sectors	Schneider, U. A., B. A. McCarl, and E. Schmid. 2007. Agricultural sector analysis on greenhouse gas mitigation in US agriculture and forestry. *Agricultural Systems* 94(2):128-140.	http://www.epa.gov/climatechange/EPAactivities/economics/modeling/peerreview_FASOM.html http://agecon2.tamu.edu/people/faculty/mccarl-bruce/FASOM.html

FAPRI (Food and Agricultural Policy Research Institute)	Develops projections for the U.S. agricultural sector and international commodity markets using comprehensive data and computer modeling systems of the world agricultural market	Meyers, W. H., P. Westhoff, J. F. Fabiosa, and D. J. Hayes. 2010. The FAPRI global modeling system and outlook process. *Journal of International Agricultural Trade and Development* 6(1):1-20.	http://www.fapri.org

Appendix C

Acronyms

ACA	Patient Protection and Affordable Care Act
AR	antibiotic resistance
b. lbs	billion pounds
BCA	benefit–cost analysis
BLS	Bureau of Labor Statistics
BMI	body mass index
CAFO	concentrated animal feeding operation
CDC	Centers for Disease Control and Prevention
CEA	cost-effectiveness analysis
CHD	coronary heart disease
CO	carbon monoxide
CPI	Consumer Price Index
CVD	cardiovascular disease
CWA	Clean Water Act
DGA	*Dietary Guidelines for Americans*
DGAC	Dietary Guidelines for Americans Committee
DNDC	Denitrification/Decomposition
DRI	Dietary Reference Intake
EIA	environmental impact assessment
EISA	Energy Independence and Security Act
EPA	Environmental Protection Agency

ERS	Economic Research Service
EU	European Union
FAFH	food away from home
FAH	food at home
FAO	Food and Agriculture Organization of the United Nations
FDA	U.S. Food and Drug Administration
FFV	flex fuel vehicle
FSMA	Food Safety Modernization Act
GDP	gross domestic product
GFSI	Global Food Security Index
GHG	greenhouse gas
GMO	genetically modified organism
H_2S	hydrogen sulfite
HACCP	Hazard Analysis and Critical Control Points
HIA	health impact assessment
IOM	Institute of Medicine
ISO	International Organization for Standardization
LCA	life cycle assessment
LEAP	Livestock Environmental Assessment and Performance Partnership
MTHFR	methylenetetrahydrofolate reductase
NH_3	ammonia
NHANES	National Health and Nutrition Examination Survey
NIOSH	National Institute for Occupational Safety and Health
NO_2	nitrogen dioxide
NORS	National Outbreak Reporting System
NPS	non-point source pollution
NRC	National Research Council
NRCS	Natural Resources Conservation Service
O_3	ozone
PM	particulate matter
QALY	quality-adjusted life year

RCT	randomized controlled trial
RDA	Recommended Dietary Allowance
RFS	Renewable Fuel Standard
SES	socioeconomic status
SLP	School Lunch Program
SNAP	Supplemental Nutrition Assistance Program
SO_2	sulfur dioxide
STEC	Shiga toxin-producing *Escherichia coli*
SWF	social welfare function
TFP	Thrifty Food Plan
USDA	U.S. Department of Agriculture
USGS	U.S. Geological Survey
VOC	volatile organic compound
WDR	waste discharge requirement
WIC	Special Supplemental Nutrition Program for Women, Infants, and Children

Appendix D

Committee Member Biographical Sketches

Malden C. Nesheim, Ph.D. (*Chair*) is provost emeritus and professor of nutrition emeritus at Cornell University. His previous positions have included director of the Division of Nutritional Sciences and vice president for planning and budgeting at Cornell University. He has also served as chair of the Board of Trustees of the Pan American Health and Education Foundation, President of the American Institute of Nutrition, chair of the National Institutes of Health Nutrition Study Section, and chair of the National Nutrition Consortium. He also chaired the 1990 U.S. Department of Agriculture (USDA)/Department of Health and Human Services Dietary Guidelines Advisory Committee and has been on the USDA Board of Scientific Counselors. Dr. Nesheim has served as an advisor to the Office of Science and Technology Policy and chaired the Presidential Commission on Dietary Supplement Labels, appointed in 1996-98 to consider regulatory matters relative to marketing dietary supplements. He is a Fellow of the American Society for Nutritional Sciences and of the American Academy of Arts and Sciences. Dr. Nesheim is the recipient of numerous awards, including the Conrad A. Elvejhem Award for Distinguished Service to the Public Through the Science of Nutrition. His research interests are in human and animal nutrition, and nutritional assessment and nutrition policy. He has written extensively on animal and human nutrition and agriculture production. His research has focused on both domestic and international matters. He has contributed to many National Academy of Sciences (NAS) activities. Dr. Nesheim is a past member of the Institute of Medicine (IOM) Food and Nutrition Board. He previously served as chair of the IOM Committee on Nutrient Relationships in Seafood: Selections to Balance Benefits and Risks, and served as the vice chair and chair of the IOM Committee on International Nutrition Programs. He was also a member of the Subcommittee on the 10th Edition of the Recommended Dietary Allowances and an ex officio member of the U.S. National Committee of the International Union of Nutritional Sciences. Dr. Nesheim was elected a National Associate of the NAS in 2008. He received a Ph.D. in nutrition from Cornell University as well as an M.S. in animal nutrition and a B.S. in agricultural science.

Katherine (Kate) Clancy, Ph.D., is currently a food systems consultant, visiting scholar at the Center for a Livable Future Johns Hopkins Bloomberg School of Public Health, adjunct professor at Tufts University, and Senior Fellow in the Minnesota Institute for Sustainable Agriculture, University of Minnesota (she resides in University Park, Maryland). She has held faculty positions at Cornell University and Syracuse University, the Federal Trade Commission, and nonprofits such as the Wallace Center for Agricultural and Environmental Policy, the Union of Concerned Scientists, and the National Center for Food and Agricultural Policy. She has served on numerous boards (Society for Nutrition Education, Bread for the World, Wallace Institute for Alternative Agriculture, Consortium for Sustainable Agriculture Research and Education, Michael Fields Agricultural Institute, and the Agriculture Food and Human Values Society, among others). Her current interests are the research and policy facets of Agriculture of the Middle, the development of regional food systems, food supply chain analyses, the connections between community food security and regional food security, and the research needed to advance sustainable agriculture and food systems policy. Dr. Clancy is a member of the IOM Planning Committee on Sustainable Diets: Food and Healthy People and a Healthy Planet: A Workshop. She received her Ph.D. in nutrition sciences from the University of California (UC), Berkeley.

James K. Hammitt, Ph.D., is professor of economics and decision sciences and director of the Center for Risk Analysis at the Harvard School of Public Health. His research and teaching concern the development of decision analysis, benefit–cost analysis, and other quantitative methods and their application to health and environmental policy. Dr. Hammitt is particularly interested in comprehensive evaluation of risk control measures (including ancillary benefits and countervailing risks) and alternative methods for measuring the value of reducing health risks, including monetary and health-adjusted life-year metrics. He served as a member of the Environmental Protection Agency (EPA) Science Advisory Board and its Environmental Economics Advisory Committee and chaired the EPA Advisory Council on Clear Air Compliance Analysis. He also served as a member of the American Statistical Association Committee on Energy Statistics

(Advisory Committee to the U.S. Energy Information Administration) and on the National Research Council (NRC) and the IOM panels on dioxin in the food supply, external costs and benefits of energy production and consumption, and measures of health benefits for environmental, health, and safety regulation. He held the Pierre-de-Fermat Chaire d'Éxcellence at the Toulouse School of Economics and served as senior mathematician at the RAND Corporation. Dr. Hammitt received his Ph.D. in public policy from Harvard University.

Ross A. Hammond, Ph.D., is senior fellow in economic studies at The Brookings Institution, where he is also director of the Center on Social Dynamics and Policy. His primary area of expertise is modeling complex social dynamics in economic, political, and public health systems. Dr. Hammond has more than 15 years of experience with mathematical and computational modeling techniques from complex systems science. His current research topics include obesity, behavioral epidemiology, food systems, tobacco control, corruption, segregation, trust, and decision making. He has authored numerous scientific articles, and his work has been featured in *New Scientist*, *Salon*, *The Atlantic Monthly*, *Scientific American*, and major news media. Dr. Hammond currently serves on the editorial board of the journal *Childhood Obesity*; on the steering committee for the National Institutes of Health (NIH) Comparative Modeling Network of the National Collaborative on Childhood Obesity Research; and as a member of the NIH MIDAS (Models of Infectious Disease Agent Study) and NICH (Network on Inequality, Complexity, and Health) networks. Dr. Hammond has been a consultant to the World Bank, the Asian Development Bank, the IOM, and NIH. He has taught computational modeling at Harvard School of Public Health, the University of Michigan, Washington University, and the NIH/Centers for Disease Control and Prevention Institute on Systems Science and Health. He has previously held positions as the Okun-Model Fellow in Economics, a National Science Foundation Fellow in the Center for the Study of Complex Systems at University of Michigan, a visiting scholar at The Santa Fe Institute, and a consultant at PricewaterhouseCoopers, LLP. Dr. Hammond received his B.A. from Williams College and his Ph.D. from the University of Michigan.

Darren L. Haver, Ph.D., is the water resources/water quality advisor and county director for the UC Cooperative Extension in Orange County and center director of the South Coast Research and Extension Center in Orange County. His research and extension efforts focus on protecting local water resources and water quality through pollutant source identification and transport; identification and implementation of pollutant mitigation management methods and practices; and reduced water consumption in agricultural, urban, and natural environments. He earned his Ph.D. in botany and plant physiology from UC Irvine.

Douglas Jackson-Smith, Ph.D., is professor and director of graduate studies in the Department of Sociology, Social Work, and Anthropology at Utah State University (USU). His principal teaching and research interests include the sociology of agriculture, natural resources and the environment, rural community studies, human dimensions of water systems, and applied research methods. Dr. Jackson-Smith is also interested in international development, social studies of science and technology, and political and economic sociology. Currently, he is engaged in research focusing on the social, cultural, and institutional drivers of environmental behaviors; interdisciplinary studies of coupled human–natural systems; and dynamics of economic and technological change in agriculture and their effects on farm families, rural communities, and the environment. He is also developing methods to track the spatial patterns of rural and agricultural land-use changes to evaluate the effectiveness and impacts of exurban land-use planning in the Intermountain West. Dr. Jackson-Smith recently served on the NRC Committee to Study 21st Century Agricultural Systems. Before coming to USU, he served as assistant professor of rural sociology and urban and regional planning at the University of Wisconsin–Madison. He previously served as codirector of the Program on Agricultural Technology Studies (a research and extension unit of the College of Agriculture), which examined the impacts of technological change and public policies on farm families in Wisconsin. Dr. Jackson-Smith received his M.A. in agricultural economics and his Ph.D. in sociology from the University of Wisconsin–Madison.

Robbin S. Johnson, B.S., is senior policy advisor for global policy studies at the Humphrey School of Public Affairs of the University of Minnesota. He previously served as president of the Cargill Foundation until he retired in 2007. He was elected senior vice president of corporate affairs, working with Cargill's senior leadership team on public policy and communications strategies. Mr. Johnson currently teaches a course at the Humphrey School on "The Role of Food in the World Economy," which covers the entire food supply chain from production agriculture to farm, trade, nutrition, climate change, and biotechnology issues. He is a current member of the NRC Board on Agriculture and Natural Resources. He also serves on the boards of Parent Aware for School Readiness and Second Harvest Heartland, and he is a member of the International Policy Council on Food, Agriculture and Trade and the Council on Foreign Relations. Mr. Johnson writes on topics of food security, food trade, sustainability, and the global food system. He is a past chair of the U.S. Feed Grains Council and the

Canada-Minnesota Business Council. Mr. Johnson received his B.S. from Yale University and he completed graduate study as a Rhodes Scholar at Oxford University in England.

Jean D. Kinsey, Ph.D., is professor emeritus of applied economics in the Department of Applied Economics in the College of Agricultural, Food and Environmental Sciences at the University of Minnesota. Dr. Kinsey is also the director emeritus of The Food Industry Center, which focuses on how various retailers in the food industry serve consumers and how retailers and suppliers interact in food distribution channels. The Food Industry Center at the University of Minnesota is 1 of 13 industry study centers funded by the nonprofit Sloan Foundation. Dr. Kinsey's research interests include food consumption trends, consumer buying behavior, food safety and consumer confidence, demographic changes in households, food industry structure, trends in food distribution and retail sales, effects of electronic technology on efficiency in retail outlets, economic effects of health and safety regulations, and regulation in the food industry. Dr. Kinsey was appointed as a Resident Fellow at the National Center for Food and Agricultural Policy, Resources for the Future, a Distinguished Fellow of the American Council on Consumer Interests, and a Fellow of the American Agricultural Economics Association. She previously served as a member of the IOM Committee to Review the Special Supplemental Nutrition Program for Women, Infants, and Children Food Packages. Dr. Kinsey received her Ph.D. in agricultural economics from UC Davis.

Susan M. Krebs-Smith, M.P.H., Ph.D., is chief of the Risk Factor Monitoring and Methods Branch, in the Division of Cancer Control and Population Sciences at the National Cancer Institute. She oversees a program of research on the surveillance of risk factors related to cancer, including diet, physical activity, weight status, tobacco use, and sun exposure; methodological issues to improve the assessment of those factors; and issues related to guidance and food policy. Her own surveillance research has emphasized trends in intake of foods and nutrients, especially fruits and vegetables; food sources of nutrients; and factors associated with the intake of foods and/or nutrients, using data from the National Nutrition Monitoring and Related Research Program. Her contributions in the area of dietary assessment methodology have focused on developing methods to assess dietary patterns, the usual intake of foods, overall diet quality, and conformance to dietary guidelines. Her efforts in dietary guidance and food policy include evaluation of the U.S. food supply and estimating future demand for food commodities, based on population-wide adoption of the *Dietary Guidelines for Americans* and Census projections. Dr. Krebs-Smith is a member of the Advisory Committee for the International Conference on Dietary Assessment Methods, and she has served on the editorial boards for the *Journal of the American Dietetic Association* and the *Journal of Nutrition Education and Behavior*, and on the Governing Council of the American Public Health Association. She previously served as a member of the IOM Committee on Nutrient Relationships in Seafood: Selections to Balance Benefits and Risks. Dr. Krebs-Smith received a B.S. in home economics from Bradley University, an M.P.H. from the University of Minnesota, and a Ph.D. in nutrition from Pennsylvania State University.

Matthew (Matt) Liebman, Ph.D., is a professor of agronomy, the Henry A. Wallace Chair for Sustainable Agriculture, and a member of the graduate faculties in Sustainable Agriculture, Ecology and Evolutionary Biology, Biorenewable Resources and Technology, and Crop Production and Physiology at Iowa State University. In 2009, he was selected as a Fellow of the American Society of Agronomy. He was awarded the Sustainable Agriculture Achievement Award from Practical Farmers of Iowa in 2013. His scientific research focuses on cropping system diversification, conservation systems, and weed ecology and management. Dr. Liebman is a graduate of Harvard University and obtained his Ph.D. in botany from UC Berkeley.

Frank Mitloehner, Ph.D., is professor and air quality specialist in cooperative extension at UC Davis. He is an expert in agricultural air quality, animal-environmental interactions, and agricultural engineering. Dr. Mitloehner is principal investigator of a broad range of studies, and since appointed to the UC faculty in 2002, he has authored 70 publications in refereed journals and obtained approximately $12 million in extramural grants. Dr. Mitloehner has recently been elected chair of a global United Nations Food and Agriculture Organization project to benchmark the environmental footprint of livestock production. In 2007, he served as the livestock production specialist on a national panel appointed by the White House Office of the Chief Economist to review the USDA Report titled *The Effects of Climate Change on Agriculture, Land Resources, Water Resources, and Biodiversity*. He serves as work group member on the President's Council of Advisors on Science and Technology and is the director of the UC Davis Agricultural Air Quality Center. Dr. Mitloehner was the 2006 recipient of the UC Davis Academic Federation Excellence in Research Award, the 2009 UC Distinguished Service Award for Outstanding Research, and the 2010 EPA Region IX Environmental Award. Dr. Mitloehner received his Ph.D. in animal science from Texas Technical University.

Keshia M. Pollack, M.P.H., Ph.D., is associate professor and director of the Occupational Injury Epidemiology and Prevention Training Program at the Johns Hopkins Bloomberg School of Public Health. Dr. Pollack uses injury epidemiology, translational research, and health impact assessment to advance policies that create safe and healthy environments where people—particularly the most vulnerable—live, work, play, and travel. Her research focuses on identifying risk factors for, and strategies to prevent, injuries related to occupation, obesity, sports and recreation, physical activity, and the built environment. She is also engaged in research that seeks to strengthen food policy councils and promote safe opportunities for play and physical activity to prevent childhood obesity. Dr. Pollack received the 2012 American Public Health Association Injury Control and Emergency Health Services Mid-Career Outstanding Service Award, and she is the 2011 recipient of The Daily Record's Very Important Professionals Successful by 40. Dr. Pollack received her M.P.H. from Yale University School of Public Health and her Ph.D. from Johns Hopkins University.

Patrick J. Stover, Ph.D., is professor and director of the Division of Nutritional Sciences at Cornell University. He is also director of the United Nations Food and Nutrition Program for Human and Social Development at Cornell University and vice president elect of the American Society for Nutritional Sciences. Dr. Stover's research interests focus on the biochemical, genetic, and epigenetic mechanisms that underlie the relationships between folic acid and human pathologies, including neural tube defects and other developmental anomalies, cardiovascular disease, and cancer. Specific interests include the regulation of folate-mediated one-carbon metabolism and cellular methylation reactions, molecular basis of the fetal origins hypothesis, development of mouse models to elucidate mechanisms of folate-related pathologies, and translational control of gene expression by ferritin. In 1976, he received the Presidential Early Career Award for Scientists and Engineers, the highest honor bestowed by the U.S. government on outstanding scientists and engineers beginning their independent careers. He received the ERL Stokstad Award in Nutritional Biochemistry from the American Society for Nutritional Sciences and has been selected as an Outstanding Educator four times by Cornell Merrill Presidential Scholars. Dr. Stover is a member of the IOM Food and Nutrition Board (FNB) and he served on the FNB Nutrigenomics Workshop Planning Group. Dr. Stover received his Ph.D. in biochemistry and molecular biophysics from the Medical College of Virginia.

Katherine M. J. Swanson, Ph.D., is president of KMJ Swanson Food Safety, Inc., a consulting firm based in St. Paul, Minnesota. Previously, Dr. Swanson served as vice president of food safety at Ecolab, Inc., in St. Paul. She has 30 years of food safety management and quality experience, including a focus on preventive microbiological and allergen controls. Currently, she is executive editor for the Food Safety Preventive Controls Alliance Curriculum, and she is working with the Food and Drug Administration (FDA), industry, academics, and state and local regulators on developing the training curriculum that will be recognized by FDA for compliance with the Food Safety Preventive Controls regulation requirements. Previously, as director of microbiology and food safety for the Pillsbury Company, Dr. Swanson developed and implemented Hazard Analysis and Critical Control Points and food allergen training and programs for research and development and operations; managed development of electronic specification systems; oversaw food quality system audits; and developed corporate product quality management systems. Dr. Swanson served on two NRC and IOM committees, including the Committee for the Review of Food Safety and Defense Risk Assessments, Analyses, and Data. In 2009, she was elected to the International Association for Food Protection Executive Board. Dr. Swanson is a member of the International Commission on Microbiological Specifications for Foods and chaired the editorial committee for *Microorganisms in Food 8—Use of Data for Assessing Process Control and Product Acceptance*. She served on the *Journal of Food Protection* editorial board from 1988 to 1999 and the *Food Protection Trends* editorial board from 2005 to 2007. Dr. Swanson has received numerous awards, including the 2003 National Food Processors Association Food Safety Award and the 2008 National Center for Food Safety and Technology Food Safety Award. Dr. Swanson received a Ph.D. in food science from the University of Minnesota.

Scott M. Swinton, Ph.D., is professor and associate chairperson of the Department of Agricultural, Food, and Resource Economics at Michigan State University in East Lansing. Dr. Swinton directs the department's graduate program and teaches applied microeconomics at the graduate level. His economic research explores how people manage agricultural ecosystems, and how changes in policy and technology can encourage better environmental stewardship while sustaining farm livelihoods. He collaborates closely with biologists, engineers, and other social scientists in analyzing food and energy biomass production systems, particularly in the Americas and in Africa. Dr. Swinton has published more than 70 journal articles and edited 3 books. He is currently a director of the Agricultural and Applied Economics Association as well as an Aldo Leopold Fellow and past associate editor of the *American Journal of Agricultural Economics*, *Frontiers in Ecology and Environment*, the *Review of Agricultural Economics*, and the *Journal of Production Agriculture*. Dr. Swinton served on the NRC's Committee on Status of Pollinators: Monitoring and Prevention of their Decline in North America. He received his Ph.D. from the University of Minnesota.